U0944826

光散射技术
及其在生化药物分析中的应用

Light Scattering Techniques and Their Applications in Biochemical and Pharmaceutical Analysis

黄承志 谭克俊 李原芳 编

西南师范大学出版社
XINAN SHIFAN DAXUE CHUBANSHE

图书在版编目（CIP）数据

光散射技术及其在生化药物分析中的应用／黄承志，谭克俊，李原芳编.－重庆：西南师范大学出版社，2007.10
ISBN 978-7-5621-3983-6

Ⅰ.光… Ⅱ.①黄…②谭…③李… Ⅲ.光散射－应用－生物制品－药物分析 Ⅳ.R977

中国版本图书馆 CIP 数据核字(2007)第 165296 号

Light Scattering Techniques and Applications in Biochemical and Pharmaceutical Analysis

光散射技术及其在生化药物分析中的应用

黄承志 谭克俊 李原芳 编

责任编辑：杨光明 杨浩宇
特约编辑：张迎雪
封面设计：CASTALY 尚品视觉 周 娟 钟 琛
出版发行：西南师范大学出版社
地址：重庆市北碚区天生路 2 号
网址：www.xscbs.com
邮编：400715
印 刷：四川外语学院印刷厂
开 本：889mm × 1194mm 1/16
印 张：16.75
字 数：520 千字
版 次：2007 年 10 月第 1 版
印 次：2007 年 10 月第 1 次印刷
书 号：ISBN 978-7-5621-3983-6
定 价：35.00 元

前 言

散射光产生于光子与微小粒子的相互作用。当光子作用于任何不均匀介质时，都有散射光产生。结合激光技术，散射光已在胶体化学、高分子化学等粒子大小表征和分子量测定方面得到了应用，但在吸收和发射(荧光)光谱分析中，散射光却是严重的干扰因素。1993年，美国学者Pasternack及其合作者发现使用普通荧光光度计获得的光散射信号可应用于生物色素聚集体研究。在此基础上，我们把普通荧光光度计测定的光散射信号与物质的量联系起来，建立了以散射发光为检测信号的光谱分析法。近十年来，基于散射光信号的光谱分析法已为分析工作者广泛应用于无机离子、蛋白质和核酸、药物的测定中，发展十分迅速，并随着纳米科学的发展取得了新成就。

作为近年来工作的总结，我们选编了本论文集。内容主要涉及到我攻读博士学位期间完成的工作和我在西南大学所指导的研究生的论文。在此，感谢我的恩师北京大学童沈阳教授及其课题组的李克安教授、刘锋教授、赵凤林教授和李娜教授等的指导和帮助，感谢我的研究生们近年来为光散射分析所付出的努力，并希望他们在今后的工作中取得优异成绩。

上述研究工作得到了国家杰出青年科学基金（No: 20425517）、国家自然科学基金面上项目（No: 30570465、No: 20675065、No: 20275032和No: 2987519）、科技部重大研究计划课题(No: 2006CB9331003)、教育部优秀人才计划（教人司2000-11-123）、重庆市科委（发光与实时分析重庆市重点实验室）、重庆市教委(重庆市高校现代分析化学重点实验室)和西南大学（原西南师范大学博士启动基金、光散射分析化学创新研究群体基金和分析化学重点学科建设基金）的大力支持，在此一并致谢！感谢西南师范大学出版社的领导及编辑杨光明同志为本论文集的出版付出的辛勤劳动。

黄承志

2007-10-22

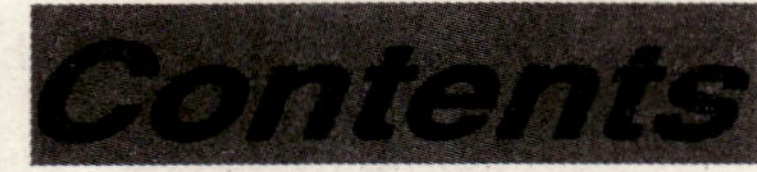

Chapter 1

Developing Process of Light Scattering Technique Analysis

1.1 Resonance Light Scattering Technique Used for Biochemical and Pharmaceutical Analysis

Abstract: By coupling and scanning simultaneously excitation and the emission monochromators of a common spectrofluorometer, enhanced resonance light scattering (RLS) signals could be obtained. The enhanced RLS signals could be used for designating bio-assemblies, aggregation species, and analytical purposes. Herein, we review the reports since the year of 2000 concerning the biochemical and pharmaceutical analysis with the RLS measurements, and discuss the possible developments of this technique.

Keywords: Resonance light scattering (RLS) technique; Biomolecule; Biochemical analysis; Pharmaceutical analysis

1.1.1 Introduction

Light scattering exists starting from our daily life to universal space. Beautiful unforgettable views of rainbows, sunrises and sunsets originate from scattered rays of photons interacting with particles such as dust, cloud and smog in the medium like air[1]. Scattered lights can emit in all directions except that of the incident light beams propagated, and are strongly related to the inhomogeneity of the medium. Observations of scattered lights are very common since all media except vacuum are relatively inhomogenous[2,3]. Depending on the size of the photon-interacted particles *(d)* and the wavelength of incident light beams (λ_0), light scattering can be classified into Mie ($d >> \lambda_0$), Tyndall ($d \approx \lambda_0$), and Rayleigh scattering ($d \le 0.05\lambda_0$) [2]. In terms of the wavelength, difference of the incident and the scattered beams, light scattering can also be divided into elastic scattering, inelastic scattering and quasi-elastic scattering[3,4]. Rayleigh scattering is elastic scattering, while Raman scattering and Brillouin scattering belong to inelastic scattering. Quasi-elastic scattering results from the Brownian movement of the scatterers, and can be named as dynamic light scattering[3,4].

These light scattering phenomena, if coupled with laser technique, have been extensively applied to polymer, colloidal and pharmaceutical sciences including measuring the size and distributions of polymer particles[5,6], colloids[6~8], drug powders[9] and selfassemblies of biopolymers [10]. In analytical chemistry, light scattering detectors have been developed in chromatographic determinations based on measuring the signals of multiple light scattering[11,12] and multi-angle light scattering (MALS) [13,14]. Evaporative light scattering detections (ELSD) have been developed for aerosol converted from the effluent of the separation in capillary electrophoresis[15] and HPLC[16], acting as complementary methods in terms of universality ensuring that LC–MS–ELSD run can provide sufficient MS and retention time data for identification of known present. ELSD also supplies quantification with a great degree of accuracy than UV detection for the analysis of combinatorial libraries[17].

On the contrary, light scattering is one of key interference sources in spectrophotometry and spectrofluorometry. Techniques such as low temperature and magnetic field-resolved techniques have been proposed to reduce their effects[18], and mathematical methods have been put out for separating the scattering and absorptions in the geometrical arrangement of interacting chromophores in order to avoid misleading investigations of the experimental spectroscopic parameters[19,20]. However, the establishment of resonance light scattering (RLS) technique, which measures light scattering signals on a common spectrofluorometer, has greatly changed the situation of the light scattering in spectral measurements [21]. Due to the simplicity of the technique, its applications have been developed greatly in recent years, and there have been several mini-views standing at different positions displayed[22–25] based on the reports before the year of 2000. Considering that analytical methods are basically established on the enhanced RLS signals resulting from the aggregations or assembly of chromophores on biomolecule template, starting from that point herein we make a mini-view with the reports since the year of 2000.

1.1.2 Basic theory

For particles with their size less than 20-fold of the wavelength of incident beams ($20\,d \le \lambda_0$), their scattered light could be described by Rayleigh theory, which assumes that all of the electrons in a particle *oscillate* with the same phase and frequency as the incident electromagnetic wave, and this collective oscillation results in a large oscillating electric dipole moment that produces scattered light. The produced light scattering intensity could be expressed by Rayleigh equation [21,22,26]:

$$I = I_0 \frac{8000(2.303)^2 \pi V n^2 c}{3\lambda_0^4 N_A} \left\{ \frac{\varepsilon^2(\lambda_0)}{4\lambda_0^2} + \left[\frac{1}{\pi} \int_0^\infty \frac{\varepsilon(\lambda) d\lambda}{\lambda_0^2 - \lambda^2} \right]^2 \right\} = Kc \quad (1)$$

where I is the intensity of the light scattering, I_0 the intensity of incident light beam, λ_0 and λ the wavelength of the incident and scattered light beams, respectively, c the concentration of the scatterers, and N_A the Avogadro constant. The terms in brackets indicate the real and imaginary parts of the refractive index, respectively.

Eq. (1) shows that in the non-absorption medium, the light scattering is mainly dependent on the real part of the refractive index *(n);* while if the excitation wavelength is near to the absorption bands, both the real and imaginary parts of the index make the contributions to the light scattering. If the absorption is strong, the contribution of the imaginary part is very significant since the fluctuation of the complicate index is very steep, strong enhanced Rayleigh scattering signals could be expected[21]. The enhanced light scattering could reach the maximum when the real part of the refractive index is zero and the imaginary part relative to the medium is 1.414[27]. These enhanced light scattering signals can be measured by using a common spectrofluorometer through simultaneously scanning the excitation and emission monochromators of a common spectrofluorometer with the wavelengths of the two monochromators being equal (namely $\Delta\lambda = 0$)[21].

It should be noted that electrons in different parts of the particle oscillate with different phase when the particle is comparable to or larger than the wavelength of incident beams. This leads to interference of the light scattered by electrons in different parts of the particle, and the magnitude and angular distribution of the scattered light intensity then deviates from that of an oscillating electric dipole [1]. However, according to theoretical calculation, Eq. (1) could be extended to the Mie scattering at some proximity, for example, to the light scattering of 40 nm gold particles excited by 500 nm incident beams [27]. In addition, the RLS measurements by using a common spectrofluorometer are generally operated with comparatively large slit-width for excitation and emission (≥ 5 nm). It has proved that $\Delta\lambda$ is not always zero if maximal RLS signals are available when large slit-widths (≥ 10 nm) are employed[28]. Without optical correction, the stray lights in the optical system of the spectrofluorometer obviously exist. Thus, RLS signals, obtained by using a common spectrofluorometer, involve in not only pure Rayleigh scattering, but also other light scattering signals including Mie, Tyndall, and Brillouin light scattering. Even though, as following will demonstrate, RLS is a valuable technique for detecting and characterizing self-assemblies and extended aggregates of chromophores since the assemblies or aggregations lead to formation of large fractal structures exhibiting strong RLS signals [29].

1.1.3 RLS measurements to assign assemblies

1.1.3.1 Self-assemblies of chromophores

Self-assemblies of porphyrins stand out of supramolecular chemistry since monomers of porphyrins can spontaneously self-assemble into dimers or higher aggregates through π-π stacking interactions and σ-π attractions, supplying the possibilities to mimic complicate physicochemical processes[30], and to build blocks for the rational design of self-assembled supramolecular structures in nanoelectronics applications, and the synthesis of materials capable of exhibiting specific properties and functions[31].

Water-soluble porphyrins bearing charged groups could be fostered to aggregate by simply screening the repulsive interactions between side-groups with the same charge, thus aggregation of porphyrins in variety of media have been investigated by spectroscopic techniques including RLS[32]. The dimers or higher aggregates of anion porphyrins such as tetraphenyl sulfonate porphyrins ($TPPS_4$), and tetraphenyl carboxylic porphyrins (TCPP) formed in aqueous media generally display enhanced RLS signals around the absorption bands of the J- and H-aggregate species since the absorptions of the J- and H-aggregate species are strong, and the contribution of the imaginary part of the complicate index of the aggregates is very significant[22,33]. The amount of RLS signals increases with a "good" electronic coupling among the porphyrin chromophores, whereas corresponding signals were absent in monomers [34]. Furthermore, RLS measurements have shown that H^+ and Na^+ in aqueous medium have displayed different driving ability to the final mesoscopic structure formed from the J-aggregation of $TPPS_4$ disclosing that the aggregation number ranges between 6 and 32, and even if a aggregation number range of $10^5 \sim 10^6$ in the case of the large clusters[35]. Similarly, nanoscale self-assembled complexes of chlorophyll in organic solvents could also be investigated by RLS measurements, and it was found that the formation of spherical-shape aggregates in which the phyil-chain is segregated in the inner part could foster the pigments so as to expose the macrocylic heads toward the bulk water solvent[36].

Since the π-π and σ-π interactions of porphyrins depending on the molecular structure mainly involve the substitute at the periphery, a variety of cationic and anonic porphyrins have been synthesized in order to clarify the factors influencing self-aggregation tendency. By means of absorption and RLS spectroscopy, Pasternack and co-workers proved that the aggregation of water-soluble porphyrins is dependent on the peripheral mesosubstituents[37]. Thus, it is easily understand, as derived from depolarized RLS measurements, that the half neutralization of carboxylic acid side chain of Protoporphyrin IX, the iron-free form of hemin, is responsible for the occurrence of a network of intermolecular hydrogen bonds contributing to a better stabilization of a supramolecular assembly, which display a prolate shape with an average of 200～500 nm and a medium height of 60 nm by evaporating solutions of the Protoporphyrin IX dimers[31].

1.1.3.2 Assembly of chromophores on charged polymeric template

By coupling the absorption, fluorescence, circular dichroism (CD) spectra and RLS measurements, a different approach could be made based on the electrostatic interaction between charged porphyrins and oppositely charged polymeric matrices including surfactants, nucleic acids, proteins [38], and hindered oppositely charged porphryins, where they act as template supports [39]. Pigment-surfactant aggregate of chlorophyll could be designated with induced RLS spectra in the micellar solution, in which the positive charge of the surfactant interacts with the C-13[2] ketoester group of monomeric porphyrin and form a delocalized exciton state[40].

Unlike free base porphyrin, such as $TPPS_4$, TCPP, and Protoporphyrin IX, metalloporphyrins display different aggregation features induced by ionic and nonionic surfactants. Metalloporphyrin including $FeTPPS_4$ and $ZnTPPS_4$, either monomers or aggregates, could bind to micelles, forming non-micellar metalloporphyrin/surfactant aggregates, and the binding ratio and constant of metalloporphyrin/$TPPS_4$, which could be made with UV, fluorescence and RLS measurements, are varied depending on the metal ions since the metalloporphyrins are incorporated into the micelles near the terminal part of their hydrocarbon chains[41,42]. Copper(II) porphyrins, if differing in peripheral substituents when interacting to DNA template, are either intercalated, bound externally or form extended electronically coupled arrays, and the extended electronically coupled arrays have characteristic RLS spectra corresponding to their absorption bands[43]. Similarly, induced RLS signals concerning the binding and self-organization cation porphyrin onto the long-range assemblies on $poly(dA\text{-}dT)_2$ or $poly(dG\text{-}dC)_2$ indicate that exciton coupling occurs between adjacent porphyrins moieties, and higher hydrophobicity of porphyrin is manifested by more extensive self-organization[44].

Depending on the substituted β-cyclodextrins (β-CDs), 2:1 supramolecular inclusion of the β-CDs with tetrakis(4-methoxyphenyl)porphyrin follows obvious RLS enhancement of the porphyrin, and is related to the size of the alkylated substituents interactions[45]. On the contrary, trans-bis (*N*-methylpyridnium-4-yl) diphenylporphyrin forms extended and organized assemblies on DNA template, but the addition of β-CD to these arrays leads to their disassembly as evidenced by the changes in extinction, CD and RLS spectra since β-CD attack the interior of the porphyrin assemblies as well as the ends [46]. Similar to the inclusion of β-CDs with porphyrins, induced RLS signals have been employed to designate the 1:1 inclusion complex of procaine hydrochloride into β-CD with the formation constant at 1.2×10^2 $mol\cdot L^{-1}$[47,48].

RLS measurements show that the aggregation of $TPPS_4$ induced by cationic cyanines with different substituents results from the hexyl-chain, indicating that it is the chain length of the alkyl group attached to the benzoxazole in the cyanine dyes for stabilizing the structure of the aggregate[49] that induced the aggregation of $TPPS_4$. The porphyrin's aggregation kinetics display an induction period unlike that of the cyanine dye[50], while the assemblies of carbocyanine dyes display a dependence on the substituents differing complex supramolecular structures of nanometer-to-micrometer size, that could be detected by coupling RLS and cryo-TEM [51]. In addition, G-quadruplex DNA could selectively bind to perylene diimide depending on the pH-dependent aggregation of chromophores[52,53]. The pH-dependent assemblies of chromophores can be used as pH sensors, and these supramolecular aggregates can also be employed as sensors for DNA [54].

1.1.4 Factors deciding enhanced RLS intensity

As shown in Section 3, RLS technique is powerful to designate the assemblies or aggregations, and it is generally combined with the absorption, fluorescence, and CD measurements in order to assign spectral features. Besides that, we can establish analytical methods through Eq. (1) by measuring enhanced RLS intensity in the aggregation and assembly process as stated above. Tables 1～3 list the RLS methods of biochemical and pharmaceutical analysis since the year 2000[55～136]. However, here we only stress on common features of the RLS signals extracted from these numerous reports, and will not fall in to the diversity of the interaction system even if these methods are generally established based on the interaction of the analytes with chromophores holding with different molecular structures, since a general summary of these interactions is beneficial to developing new analytical methods regarding the choice and synthesis of new chromophores. Based on extensive studies from the molecular recognition, assemblies and aggregations of chromophores induced by biomolecules, we suppose that enhanced RLS signals at least depend on following factors on the basis of the formation of delocalized exciton state of the assemblies.

1.1.4.1 Structural compatibility of the interacting components

The factors of structural compatibility include the interacting components' size, symmetry, charges and the solubility in appropriate solvents[36,37,55]. The interaction-induced enhanced RLS signals were thought to result from the size difference and the charge-coupled transfer of the scatterers before and after the interaction due to the electrostatic or hydrophobic interactions[66～68]. That is, the enhanced RLS intensities are related to the charge properties of chromophores, the charge-coupled degree of the formed species related to the intramolecular electronic interaction, and the size of the formed species. Thus, the strong electrostatic interaction between the two interacting components inducing high electronic delocation, and the formation of large particles are compulsory to display characteristic RLS spectra[33,63]. For the interactions between chromophores with proteins[66～97] or nucleic acids[103～117,122～128], the general rule is that positively charged chromophores interact with nucleic acids while negatively chromophores with proteins.

Table 1 Determinations of saccharides and medicines with enhanced RLS signals

Saccharide, medicines	pH	λ^a (nm)	Linear range ($\mu g \cdot mL^{-1}$)	LOD (3σ, $ng \cdot mL^{-1}$)	Reference
Heparin-Victoria blue 4R (VB-4R)[b]	5.0～7.6	523	0～0.4	3.35	[55]
Heparin-Victoria blue B (VBB)	5.0～6.4	534	0～0.4	6.62	[55]
Heparin-Night blue 4R (NB)	5.0～6.4	554	0～0.4	6.69	[55]
Heparin-Crystal violet (CV)	6.0～11.2	492	0～1.2	2.9	[56]
Heparin- Methylene blue (MB)	5.0～6.0	346	0～0.6	9.0	[57]
Heparin-Azure B	4.0～7.0	338	0～1.2	14.5	[57]
Heparin-Toluidine blue (TB)	4.0～7.0	329	0～0.8	26.0	[57]
Heparin-Brillint cresol blue (BCB)	6.0～6.5	348, 545	0～5.0	/	[58]

Continued

Saccharide, medicines	pH	λ^a (nm)	Linear range ($\mu g\cdot mL^{-1}$)	LOD (3σ, $ng\cdot mL^{-1}$)	Reference
Chondroitin 4-sulfate (CS)- Brillint cresol blue (BCB)	6.0～6.5	360, 544	0～5.0	/	[58]
Glycogen-Concanavalin A	7.4	400	0.32～24.0	/	[59]
Glycogen-Aqueous solution	2.5～11.5	350	0.8～4000	/	[60]
Thiamine (VB1)-Sodium dodecylbenzene sulonate	3.29	375, TIR-RLS	0.12～0.8	0.12	[61]
Chlortetracycline (CTC)-Eu-Trioctyl phosphine oxide (TOPO)	7.54～8.14	340, TIR-RLS	0.98～20.0×10^{-7}M	9.8×10^{-9}M	[62]
Berberine-Acidic xanthene (Eosine Y, Erythrosine, Ethyl eosin, Phloxin, Rose bengal)	4～5	576,578,572,384,464	0～5.0×10^{-6}M	14.3,30.8	[63]
Raloxifene-Evans blue (EB)	1.8	470,400	0～8.3	18.9	[64]
Vitamin B1(VB1)-Methyl orange	2.3～3.0	588	0～0.4	7.2	[65]

[a], Maximal RLS wavelength; [b], analytes were listed before the dash and after that the chromophores were presented.

1.1.4.2 Environmental conditions

If the interaction results from electrostatic attraction between biomolecules and chromophores, it is necessary that they should have opposite charges. Thus, these interactions originating from the negative charges of phosphate in the molecules of nucleic acids and the positive charges of proteins should be controlled under appropriate acidity and ionic strength, since the change of acidity and ionic strength of the medium would change the charges of both interacting components and the conformation of the biological molecules[73～78].

Different RLS signals could be obtained when different proteins bind to same chromophores since the number of $-NH_3^+$ of different proteins are greatly different[23,24]. For example, the number of the alkali amino acids residue in protamine sulfate is much more than that in bovine serum albumin (BSA), and the obtained RLS signals concerning the interaction of negatively chromophores with protamine sulfate are much stronger than that with bovine serum albumin [24]. On the contrary, the isoelectric point of pepsin is 1.0, and its interaction with negatively charged dyes seems impossible in common acidic medium [93]. For the interaction of proteins with chromophores, suitable pH for the interaction is generally lower than the isoelectric point of proteins[68]; while the appropriate pH for the interaction between nucleic acids with chromophores mainly depends on the protonization constant of chromophores[108,109]. As to these interactions of proteins with chromophores mainly through electrostatic force, RLS intensity is in proportional to molecular weight of proteins in Dalton[93]. That finding could be used for molecular weight measurements.

Besides acidity and ionic strength of the medium, temperature has effect also. With the increase of temperature, Brownian movements of molecules are encouraged, that induces more dynamic light scattering signals since RLS signals were measured generally with large slit-width (≥ 5 nm), and the direct outcome is the instability of the RLS signals[28].

Table 2 Determinations of bovine serum albumin on its enhanced RLS signals on chromophores

Chromophores	pH	RLS peak (nm)	Linear range ($\mu g\cdot mL^{-1}$)	LOD (3σ, $ng\cdot mL^{-1}$)	Reference
Anion porphyrins					
$\alpha, \beta, \gamma, \delta$-tetrakis(4-sulfophenyl)porphine ($TPPS_4$)	1.86	490.2	0.15~0.8	18	[66]
Triphenylmethane					
Fuchsine Acid (FSA)	4.10	277	0~3.8	0.47	[67]

Continued

Chromophores	pH	RLS peak (nm)	Linear range ($\mu g \cdot mL^{-1}$)	LOD (3σ, $ng \cdot mL^{-1}$)	Reference
Fast Green FCF(FCF)	4.10	279	0.02~2.0	1.86	[68]
Xanthene dyes					
Pyrogallol red (PR)	3.6~4.2	347	0.25~13.0	51.0	[69]
Azo dyes					
4-Azochromotoropic acid phenylfluorone (ACAP)	0.5~1.8	337	0.2~4.0	68.0	[70]
Dibromochloroarsenazo (DBC-Arsenazo)	/	/	2.5~6.0	88.1	[71]
Dibromomethyl-Arsenazo-Al(III)	5.6~7.2	410	2.5~50	135.0	[72]
Dibromomethylchlorophosphonazo (DBM-CPA)	3.78~4.35	411.6	0.065~40.05	30	[73]
Amaranth	3.87	364	0.5~5.0	/	[74]
Monoazo dyes (Chromazol KS, Acid chrome dark blue, Chrome blue SE, Acid chrome blue K, Chlorophosphonazo I, Arsennazo I, Chromotrope ZR)	3.8,3.2~4.2, 3.4~4.2	338, 314, 330, 336, 338	1.0~7.0	10	[75]
Th(IV)-Bisazo dyes of chromotropic acids:					[76]
arsenazo III (AA Ell),	Acidic medium	470	0~2.0	13.6	[76]
arsenazo M (AA M),	Acidic medium	470	0~2.8	22.1	
chlorophosphonazo HI (CPA III),	Acidic medium	470	0~1.6	10.7	
chlorosulphonphenol S (CSP S)	Acidic medium	470	0~0.28	6.3	
Orange G	0.6~2.0	548	0.5~5.0	2.6	[77]
3-(4-Sulphophenylazo)-4,5-dihydroxy-2,7-naphthalene disulfonic acid (SPADNS)	2.6	340	0.125~14.9	/	[78]
Beryllon II	3.80	/	0.10~32.40	/	[79]
Beryllon II-Al(III)	5.6~7.2	400~420	0.2~41.2	87.0	[80]
m-Acetylchlorophosphonazo (CPA-mA)	4.1	408	0.50~30.0	52.7	[81]
m-carboxychlorophosphonazo(CPA-mK)	4.1	410	0.5~35.0	104	[82]
Fast red VR(FRV)	3.52	287.0	0.1~8.0	7.1	[83]
Titan yellow(TY)	4.1	/	0.1~5.0	12.7	[84]
Dibromochloro-arsenazo-Al^{3+}	5.0~7.0	405~420	2.5~50.0	123.4	[85]
Arsenazo-DBS		400~420		77.0	[86]
Arsenazo-DBN-Al(III)	5.3~7.0	420~440	0.34~41.71		[87]
Resorcinol yellow(RY)-OP	2.35		0.02~4.0	10.4	[88]
Arsenazo I	3.29	400	0~18	60	[89]
Thorin			1.8~4.7	52.0	[90]
Arsenazo M (AA M), Chlorophosphonazo III (CPA III), Chlorosulphonphenol S (CSP S)	3.4~4.0	470	0~4.8	18.5	[91]
Eriochrome black T(EBT)	4.1	375	0~15.0	39.0	[92]
Other chromophores					
Alcian blue 8GX (ABGX)	7.24	398	0.1~3.0	8.2	[93]
Tetra-substituted sulphonated aluminum phthalocyanine (AlS_4Pc)	3.0	413	0.050-2.0 (HSA)	12.7	[94]
PsbMo heteropoly blue (PSbMo)	Acidic medium	470	0~6.0	21.0	[95]
Morin-CTMAB	7.8~8.0	305/610	0.075~10.0	66.0	[96]
Pyrocatechol violet (PV)-Triton X-100	1.4~2.0	341	0~8.0	0.05	[97]
$K_3[Fe(CN)_6]$	2.7	351	0~12((HSA)	100	[98]
Nanoparticles					
Colloidal silver chloride	3.0~9.0	398, 475	0.001~0.4	8	[99]
Reagents without absorption in VIS region					
Sodium lauryl sulfate (SLS)	1.81~4.1	470	/	/	[100]
Sodium dodecane sulfonate (SDS)	1.98	470	0.023~6.0	23.7	[101]
Sodium dodecylbenzene sulfonate- Thorium	6.37~6.59	340~370	0.15~1.0(HSA)	14.4	[102]

Table 3 Determinations of calf thymus DNA with its enhanced RLS signals on chromophores

Chromophores	pH	RLS peak (nm)	Linear ranges ($\mu g \cdot mL^{-1}$)	LOD (3σ, $ng \cdot mL^{-1}$)	Reference
Cation porphyrins & phthalocyanines					
Tetra-amino aluminum phthalocyanine (TAA1Pc)	6.0	400	0~0.25	1.4	[103]
Quinone-imines					
Brilliant cresol blue (BCB)	4.1~9.0	364	0.12~4.70	118.0	[104]
Brilliant cresyl blue	11.0~11.5	347	0.08~1.0	2.3	[105]
Neutral Red (NR)	7.63	535.0	0~1.5	10.32	[106]
Neutral Red (NR)	5.0~7.0	335.0	0~0.6	12.8	[107]
Azur A (AA)	3.29	398	0~2.0	10.9	[108]
Azur B (AB)	1.98~2.56	359.7	0~3.0	8.7	[109]
Methylene blue (MB)	5.5~7.5	350	0.2~1.4	1.5	[110]
Janus green B (JGB)	6.37	416.0	0~3.5	9.9	[111]
Basic triphenylmethanes					
Methyl violet (MV)	7.51	651.0	0~3.0	404.5	[112]
Crystal Violet	5.03	666.0	0~4.5	36.8	[113]
Brilliant Green (BG)-CTMAB	10.4~11.8	398.0	0~1.2	3.9	[114]
Methyl green (MG)-CTMAB	6.9~7.2	414.0	0.025~1.0	7.8	[115]
Rosaniline	10.5~10.8	485.0	0~1.0	14.2	[116]
Butyl rhodantine B	1.1	335.0			[117]
Drugs					
Dequalinium chloride (DC)	7.0	362	0.04~10	6.2	[118]
Thiamine Hydrochloride (TH)-CTMAB	/	406	0.02~10	11.0	[119]
Berberine-CTMAB	7.30	416.5	0.0075~75	2.1	[120]
Berberine	2.0~2.8	308	0~600	20	[121]
Other chromophores					
Pd(II)/5-Br-PADAP)	5.9~7.5	582	0~5.0	44	[122]
Pd(II)/2-(2-thiazolylazo)-5-dimethylamino-benzoic acid (TAMB)	5.9	675	0~3.5	22	[123]
Alcian blue 8GX	7.54	398.8	0.25~2.0	7.1	[124]
Histone	4.5~6.5	551	0.05~1.5	2.0	[125]
Morin-CTMAB	7.30	462.2	0.0075~10.0	3.4	[126]
Morin-CTMAB	7.30		0.025~5.0	16.7	[127]
Acridine red (AR)-CTMAB	6.40~7.10	555	0.05~1.2	8.53	[128]
Cetyl Trimethyl Ammonium Bromide (CTMAB)	2.21	470	0.05~2.5	4.9	[129]
CTMAB	8.5	414	0.025~20.0	8.3	[130]
CTMAB, Cetylpyridine bromide (CPB)	2.0~8	470	0~3.0	13.3, 7.30	[131]
Cetylpyridine bromide (CPB)		310~400	0.005~50	4.3	[132]
Eu-Trioctyl phosphine oxide (TOPO)	8.69	348, TIR-RLS	0.002~2.5	0.16	[133]
Al^{3+}	2.21	291.0	0~5.0	6.1	[134]
HCl	0.1 $mol \cdot L^{-1}$	310	0.06~100	18.0	[135]
H_2SO_4	0.1 $mol \cdot L^{-1}$	343	0.08~70	17.8	[135]
HNO_3	0.1 $mol \cdot L^{-1}$	310	0.1~100	18.4	[135]
AgCl sol	4.0	398	0~20	0.65	[136]

1.1.4.3 Molar ratio of the interacting components

It was found that enhanced RLS signals are generally available at low ionic strength and high molecular ratio of chromophores to biomolecules. Under such conditions, UV and fluorescence detections are insensitive, but the long-range assembly of dyes along the biomolecular surfaces can induce strong RLS signals since the change of biomolecular conformations induced by the large concentrated amount of dyes. For example, superhelical helixes of nucleic acids could be induced when the long-range assembly of positively charged porphyrin occurs, displaying strong enhanced RLS signals near the Soret absorption region[137]. With decrease in the molar ratio, which is very common in the study of pharmacology, RLS signals begin reducing, indicating chromophores intercalate into the interior of the double stranded structure. Thus, the change of the RLS signals could be used to assign the binding mode of the chromophores with nucleic acids, and correspondingly, the chromophores act as molecular structural probes of nucleic acids.

1.1.4.4 Molecular absorption in the medium

Unlike conventional light scattering techniques in which the absorption wavelength region of chromophores is avoided, RLS measurements focus on this portion of the electromagnetic spectrum. Since the molecular absorption species should absorb both the excitation and the light scattering, the available RLS signals corresponding the absorption band are reduced, inducing distortion of the real RLS spectrum[138]. Thus, similar to the corrections needed in fluorescence spectroscopy for primary and secondary absorption processes, Pasternack and co-workers proposed that RLS spectra need to be corrected for the absorption of the incident and the scattered light in order to extract useful information from the spectroscopy experiments on aggregates of the chromophores[139]. The basic theory of the correction is to combine the extinction and RLS measurements for the same samples by introducing a correction factor to compensate for the absorption loss of the enhanced light scattering signals[22,139,140].

1.1.4.5 Sensitivity of RLS methods

The sensitivity of RLS methods depends on the properties of the molecular structures of the interacting components, and the environmental conditions. As displayed above, the RLS signals resulting from the interactions of chromophores with proteins or nucleic acids are strongly dependent on the molecular structures, pH and ionic strength of the aqueous medium. If the size is the main factor responsible for the enhanced RLS signals, the enhanced RLS intensity is proportional to the molecular weight of proteins [93]. Besides these factors, the concentrations of the chromophores used for the determination are dependent also [141,142]. In addition, some interactions, especially the interaction of quinone-imines with nucleic acids, display several RLS peaks. The sum of the RLS intensities at these peaks can be used for the determination of nucleic acid, and the sensitivity can be improved [143].

Although the cmc value of a surfactant could be determined by measuring the RLS signals of micelle in aqueous medium[144], it has been proved that cation surfactants are able to sensitize the interactions between chromophores and DNA[114]. The RLS intensities of chromophores–surfactants–buffer are easily affected with pH variation, so pH control should be specially considered when discussing these interactions of chromophores–DNA–surfactants. The interaction of CTMAB–DNA, for example, has strongly enhanced RLS signals at pH 2.21, but the signals decrease steeply when pH is higher than 4.5[129]. In addition, ethanol was also found to have sensitizing effect on the determination of proteins with Titan Yellow[84].

1.1.5 RLS at liquid/liquid interfaces

As stated above, RLS technique ($\lambda_{em} = \lambda_{ex}$) is simple, sensitive, and has broadly practiced in analytical chemistry. However, the technique has poor selectivity, and its tolerance of coexisting foreign substances is scarcely at the same level as the analytes. The reason is that RLS signals of scatterers are related to the absorption features of the medium, size, shape, concentration, and refractive index compared to the scatterers' environments [21,145~147]. Thus, particles or colloidal scatters of coexisting foreign substances can exert influences significantly[22~24]. Surfactants, metal ions, amino acids, and sugars have different interference on the RLS methods since they can interact with the biomolecules through electrostatic attraction or hydrophobic interactions, thus measures should be taken, such as adjusting pH value[129], diluting the sample[94] or using standard addition method[67] to reduce the effect of foreign materials or the background in turbid medium.

Since RLS technique is established on the basis of the fluctuation of the refractive indexes in an aqueous solution where a steep change occurs between the refractive index of the inner scattered particles and that of their outer atmosphere[21,145], a total internal reflected resonance light scattering (TIR-RLS) technique has been developed[62]. It has been proved that TIR-RLS holds following advantages: (1) TIR-RLS will easily bring about a sharp fluctuation of refractive indexes at the interfacial region due to the formation of an evanescent field, leading to much stronger enhanced RLS signals. The liquid/liquid interface is somewhat similar to an enlarged surface of a scattered particle and the refractive indexes play the same role as they do in a bulk phase according to Eq. (1); (2) the analytes can be adsorbed to the oil/water interface to acquire a good separation of the analytes with coexisting foreign substances, during which enrichment of the analytes at the oil/water interface also occurs, and high selectivity and sensitivity can be expected as well[62]. Compared to the methods based on RLS measurements and spectrofluorometry[148], the sensitivity of TIR-RLS methods for clinical drugs is about 100–1000-fold higher[61,62,102]. In addition, it has been found that enhanced RLS signals of the interaction of nucleic acids with dyes can be observed only in a medium of low ionic strength in an bulk aqueousmedium, while, however, the interaction can proceed or enhanced RLS signals can be observed in a medium of ionic strength higher than 0.2 M in the TIR-RLS system[133]; (3) hosts and guests with immiscible property can encounter and interact at an oil/water interface, thus corresponding amphiphilic species can be separated from the bulk phases, adsorbed and enriched by the oil/water interface [62,149], leading to that the recognition and interaction of hosts and guests with immiscible property can be carried out easily at the liquid/liquid interfaces that are lower than 200 nm in thickness[66,150]; (4) oil-soluble chromophores can be used as reagents conveniently owing to the existence of the oil phase [102]; (5) the interfacial region presents a good chance to study orientation of molecules by means of polarized incident light beams as a result of the relatively simplex components in it. Therefore, TIR-RLS technique is not only applied to analytical purposes, but also shows high promise in the characterization of the molecular assembly, recognition, drug extraction and transport at liquid/liquid and liquid/vapor interfaces.

1.1.6 Future of RLS technique

As a new spectral analysis technique, the light scattering measurements by using a common spectrofluorometer are very simple, and sensitive. This technique is generally coupled to other spectral analysis techniques such as absorption, fluorescence and CD, and can compensate for the drawbacks of spectrophotometric and spectrofluorometric measurements. Hyperchromism and hypochromism are generally found in the interaction between chromophores with proteins or nucleic acids, thus the spectrophotometry or spectrofluorometry based on them have low sensitivities. On the contrary, methods based on measuring enhanced RLS signals that are generally related to hyperchromism and hypochromism are much more sensitive. Furthermore, RLS methods could be established in a turbid system without UV-Vis absorption properties, extending the usefulness of reagents in the quantitative analysis of medicines, proteins and nucleic acids [93,130,135]. Even though we believe that there still is an extensive space for further development of light scattering techniques in terms of analytical proposes.

1.1.6.1 RLS as a technique for spectral assignment

RLS technique has been successfully to assign the assembly and aggregate species, and applied for analytical purposes, but as a spectral technique, it is much better if it could be used for fine spectral assignment [37]. Especially, the relationship of the RLS spectra with the molecular structure should be further assigned. For example, Methylene Blue (MB), Azure A(AA), Azure B(AB) and Lauthis Violet (LV) have similar molecular structure, but the RLS features displayed molecular structural dependent when interacting with nucleic acids are greatly diferent, and thus possibly involving in different interaction mechanism [108,109,151]. According to semi-empirical molecular calculation, the different interaction mechanism mainly results from the substitute groups and the coplanar structures. The structure dependence of the RLS signals can be seen also from the distribution variation of the charge density of basic triphenylmethane dyes before and after these dyes forming ion associates with iodide anion and metal cations[152,153].

1.1.6.2 Developing Raman light scattering technique in UV-Vis region

Bedsides RLS signals ($\lambda_{em}=\lambda_{ex}$), other light scattering signals can be detected by using a three-dimensional (3D) functioned spectrofluorometer including second-order light scattering (SLS, $\lambda_{em}=2\lambda_{ex}$), anti-second-order light scattering (ASLS, $\lambda_{em}=0.5\lambda_{ex}$) and Raman light scattering in the assembly of chromophores on the template of DNA[154]. The wavelength of light scattering signals has linear relationship with that of incident light beams. SLS and ASLS signals are weaker than RLS ones for same scatterers, and the sensitivity of SLS and ASLS methods are lower than that of RLS method[154]. Raman light scattering signals are always found along RLS, SLS, and ASLS. The weak enhanced Raman light scattering signals in UV-Vis region open new avenues of technology that could designate Raman light scattering signals in UV-Vis region. It is technically possible by using a variable-angle controlled spectrofluorometer to measure the Raman light scattering signals in UV-Vis region under a high sensitivity function mode.

1.1.6.3 Developing new clinical instrument for cancer diagnosis

Compared to the diagnostic techniques of high energy X-rays and expensive magnetic resonance images, light rays in UV-Vis region is much safer and cheaper for diagnosis of tissue problem. Thus, light scattering image techniques have begun to find applications in clinical test and diagnostics. One big finding is that cancer cells generally have high density of cell matrix, and have stronger light scattering signals than normal cells, so back light scattering technique, if coupled with image facilities, could be applied to the forepart diagnosis of cancers[155,156].

1.1.6.4 RLS particles as novel reagents

RLS particles have the size between 40 and 120 nm in diameter, and it could be used as fluorescent analogs[27,157]. These particles have been used for fluorescence tracers in immuno-, DNA[158,159] and protein[160] assays as well as in cell and molecular biology studies [161]. Similarly, nanoparticles with different sizes have special optical and electric properties, and are promising RLS reagents in biochemical and pharmaceutical analysis. It has been reported that Au nanoparticles could be used to the sensitive determination of proteins[162], and useful probes for the biological molecules[99,136]. Based on the RLS measurements, the spectral features of new nanoparticles can be characterized[163~165]. Both Au and Ag nanoparticles have visible absorption, and these absorptions bathochromicly shift with the size increasing in the range of 10~95 nm, displaying that the RLS intensity is proportional to cube of the size of the nanoparticles[166~169].

Due to its high sensitivity, RLS technique shows high promise in the hybridization study of nucleic acids and genetic diagnosis[158,159]. With the development of new instruments by introducing laser techniques[170~171], immunoassay of resonance light scattering, and time-resolved resonance light scattering techniques are expected, displaying high promise not only in biochemical and pharmaceutical analysis, but also in the study of molecular biology and cell biology.

Acknowledgements

This work has received the support of the National Natural Science Foundation of China (NSFC, No. 20275032), to which all the authors here are grateful.

References

[1] C.F. Bohren, D.R. Huffman, Absorption and Scattering of Light by Small Particles, Wiley, New York, 1998.
[2] W.Z. Yang, Physical Chemistry Techniques, Peking University Press, Beijing, 1992.
[3] R. Pecora, Dynamic Light Scattering, Plenum Press, New York, 1985.
[4] Q. Zuo, Laser Light Scattering and its Application in Polymer Science, Henan Science and Technology Press, Zhengzhou, 1994.
[5] M.R. Schure, S.A. Palkar, Anal. Chem. 74 (2002) 684.
[6] M. Andersson, B. Wittgren, K.G. Wahlund, Anal. Chem. 73 (2001) 4852.
[7] A. Yethiraj, A. van Blaaderen, Nature 421 (2003) 513.
[8] M.L. Magnuson, D.A. Lytle, C.M. Frietch, C.A. Kelty, Anal. Chem. 73 (2001) 4815.
[9] T. Pan, E.M. Sevick-Muraca, Anal. Chem. 74 (2002) 4228.
[10] H. Lee, S.K.R. Williams, S.D. Allison, T.J. Anchordoquy, Anal. Chem. 73 (2001) 837.
[11] P.K. Owens, J. Johansson, Anal. Chem. 72 (2000) 740.
[12] W.H. Yokoyama, B.E. Knuckles, P.A. Davis, B.P. Daggy, J. Agric. Food Chem. 50 (2002) 7726.
[13] C. Viebke, P.A. Williams, Anal. Chem. 72 (2000) 3896.
[14] A.R. Clapp, R.B. Dickinson, Langmuir 17 (2001) 2182.
[15] B. Szostek, J.A. Koropchak, Anal. Chem. 68 (1996) 2744.
[16] D.S. Risley, M.A. Strege, Anal. Chem. 72 (2000) 1736.
[17] P.A. Cremin, L. Zeng, Anal. Chem. 74 (2002) 5492.
[18] L.J. Yu, Y.Q. Li, W. Sui, Spectrosc. Spect. Anal. 22 (2002) 819.

[19] N. Micali, F. Mallamace, M. Castriciano, A. Romeco, L.M. Scolaro, Anal. Chem. 73 (2001) 4958.
[20] H. Martens, J.P. Nielsen, S.B. Engelsen, Anal. Chem. 74 (2003) 394.
[21] R.F. Pasternack, C. Bustamane, P.J. Collings, A. Giannetteo,E.J. Gibbs, J. Am. Chem. Soc. 115 (1993) 5393.
[22] Y.F. Li, C.Z. Huang, X.L. Hu, Chin. J. Anal. Chem. 26(1998) 1508.
[23] K.A. Li, C.Q. Ma, Y. Liu, S.Y. Tong, Chin. Sci. Bull. 44 (2000) 682.
[24] Y.T. Wang, F.L. Zhao, K.A. Li, S.Y. Tong, Chem. J. Chin. Univ. 21 (2000) 1491.
[25] R. Yang, S.P. Liu, Chin. J. Anal. Chem. 29 (2001) 232.
[26] J. Anglister, I.Z. Steinberg, J. Chem. Phys. 78 (1983) 5358.
[27] J. Yguerabide, E.E. Yguerabide, Anal Biochem. 262 (1998) 137.
[28] Y.J. Wei, Molecular absorption and scattering spectroscopic probes of proteins, Ph.D. Dissertation, Peking University, Beijing, 1997.
[29] F. Mallamace, N. Micali, A. Romeo, L.M. Scolaro, Curr. Opin. Coll. Interf. Sci. 5 (2000) 49.
[30] J.M. Ribo, J. Crusats, F. Sagues, J. Claret, R. Rubires, Science 292 (2001) 2063.
[31] L.M. Scolaro, M. Castriciano, A. Romeo, S. Patane, E. Cefali, M. Allegrini, J. Phys. Chem. 106 (2002) 2453.
[32] L.M.M. Castriciano, A. Romeo, A. Mazzaglia, A. Scolaro, F. Mallamace, N. Micali, Physica A 304 (2002) 158.
[33] M.Y. Choi, J.A. Pollard, M.A. Webb, J.L. McHale, J. Am. Chem. Soc. 125 (2003) 810.
[34] K. Kano, K. Fukuda, H. Wakami, R. Nishiyabu, R.F. Pasternack, J. Am. Chem. Soc. 122 (2000) 7494.
[35] N. Micali, F. Mallamace, A. Romeo, R. Purrello, L.M. Scolaro, J. Phys. Chem. B 104 (2000) 5897.
[36] A. Agostiano, P. Cosma, M. Trotta, L. Monsu-Scolaro, N. Micali, J. Chem. Phys. B 106 (2002) 12820.
[37] K. Kano, K. Fukuda, H. Wakami, R. Nishiyabu, R.F. Pasternack, J. Am. Chem. Soc. 122 (2000) 7494.
[38] A.K. Bordbar, A. Eslami, S. Tangestaninejad, J. Porphyr. Phthaloc. 6 (2002) 225.
[39] R. Lauceri, S. Gurrieri, E. Bellacchio, A. Contino, L. Monsuscolaro, A. Romeo, A. Toscano, R. Purrello, Supramol. Chem. 12 (2002) 193.
[40] A. Agostiano, L. Catucci, G. Colafemmina, H. Scheer, J. Phys. Chem. 106 (2002) 1446.
[41] S.C.M. Grandini, V.E. Yushmanov, M. Tabak, J. Inorg. Biochem. 85 (2001) 263.
[42] L.M. Scolaro, C. Donato, M. Castriciano, A. Rameo, R. Romeo, Inorg. Chim. Acta 300 (2000) 978.
[43] R.F. Pasternack, S. Ewen, A. Rao, A.S. Meyer, M.A. Freedman, P.J. Collings, S.L. Frey, M.C. Ranen, J.C. De Paula, Inorg. Chim. Acta 317 (2001) 59.
[44] K. Lang, P. Anzenbacher, P. Kapusta, V. Kral, P. Kubat, D.M. Wagnerova, J. Photochem. Photobiol. B 57 (2000) 51.
[45] R. Yang, K.A. Li, K. Wang, F. Liu, N. Li, F.L. Zhao, Spectrochim. Acta A 59 (2003) 153.
[46] R.F. Pasternack, E.J. Gibbs, D. Bruzewicz, D. Stewart, K.S. Engstrom, J. Am. Chem. Soc. 124 (2002) 3533.
[47] N.B. Li, H.Q. Luo, S.P. Liu, G.N. Chen, Spectrochim. Acta A 58 (2002) 501.
[48] N.B. Li, S.P. Liu, H.Q. Luo, Anal. Chim. Acta 472 (2002) 89.
[49] A.S.R. Koti, N. Periasamy, J. Mater. Chem. 12 (2002) 2312.
[50] R.F. Pasternack, C. Fleming, S. Herring, P.J. Collings, J. dePaula, G. DeCastreo, E.J. Gibbs, Biophys. J. 79 (2000)550.
[51] H. vo Berlepsch, C. Bottcher, A. Ouart, C. Burger, S. Dahne, S. Kirsteins, J. Phys. Chem. 104 (2002) 5255.
[52] S.M. Kerwin, G. Chen, J.T. Kern, P.W. Thomas, Bioorg. Med. Chem. Lett. 12 (2002) 447.
[53] J.T. Kern, S.M. Kerwin, Bioorg. Med. Chem. Lett. 12 (2002) 3395.
[54] R. Purrello, S. Gurrieri, R. Lauceri, Coord. Chem. Rev. 192 (1999) 683.
[55] S.P. Liu, H.Q. Luo, N.B. Li, Z.F. Liu, W.X. Zheng, Anal. Chem. 73 (2001) 3907.
[56] H.Q. Luo, S.P. Liu, N.B. Li, Z.F. Liu, Anal. Chim. Acta 468 (2002) 275.
[57] H.Q. Luo, S.P. Liu, Z.F. Liu, Q. Liu, N.B. Li, Anal. Chim. Acta 449 (2002) 261.
[58] S.Z. Zhang, N. Li, F.L. Zhao, K.A. Li, S.Y. Tong, Spectrochim. Acta A 58 (2002) 273.
[59] S.Z. Zhang, F.L. Zhao, K.A. Li, S.Y. Tong, Talanta 54 (2001) 333.
[60] S.Z. Zhang, F.L. Zhao, K.A. Li, S.Y. Tong, Anal. Chim. Acta 431 (2001) 133.
[61] W. Lu, C.Z. Huang, Y.F. Li, Anal. Chim. Acta 475 (2003) 151.
[62] P. Feng, W.Q. Shu, C.Z. Huang, Y.F. Li, Anal. Chem. 73 (2001) 4307.
[63] S.P. Liu, P. Feng, Microchim. Acta 140 (2002) 189.

[64] L. Fan, S.P. Liu, D.C. Yang, X.L. Hu, Chin. J. Chem. 20 (2002) 1552.
[65] S.P. Liu, Z.Y. Zhang, H.Q. Luo, K. Ling, Anal. Sci. 18 (2002) 971.
[66] C.Z. Huang, Y.F. Li, P. Feng, Anal. Chim. Acta 443 (2001) 73.
[67] C.Z. Huang, Y.F. Li, M. Li, Fresenius J. Anal. Chem. 371 (2001) 1034.
[68] Y.F. Li, C.Z. Huang, M. Li, Anal. Sci. 18 (2002) 177.
[69] Q.E. Cao, Z.T. Ding, R.B. Fang, X. Zhao, Analyst 126 (2001) 1444.
[70] Z.X. Guo, H.X. Shen, Anal. Chim. Acta 408 (2000) 177.
[71] Q.F. Li, L.J. Dong, R.P. Jia, X.G. Chen, Z.D. Hu, Spectrosc. Lett. 34 (2001) 407.
[72] R.P. Jia, L.J. Dong, Q.F. Li, X.G. Chen, Z.D. Hu, Y. Nagaosa, Anal. Chim. Acta 442 (2001) 249.
[73] Q.F. Li, H.Y. Zhang, C.X. Xue, X.G. Chen, Z.D. Hu, Spectrochim. Acta A 56 (2000) 2465.
[74] X.X. Wang, H.X. Shen, Y.M. Hao, Chin. J. Anal. Chem. 28 (2000) 1388.
[75] S.P. Liu, Q. Liu, Anal. Sci. 17 (2001) 239.
[76] L. Fan, S.P. Liu, D.C. Yang, H.Q. Luo, Chin. J. Chem. 21 (2003) 56.
[77] S.P. Liu, R. Yang, Q. Liu, Anal. Sci. 17 (2001) 243.
[78] Y.T. Wang, F.L. Zhao, K.A. Li, S.Y. Tong, Anal. Lett. 33 (2000) 221.
[79] H. Zhang, F.L. Zhao, K.A. Li, Anal. Lett. 34 (2001) 701.
[80] L.J. Dong, R.P. Jia, Q.F. Li, X.G. Chen, Z.D. Hu, Analyst 126 (2001) 707.
[81] Q.F. Li, S.H. Liu, H.Y. Zhang, X.G. Chen, Z.D. Hu, Anal. Lett. 34 (2001) 1133.
[82] Q.F. Li, X.G. Chen, H.Y. Zhang, C.X. Xue, Y.Q. Fan, Z.D. Hu, Fresenius J. Anal. Chem. 368 (2000) 715.
[83] C.X. Yang, Y.F. Li, C.Z. Huang, Anal. Lett. 35 (2002) 1945.
[84] H.L. Wu, W.Y. Li, X.W. He, Acta Chim. Sin. 60 (2002) 1822.
[85] R.P. Jia, L.J. Dong, Q.F. Li, X.G. Chen, Z.D. Hu, Talanta 57 (2002) 693.
[86] L.J. Dong, R.P. Jia, Q.F. Li, X.G. Chen, Z.D. Hu, Anal. Chim. Acta 459 (2002) 313.
[87] L.J. Dong, R.P. Jia, Q.F. Li, X.G. Chen, Z.D. Hu, M.A.Hooper, Fresenius J. Anal. Chem. 370 (2001) 1009.
[88] Y.J. Chen, J.H. Yang, X. Wu, T. Wu, Y.X. Luan, Talanta 58 (2002) 869.
[89] S.W. Li, N. Li, F.L. Zhao, K.A. Li, Spectrosc. Spect. Anal. 22 (2002) 619.
[90] L.H. Chen, F.L. Zhao, K.A. Li, Chin. J. Chem. 20 (2002) 368.
[91] L. Fan, S.P. Liu, X.F. Long, X.L. Hu, Chin. J. Chem. Anal. 30 (2002) 81.
[92] S.W. Li, N. Li, F.L. Zhao, K.A. Li, Chin. J. Chem. Anal. 30 (2002) 732.
[93] Y.F. Li, C.Z. Huang, X.H. Huang, M. Li, Anal. Sci. 16 (2000) 1247.
[94] X.L. Chen, D.H. Li, Q.Z. Zhu, H.H. Yang, H. Zheng, Z.H. Wang, J.G. Xu, Talanta 53 (2001) 1205.
[95] X.F. Long, S.P. Liu, J. Southwest Norm. Univ. (Nat. Sci. Ed.) 25 (2000) 155.
[96] R.T. Liu, J.H. Yang, X. Wu, Z.J. Lan, Spectrochim. Acta A 58 (2002) 3077.
[97] X. Cong, Z.X. Guo, X.X. Wang, H.X. Shen, Anal. Chim. Acta 444 (2001) 205.
[98] Z.L. Jiang, Z.L. Peng, S.P. Liu, Chin. J. Chem. 20 (2002) 1566.
[99] C.Q. Zhu, D.H. Li, Q.Z. Zhu, H. Zheng, Q.Y. Chen, H.H. Yang, J.G. Xu, Fresenius J. Anal. Chem. 366 (2000) 863.
[100] P. Feng, W.Q. Shu, C.Z. Huang, Environ. Chem. 20 (2001) 497.
[101] W. Lu, P. Feng, Y.F. Li, C.Z. Huang, Anal. Lett. 35 (2002) 227.
[102] P. Feng, C.Z. Huang, Y.F. Li, Anal. Biochem. 308 (2002) 83.
[103] X.L. Chen, D.H. Li, Q.Z. Zhu, H.H. Yang, H. Zheng, J.G. Xu, Chem. J. Chin. Univ. 22 (2001) 901.
[104] Y.T. Wang, F.L. Zhao, K.A. Li, S.Y. Tong, Spectrochim. Acta A 56 (2000) 1827.
[105] C. Liu, X.M. Chen, Chin. J. Anal. Chem. 29 (2001) 685.
[106] X.H. Huang, C.Z. Huang, Y.M. Huang, J. Southwest Norm. Univ. (Nat. Sci. Ed.) 25 (2000) 273.
[107] H.Y. Xiang, X.M. Chen, S.Q. Li, S. Xia, A.X. Liu, Spectrosc. Spect. Anal. 21 (2001) 822.
[108] Y.F. Li, C.Z. Huang, X.H. Huang, M. Li, Anal. Chim. Acta 429 (2001) 311.
[109] Y.F. Li, C.Z. Huang, M. Li, Anal. Chim. Acta 452 (2002) 285.
[110] H.Y. Xiang, X.M. Chen, S.Q. Li, S. Xia, A.X. Liu, Chin. J. Anal Chem. 28 (2000) 1398.
[111] C.Z. Huang, Y.F. Li, X.H. Huang, M. Li, Analyst 125 (2000) 1267.

[112] W.J. Zhang, H.P. Xu, C.X. Xue, X.G. Chen, Z.D. Hu, Anal. Lett. 34 (2001) 553.
[113] W.J. Zhang, H.P. Xu, S.Q. Wu, X.G. Chen, Z.D. Hu, Analyst 126 (2001) 513.
[114] X.H. Huang, W.Q. Shu, Y.F. Li, C.Z. Huang, Chin. J. Anal. Chem. 29 (2001) 271.
[115] R.T. Liu, J.H. Yang, X. Wu, C.X. Sun, Indian J. Chem. A 40 (2001) 1121.
[116] C. Liu, X.M. Chen, H.Y. Xiang, S.Q. Li, S. Xia, A.X. Liu, Spectrosc. Spect. Anal. 21 (2001) 697.
[117] Y. Yu, F.D. Huang, Chin. J. Chem. Anal. 30 (2002) 1234.
[118] Z.P. Li, K.A. Li, S.Y. Tong, Talanta 55 (2001) 669.
[119] R.T. Liu, J.H. Yang, X. Wu, Z.M. Li, S.X. Sun, F.J. Huang, J. Trace Microprobe Tech. 20 (2002) 363.
[120] R.T. Liu, J.H. Yang, X. Wu, C.X. Sun, Spectrochim. Acta A 58 (2002) 457.
[121] C. Liu, X.T. Chen, S.Q. Li, X.M. Chen, Chin. J. Chem. Anal. 30 (2002) 1218.
[122] Y.M. Hao, H.X. Shen, Anal. Chim. Acta 413 (2000) 87.
[123] Y.M. Hao, H.X. Shen, Anal. Chim. Acta 422 (2000) 159.
[124] Y.F. Li, C.Z. Huang, X.H. Huang, M. Li, Anal. Lett. 34 (2001) 1117.
[125] X.Y. Du, S. Sasaki, H. Nakamura, I. Karube, Talanta 55 (2001) 93.
[126] R.T. Liu, J.H. Yang, X. Wu, C.X. Sun, T. Wu, Analyst 126 (2001) 1367.
[127] R.T. Liu, J.H. Yang, X. Wu, T. Wu, Anal. Chim. Acta 448 (2001) 85.
[128] M. Wang, J.H. Yang, X. Wu, F. Huang, Anal. Chim. Acta 422 (2000) 151.
[129] Y.F. Li, W.Q. Shu, P. Feng, C.Z. Huang, M. Li, Anal. Sci. 17 (2001) 693.
[130] R.T. Liu, J.H. Yang, X. Wu, C.X. Sun, Anal. Chim. Acta 441 (2001) 303.
[131] S.P. Liu, X.L. Hu, H.Q. Luo, L. Fan, Sci. Chin. 32 (2002) 18.
[132] R.T. Liu, J.H. Yang, X. Wu, Spectrochim. Acta A 58 (2002) 1935.
[133] W. Lu, C.Z. Huang, Y.F. Li, Analyst 127 (2002) 1392.
[134] C.X. Yang, Y.F. Li, P. Feng, C.Z. Huang, Chin. J. Chem. Anal. 30 (2002) 473.
[135] Z.P. Li, K.A. Li, S.Y. Tong, Talanta 51 (2000) 63.
[136] C.Q. Zhu, D.H. Li, H. Zheng, Q.Z. Zhu, J.G. Xu, Chin. J. Anal. Chem. 28 (2000) 1485.
[137] C.Z. Huang, K.A. Li, K.A. Li, Y.T. Shen, Bull. Chem. Soc. Jpn. 70 (1997) 1843.
[138] C.Z. Huang, Y.F. Li, P. Feng, Chin. J. Anal. Chem. 29 (2001) 832.
[139] P.J. Collings, E.J. Gibbs, T.E. Starr, O. Vafek, C. Yee, L.A. Pomerance, R.F. Pasternack, J. Phys. Chem. B 103 (1999) 8474.
[140] N. Micali, F. Mallamace, A. Romeo, R. Purrello, L.M. Scolaro, J. Phys. Chem. B 104 (2000) 5897.
[141] C.X. Yang, Y.F. Li, C.Z. Huang, Anal. Sci. 19 (2003) 211.
[142] C.X. Yang, Y.F. Li, C.Z. Huang, Chin. J. Anal. Chem. 31 (2003) 148.
[143] C.Z. Huang, Y.F. Li, N.B. Li, H.Q. Luo, X.H. Huang, Chin. J. Anal. Chem. 27 (1999) 1241.
[144] N.B. Li, S.P. Liu, H.Q. Luo, Anal. Lett. 35 (2002) 1229.
[145] R.F. Pasternack, P.J. Collings, Science 269 (1995) 935.
[146] C.Z. Huang, K.A. Li, S.Y. Tong, Anal. Chem. 69 (1997) 514.
[147] C.Z. Huang, K.A. Li, S.Y. Tong, Anal. Chem. 68 (1996) 2259.
[148] J.H. Yang, C.L. Tong, N.Q. Jie, X. Wu, G.L. Zhang, H.Z. Ye, J. Pharm. Biomed. Anal. 15 (1997) 1833.
[149] H. Watarai, Y. Saitoh, Chem. Lett. (1995) 283.
[150] P. Feng, Y.F. Li, C.Z. Huang, Anal. Chim. Acta 442 (2001) 89.
[151] C.Z. Huang, Y.F. Li, S.Y. Deng, S.R. Liu, Bull. Chem. Soc. Jpn. 72 (1999) 1501.
[152] S.P. Liu, Z.F. Liu, M. Li, Acta Chim. Sin. 53 (1995) 1185.
[153] S.P. Liu, Q. Liu, Z.F. Liu, M. Li, C.Z. Huang, Anal. Chim. Acta 379 (1999) 53.
[154] C.Z. Huang, Y.F. Li, X.L. Hu, N.B. Li, Anal. Chim. Acta 395 (1999) 187.
[155] R.S. Gurjar, V. Backman, L.T. Perelman, I. Georgakoudi, K. Badizadegan, I. Itzkan, R.R. Dasari, M.S. Feld, Nat. Med. 7 (2001) 1245.
[156] V. Backman, J.A. McGilligan, Nature 408 (2000) 428.
[157] J. Yguerabide, E.E. Yguerabide, Anal. Biochem. 262 (1998) 157.
[158] P. Bao, A.G. Frutos, C. Greef, J. Lahiri, U. Muller, T.C. Peterson, L. Warden, X. Xie, Anal. Chem. 74 (2002) 1792.

[159] T. Peterson, G. Bee, J. Zhu, C. Greef, K. Rhodes, L. Korb, N. Montejano, E. Yguerabide, S. Fait, L. Warden, J. Yguerabide, Clin. Chem. 46 (2000) 1975.

[160] J. Yguerabide, E.E. Yguerabide, J. Cell Biochem. 37 (Suppl.) (2001) 71.

[161] N.A. Danielson, H.D. Holemon, E. Donaldson, K. Rhodes, L. Warden, S. LaBrie, Mol. Biol. Cell 12 (2001) 260A.

[162] G. Yao, Study on the interaction of spectroscopic probes with bioactive substances, Ph.D. Dissertation, Peking University, Beijing, 2000.

[163] Z.L. Jiang, F.X. Zhong, T.S. Li, Acta Chim. Sin. 59 (2001) 438.

[164] Z.L. Jiang, F. Li, T.S. Li, H. Liang, Chem. J. Chin. Univ. 21 (2000) 1488.

[165] Z.L. Jiang, Z.W. Feng, Q.Y. Liu, Y.M. Jiang, H. Liang, Chin. J. Inorg. Chem. 17 (2001) 355.

[166] J.Y. Xie, Z.L. Jiang, Acta Phys. Chim. Sin. 17 (2001) 406.

[167] Z.L. Jiang, F. Li, T.S. Li, H. Liang, Chem. J. Chin. Univ. 21 (2000) 1488.

[168] Z.L. Jiang, Z.W. Feng, X.C. Shen, Chin. Chem. Lett. 12 (2001) 551.

[169] H. Liang, X.C. Shen, F. Li, Z.L. Jiang, Chin. Chem. Lett. 11 (2000) 251.

[170] C.Z. Huang, Y.F. Li, W. Lu, Curr. Top. Anal. Chem. 3(3) (2002) 253.

[171] C.Z. Huang, W. Lu, Y.F. Li, Rev. Anal. Chem. 21 (2002) 267.

(Cheng Zhi Huang, Yuan Fang Li, Published in *Analytica Chimica Acta,* 2003, 500, 105～117)

1.2 The Principles and Analytical Applications of Total Internal Reflected Resonance Light Scattering Technique

Abstract: This mini-review displays the analytical applications of resonance light scattering signals at liquid/liquid interfaces. Since the deep changes of refractive indexes at liquid/liquid interface, an evanescent field is formed when a beam of light is incident from an optically dense medium to an optically rare medium at an angle greater than the critical angle. As a result, the chemical species in the interfacial region can be highly selectively excited by the evanescent wave, and the resulting total internal reflected resonance light scattering (TIR-RLS) signals can be detected and employed for sensitive and selective determination of analytes including bio-macromolecules and drugs. Possible applications of the TIR-RLS technique in the future are discussed.

Keywords: Total internal reflected-resonance light scattering (TIR-RLS) technique, liquid/liquid interface, proteins, nucleic acids, and pharmaceutical analysis.

1.2.1 Introduction

The light scattering phenomenon widely exists in the process of the interaction of photons and particles and can be observed in any direction except that the excitation light beam propagates. It has been extensively and successfully applied to measure the size and distribution of polymer particles[1]. This technique, however, suffers from the disadvantages of low signal levels and insensitivity unless laser facilities are put into use. Recent studies disclose that sensitive assays can be performed based on the measurements of enhanced light scattering signals, such as in enhanced Resonance Raman scattering[2] and nuclear magnetic resonance scattering [3]. However, expensive and complicated equipment is compulsory and seriously confines their routine analytical applications.

Similar to stray light, scattering light is one of the major interferences in fluorescent techniques and various attempts have been made to eliminate it as much as possible. With the proposal of resonance light scattering (RLS) technique[4], which was based on simultaneously scanning the excitation and emission monochromators of a common spectrofluorometer with $\Delta\lambda$=0 nm, the situation has changed, and the RLS technique has been applied to the investigations of molecular recognition, assembly[4~8], the quantification of nucleic acids and proteins[9~20] at nonogram levels, surfactants in water samples[21], metallic ions[22, 23], and pharmaceutical[24] analyses. Although sensitive and simple, RLS technique was found to suffer from bad selectivity as a general analytical method. To overcome these drawbacks, we successfully coupled RLS technique with total internal reflected light at the interface of two immiscible liquids and developed a total internal reflect resonance light scattering (TIR-RLS) technique[25], setting up a new and powerful means to investigate the liquid/liquid interface. Herein, we will demonstrate the principle of TIR-RLS techniques and its analytical applications reported in our research group. Finally, possible applications in the future are discussed.

1.2.2 Background for Proposing TIR-RLS Technique

1.2.2.1 Drawbacks of RLS as an analytical technique

As stated above, RLS technique is simple, and has been widely and fruitfully practiced in analytical chemistry. However, its drawbacks have obstructed its further analytical applications. Firstly, the technique has poor selectivity, and its tolerance levels of coexisting foreign substances are scarcely at the same level as the analytes. RLS signals of a scatterer are related to its absorption features of the medium, size, shape, concentration and refractive index compared to its environments[4~5, 9~10]. Thus, particles or colloidal scatters of coexisting foreign substances can exert significant influences. Secondly, RLS technique is still focused on the aqueous media, restricting the employment of oil-soluble reagents to the applications in recognition and interaction between hosts and guests with immiscible property, occurring possibly in complex biologic systems such as in cell matrix. Although surfactants can be introduced as emulgents to resolve this problem expediently, much more complicated interaction mechanisms are involved and it is difficult to understand the interaction processes[26]. Thirdly, researches of orientation of molecules are developed with difficulty using polarized excitation light, due to multiple light scattering components in solutions. As a result, further studies of RLS technique are essential.

1.2.2.2 Considerations for improving RLS technique

To overcome the disadvantages mentioned above, we combine the RLS technique with the liquid/liquid interface based on the following considerations: (1) RLS technique is established on the basis of the fluctuation of the refractive indexes in an aqueous solution where a steep change occurs between the refractive index of the inner scattered particles and that of their outer atmosphere[4~5], which gives rise to mini-interfaces between the inner scattered particles and their outer atmosphere. The occurrence of the adsorption will easily bring about a sharp fluctuation of refractive indexes at the interfacial region; (2) the analyte can be adsorbed to the oil/water interface to acquire a good separation of the analyte with coexisting foreign substances; during which the enrichment of the analyte at the oil/water interface also occurs, and high selectivity and sensitivity can be expected as well; (3) hosts and guests with immiscible property can encounter and interact at an oil/water interface and the corresponding amphiphilic species can be separated from the bulk phases, adsorbed and enriched by the oil/water interface[27]. Thus recognition and interaction of hosts and guests with immiscible property can be carried out easily; (4) oil-soluble reagents can be used conveniently owing to the existence of the oil phase; (5) the interfacial region presents a good chance to study orientation of molecules by means of polarized excitation light as a result of the relatively simplex components in it.

1.2.2.3 Importance to characterize liquid/liquid interfaces

Processes occurring at the interface between two immiscible liquids underlie many important phenomena in biology, pharmacology, and chemistry[28~29]. For instance, the adsorption and uptake of drugs into their target cells, and their pharmacological activities are closely relied on cellular membrane activities and the behaviors of drugs at cellular membranes, respectively[30], so the studies on cellular membranes themselves and the behaviors of drugs at them are of much importance. However, cellular membranes are structurally complex. As a result, immiscible oil/water interfaces are often used as simplified cellular membranes models, in which hydrocarbon/water interfaces are first selected as a consequence of their excellent approximation to the cellular membranes[29]. As to chemistry, the interface of two immiscible liquids is of primary importance since its chemistry is the fundamental basis for analytical and separation sciences[31, 32]. A case in point is that liquid/liquid interfaces have been most widely applied to the investigations of kinetic mechanisms of solvent extraction, including ion-pair extraction, chelate extraction and synergistic extraction, for adsorption and reaction at liquid/liquid interfaces is a significant elementary process in the solvent extraction[27, 34]. As a result, it is necessary and interesting to develop novel and powerful tools to study liquid/liquid interfaces.

In order to investigate liquid/liquid interfaces, indirect methods based essentially on bulk measurements were carried out, such as the interfacial tension method [35] and the high-speed stirring method[36, 37]. These methods, although they can yield significant information on the interfacial properties, fail to provide accurate microscopic or molecular level characteristics of the interfacial species[34, 37~40]. Therefore, to obtain greater insight into the behaviors of interfacial species, *in situ* measurements of liquid/liquid interfaces are essential: Recently, direct spectroscopic techniques have been proposed to effectively study liquid/liquid interfaces including nonlinear optical techniques such as second harmonic generation(SHG)[41,42] and sum frequency generation (SFG)[43~45], neutron specula reflectivity measurements[46], two-phase stopped flow [47], the centrifugal liquid membrane method[37], and total internal reflection fluorescence(TIRF) spectroscopy[27, 38, 48~52]. These techniques have successfully afforded valuable characteristics of liquid/liquid interfaces, such as molecular orientations at liquid/liquid interfaces, the thickness and roughness of liquid/liquid interfaces, but they have their own limitations: TIRF spectroscopy, for example, was limited for understanding the liquid/liquid interfaces when the interfacial species themselves cannot fluoresce, but TIR-RLS technique, similar to RLS technique, can be applied to characterize assembly and aggregate with no color changes or no fluorescence emission at liquid/liquid interfaces, obviously facilitating investigations of liquid/liquid interfaces. In addition, theoretical methods such as computer simulations have presented new and helpful insights into molecular level characteristics of liquid/liquid interfaces as well[53, 54]. Nonetheless, complementary studies with experiments are limited, so that predictions made from the simulations are still controversial and worth studying.

1.2.3 Principle of TIR-RLS Technique

1.2.3.1 Principle of TIR-RLS technique

TIR-RLS technique is an application of RLS technique on liquid/liquid interfaces, so RLS theory supervises how to acquire RLS signals from liquid/liquid interfaces. RLS technique is constructed on the basis of the fluctuation of the refractive index in an aqueous solution, in which the steep change of the refractive index of the inner scatterer and that of its outer atmosphere occurs[4,5,55~57]. Namely, TIR-RLS signals originate from the inhomogeneity of liquid/liquid interfaces, and its intensity can be expressed the same as RLS technique[55~57]

$$K = I_o \frac{8000(2.303)^2 \cdot \pi V n^2 \cdot c}{3\lambda_0^4 N_A} \left\{ \left[\frac{1}{\pi} \int_0^{\infty} \frac{\varepsilon(\lambda) d\lambda}{\lambda_0^2 - \lambda^2} \right]^2 + \frac{\varepsilon^2(\lambda_0)}{4\lambda_0^2} \right\} = Kc \qquad (1)$$

where N_A is Avogadro constant, $\varepsilon(\lambda)$ and (λ_0) are the molar absorbtivity at the λ and λ_0, correspondingly. If the excitation light wavelength is far away from the molecular absorption band, the first square in Eq. (1) equals zero and TIR-RLS is mainly dependent on the real part of the refractive index. However, if the excitation light wavelength is near the molecular absorption band, the first square in Eq. (1) will not be zero, and the contribution of the refractive index to TIR-RLS comes from both the real and imaginary parts. Especially, when the molecular absorption is strong, the contribution of the imaginary part is very significant, and thus it is similar to RLS strong enhanced TIR-RLS signals can be expected[1,4] when the fluctuation of the refractive index is very steep.

1.2.3.2 Total internal reflection (TIR) at liquid/liquid interfaces

Total internal reflection occurs when a beam of light is incident from an optically dense medium to an optically rare medium at an angle greater than the critical angle θ_c defined by

$$\theta_c = \sin^{-1}(\frac{n_2}{n_1}) \qquad (2)$$

where n_1, and n_2 are the refractive indexes of the dense and rare media, respectively. When the incident beam undergoes total internal reflection at the interface of the optically dense and rare media, its electromagnetic energy can be carried across the interface in the form of an evanescent wave, which follows an exponential decay with perpendicular depth from the interface and rapidly falls to undetectable levels within less than one wavelength[56]. As a result, the chemical species in the interfacial region can be highly selectively excited by the evanescent wave[34].

1.2.3.3 Detecting RLS signals at liquid/liquid interfaces

In our experiments, an optical quartz cell (10 mm) was employed after render it hydrophobic and prepare a flat organic solvent-water interface. The coating treatment was made with a toluene solution of 2% dichlorodimethylsilane. By carefully controlling the coating time and temperature, good reproducibility of coating can be achieved.

TIR-RLS spectra and intensities were measured with a common spectrofluorometer, and its sample compartment can be modified so that the species at liquid/liquid interfaces can be excited and emit the light scattering signals detected at 90° angle. Two right-angle quartz prisms (10mm × 10mm × 10 mm) were attached to the optical quartz cell walls, facing the excitation light source and the emission detector, respectively. The excitation light beam passing through the prism and the cell wall was impinged upon the water/organic solvent interface in the cell at an incidence angle of 72.6°, sufficiently greater than the critical total-reflection angle at the organic solvent-water interface (θ_c = 59 to *ca.* 70°) [52]. Therefore, this optical arrangement can be widely used for TIR-RLS studies of organic solvent-water interfaces.

As we stated above, TIR-RLS signals originate from the inhomogeneity of liquid/liquid interfaces. Therefore, we consider that chemical species adsorbing at liquid/liquid interfaces make the major contributions to the TIR-RLS signals. Because amphiphilic species, containing both hydrophilic moieties and hydrophobic moieties, are repelled from both the water and the organic solvent phases, and can be well adsorbed to the water/organic solvent interface with amphiphilic property as well, thus how to produce amphiphilic species at liquid/liquid interface is of much importance in TIR-RLS studies.

One way to create amphiphilic species is via the interfacial interaction between hydrophilic and hydrophobic substances. Tetraphenylporphyrin (TPP) is a highly hydrophobic chelate reagent and cannot adsorb at thewater/organic solvent interface. However, TPP can be protonated by the attack of hydrogen ions to produce the diprotonated species (H_2TPP^{2+}), which is sparingly soluble in water and can be adsorbed at the water/organic solvent interface[53]. Similarly, Zinc (II) can interact at pH 6.1～6.3 with α, β, γ, δ-tetrakis(4-sulfophenyl)porphine

($TPPS_4$) to form a complex, which cannot adsorb at the toluene/water interface[27]. Nevertheless, an addition of 1, 10-phenanthroline (phen) to the toluene phase induces the adsorption of the complex of Zn-$TPPS_4$ at the interface, which was interpreted by the interaction between Zn-$TPPS_4$ and phen at the interface [54].

The other way to form amphiphilic species is by using interface-active substances. Interface-active substances consist of two parts. One is surfactant, such as cationic surfactant and anionic surfactant, and the other is not surfactant but with interface-active properties, such as Rhodamine derivatives (Rhodamine B, Sulforhodamine B, and Rhodamine 110) that can adsorb at the water/organic solvent interface with the long axis of the xanthene ring tilted about 70° to surface normal. For instance, $TPPS_4$ (-4 charged) and $\alpha, \beta, \gamma, \delta$-tetrakis (N-methylpyridinium-4-yl) porphine (TMPyP) (+4 charged) were both well soluble in aqueous phase in neutral pH and cannot enter the water/organic solvent interfacial region unless cetyltrimethylammonium bromide (CTMAB) and sodium hexadecane sulfonate (SHS) were added due to the coadsorption of $TPPS_4$ and TMPyP with CTMAB and SHS, correspondingly[27].

1.2.4 Analytical Applications of TIR-RLS

By employing TIR-RLS technique, we have established highly sensitive and selective methods for determining pharmaceuticals and biomacromolecules. The assay of chlortetracycline is of interest and importance since it is widely used as a bacteriostatic and antibiotic drug in clinical medicine and food science. In the pH range of 7.54~8.14, CTC first interacts with Eu (III) to form the binary complex of Eu (III)-CTC in the aqueous phase, and then reacts with trioctyl phosphine oxide (TOPO) of the $CC1_4$ phase at the water/$CC1_4$ interface. The formed ternary amphiphiliccomplex of CTC-Eu(III)-TOPO adsorbs at the water/CCl_4 interface, giving rise to greatly enhanced TIR-RLS signals. The enhanced TIR-RLS intensity is in proportion to the CTC concentration in the range of $(0.98\sim20.0)\times10^{-7}$ mol·L^{-1}. The limit of detection can reach 9.8×10^{-9} mol·L^{-1}. The high tolerance level for coexisting materials supplies a good permission for the direct assay of CTC in body fluid samples including human urine, human serum, and fresh milk[25].

Considering the complex ability of Eu(III), we proposed a similar method of nucleic acids based on the Eu(III) complexation [58]. At pH 8.69 and ion strength 0.008, ternary amphiphilic species formed by the interaction of nucleic acids with Eu (III) in the presence of oil-soluble trioctylphosphineoxide (TOPO) are adsorbed in the water/tetrachloromethane ($H_2O/CC1_4$)interface, giving rise to significantly enhanced TIR-RLS signals. It can be used in the quantification of nucleic acids in the range of 0.002~2.5 μg·mL^{-1}, and the limit of detection can reach 0.16 ng·mL^{-1}. Complicated artificial samples with highly interfering background were determined satisfactorily.

At pH 3.29 and ionic strength 0.003, the adsorption of thiamine with anionic surfactants, such as sodium dodecyl benzene sulfonate (SDBS), sodium dodecylsulfonate (SDS) and sodium lauryl sulfate (SLS), occurs at the water/tetrachloromethane (H_2O/CCl_4) interface, giving rise to greatly enhanced TIR-RLS signals characterized at 375.0 nm. The enhanced TIR-RLS intensity at 375.0 nm is in proportion to the concentration of thiamine in the range of 0.12~850 ng·mL^{-1} and its limit of detection (3σ) is 12 pg·mL^{-1}[59]. Samples of vitamin B, tablets and injection solutions are identical with those of standard procedures[59].

Based on the TIR-RLS measurements occurring at $H_2O/CC1_4$ interfaces, we proposed a direct quantification of human serum albumin (HSA) in blood serum samples without separation of γ-IgG[60]. In a medium of pH6.37~6.59, the coadsorption of the binary complex of HSA-Th(IV) with sodium dodecylbenzene sulfonate

(SDBS) occurs at the H_2O/CCl_4 interface, forming an amphiphilic layer and displaying in greatly enhanced TIR-RLS signals with the maximum peak located at 340~370 rim. The enhanced TIR-RLS intensity is in proportion to the HSA concentration in the range 0.15~1.0 ug·mL^{-1}. The limit of detection is 14.4 ng·mL^{-1}. Common ions in fluids including Ca(II), Mg(II), NH_4^+, Mn(II) and SO_4^{2-}, amino acids, carbohydrates and urea can be allowed with high concentrations under the tolerance level of 10% (larger than 1.0×10^{-4} mol·L^{-1}. Since 1.5 fold of γ-IgG can be allowed, direct determination of trace amounts of HSA can be made in human serum samples without separating the interfering materials.

1.2.5 Prospects for TIR-RLS

From the above description concerning the analytical applications, the newly built TIR-RLS technique has higher sensitivity and selectivity than RLS techniques, indicating that the drawbacks of RLS techniques have been overcome. It can be employed not only for the determination of pharmaceuticals and biomacromolecules, but also for mechanisms at liquid/liquid interfaces, such as the thickness, polarity and roughness of liquid/liquid interfaces. At present, corresponding studies are in progress. In addition, in order to characterize further the properties of liquid/liquid interfaces, we are now beginning to consider new techniques such as polarized TIR-RLS technique, three-dimension TIR-RLS spectroscopy technique, TIR-RLS correction spectroscopy technique, TIR-RLS imaging technique, and backward light scattering technique.

Acknowledgement

We greatly appreciate the financial support of the National Natural Science Foundation of China (NSFC, 20275032).

References

[1] J. Zuo, The Principles and Applications of Laser Light Scattering in Polymer Science, Henan Science and Technology Press, Zhengzhou,1994, p. 1.

[2] H. G. M. Edwards, F. Garcia-Pichel, E. M. Newton, and D. D. Wynn-Williams, Spectrochim. Acta, Part A, 55, 193 (1999).

[3] Y. Cheng, and D. G. Cory, J. Am. Chem. Soc., 121, 7935 (1999).

[4] R. F. Pasternack, C. Bustamante, P. J. Collings, A. Giannetto, and E. J. Gibbs, J. Am. Chem. Soc., 115, 5393 (1993).

[5] R. F. Pasternack, and P. J. Collings, Science, 269, 935 (1995).

[6] R. F. Pasternack, K. S. Schaefer, and P. Hambright, Inorg. Chem., 33, 2062 (1994).

[7] J. C. de Paula, J. H. Robblee, and R. F. Pasternack, Biophys. J., 68, 335 (1995).

[8] G. Arena, L. M. Scolaro, R. F. Pasternack, and R. Romeo, Inorg. Chem., 34, 2994 (1995).

[9] C. Z. Huang, K. A. Li, and S. Y. Tong, Anal. Chem., 68, 2259 (1996).

[10] C. Z. Huang, K. A. Li, and S. Y. Tong, Anal. Chem., 69, 514 (1997).

[11] C. Z. Huang, Y. F. Li, J. G. Mao, and D. G. Tan, Analyst, 123, 1401 (1998).

[12] C. Z. Huang, K. A. Li, and S. Y. Tong, Bull. Chem. Soc. Jpn., 70, 1843 (1997).

[13] C. Z. Huang, Y. F. Li, N. Li, K. A. Li, and S: Y. Tong, Bull. Chem. Soc. Jpn., 71, 1791 (1998).

[14] Y. T. Wang, F. L Zhao, and K. A. Li, Fresen. J. Anal. Chem., 364, 560 (1999).

[15] Y. Liu, C. Q. Ma, K. A. Li, and S. Y. Tong, Anal. Biochem., 268, 187 (1999).

[16] Y. F. Li, C. Z. Huang, and M. Li, Anal. Sci., 18,177 (2002).

[17] Y. F. Li, C. Z. Huang, and M. Li, Anal. Chin. Acta, 452, 285 (2002).

[18] C. Q. Ma, K. A. Li, and S. Y. Tong, Anal. Biochem., 239, 86 (1996).

[19] Y. M. Hao, and H. X. Shen, Anal. Chim. Acta, 413, 87 (2000).
[20] C. Z. Huang,Y. F. Li, X. H. Huang, and M. Li, Analyst, 125, 1267 (2000).
[21] C. X. Yang, Y. F. Li, and C. Z. Huang, Anal. Bioanal. Chem., 374, 868 (2002).
[22] Y. K. Zhao, Q. E. Cao, Z. D. Hu, and Q. H. Xu, Anal. Chim. Acta, 388, 45 (1999).
[23] S. P. Liu, Z. F. Liu, and H. Q. Luo, Anal. Chim. Acta, 407, 255 (2000).
[24] S. P. Liu, H. Q. Luo, N. B. Li, Z. F. Liu, and W. X. Zheng, Anal. Chem., 73, 3907 (2001).
[25] P. Feng, W. Q. Shu, C. Z. Huang, and Y. F. Li, Anal. Chem., 73, 4307 (2001).
[26] J. H. Yang, C. L. Tong, N. Q. Jie, X. Wu, G. L. Zhang, and H. Z. Ye, J. Pharm. Biomed. Anal., 15, 1833 (1997).
[27] H. Watarai, and Y: Saitoh, Chem. Lett., 283, (1995).
[28] S. Haslam, S. G. Croucher, C. G. Hickman, and J. G. Frey, Phys. Chem. Chem. Phys., 2, 3235 (2000).
[29] A. Gajraj, and R. Y. Ofoli, Langmuir, 16, 4279 (2000).
[30] A. Malkia, P: Liljeroth, A. K. Kontturi, and K. Kontturi, J. Phys. Chem. B, 105, 10884 (2001).
[31] C. Shi, and F. C. Anson, Anal. Chem., 70, 3114 (1998).
[32] Y. Shao, and M. V. Mirkin, Anal. Chem., 70,3155 (1998).
[33] M. Ma, and F. F. Cantwell, Anal. Chem., 71, 388 (1999).
[34] Y. Chida, and H. Watarai, Bull. Chem. Soc. Jpn., 69, 341 (1996).
[35] T. Shioya, S. Tsukahara, and N. Teramae, Chem. Lett., 469 (1996).
[36] F. E. Cantwell, and H. Freiser, Anal. Chem., 60, 226 (1988).
[37] H. Nagatani, and H. Watarai, Anal. Chem., 70, 2860 (1998).
[38] S. Ishizaka, K. Nakatani, S. Habuchi, and N. Kitamura, Anal. Chem., 71, 419 (1999).
[39] Y. Uchiyama, I Tsuyumoto, T Kitamori, and T. Sawada, J. Phys. Chem. B, 103, 4663 (1999).
[40] N. Inger, Langmuir, 13, 2242 (1997).
[41] R. M. Corn, and D. A. Higgins, Chem. Rev., 94, 107 (1994).
[42] J. D. Byers, H. 1. Yee, and J. M. Hicks, J. Chem. Phys., 101, 6233 (1994).
[43] Q. Du, E. Freysz, and Y. R. Shen, Science, 264, 826 (1994).
[44] M. C. Messmer, J. C. Conboy, and G. L. Richmond, J. Am. Chem. Soc., 117, 8039 (1995).
[45] D. E. Gragson, and G. L. Richmond, J. Am. Chem. Soc., 120, 366 (1998).
[46] L. T. Lee, D. Langevin, and B. Farnoux, Phys. Rev. Lett., 67, 2678 (1991).
[47] H. Nagatani, and H. Watarai, Anal. Chem., 68, 1250 (1996).
[48] M. J. Wirth, and J. D. Burbage, Anal. Chem., 64, 9022 (1992).
[49] K. Bessho, T. Uchida, A. Yamauchi, T. Shioya, and N. Teramae, Chem. Phys. Lett., 264, 381 (1997).
[50] S. Ishizaka, S. Habuchi, H. B. Kim, and N. Kitamura, Anal. Chem., 71, 3382 (1999).
[51] N. Fujiwara, S. Tsukahara, and H. Watarai, Langmuir, 17, 5337 (2001).
[52] S. Ishizaka, H. B. Kim, and N. Kitamura, Anal. Chem., 73, 2421 (2001).
[53] M. Lauterbach, E. Engler, N. Muzet, L. Troxler, and G. Wipff, J. Phys. Chem., 102, 245 (1998).
[54] P. A. Fernarides, M. N. D. S. Corderiro, and J. A. N. F. Gomes, J. Phys. Chem. B, 103, 6290 (1999).
[55] M. A. S. Vigeant, M. Wagner, L. K. Tamm, and R. M. Ford, Langmuir, 17, 2235 (2001).
[56] J. Anglister, and I. Z. Steinberg, J. Chem. Phys., 74, 786 (1981).
[57] Y. F. Li, C. Z. Huang, and X. L. Hu, Chinese J. Anal. Chem., 26, 1508 (1998).
[58] W. Lu, C. Z. Huang, and Y. F. Li, Analyst, 127, 1932 (2002)
[59] W. Lu, C. Z. Huang, and Y. F. Li, Anal. Chim. Acta, 475,151 (2003)
[60] P. Feng, C. Z. Huang, and Y. F. Li, Anal. Biochem., 308, 83 (2002).

(Cheng Zhi Huang, Wei Lu and Yuan Fang Li,
published in *Reviews in Analytical Chemistry,* 2002, 21, 267～278)

1.3 Recent Developments of the Resonance Light Scattering Technique: Technical Evolution, New Probes and Applications

Abstract: The resonance light scattering (RLS) technique, scanning simultaneously the excitation and emission monochromators of a common spectrofluorometer to detect enhanced RLS signals, has been used for designating bio-assemblies, aggregation species, and analytical purposes. Herein, we review the reports since our last mini-review in 2003 concerning the new derived RLS techniques, RLS probes, and their applications.

Keywords: Resonance light scattering (RLS), RLS probe, applications

1.3.1 Introduction

Light scattering exists from our daily life to universal space, including the light beams through the black night when one uses an electric torch, beautiful unforgettable views of rainbows, sunrises and sunsets originating from scattered rays of photons interacting with particles such as dust, clouds, and smog in a medium like air[1]. Observations of scattered lights are very common since all media except vacuum are relatively inhomogeneous[2,3]. Based on these light-scattering phenomena, laser-induced light-scattering techniques have been extensively applied to the measurements of size and distribution of polymer particles[4], colloid[5], drug powder[6], and self-assembled biopolymers[7]. In analytical chemistry, light-scattering detectors have been developed in chromatographic determinations based on measuring the signals of light scattering[8,9], multi-angle light scattering (MALS) [10~12], and evaporative light-scattering detections (ELSD)[13,14].

Resonance light-scattering (RLS) techniques[15,16], developed by using a common spectrofluorometer to measure the enhanced RLS signals that occur when a light beam with the wavelength close to the absorption region of species is applied to excite the species and has found wide applications in the designation of bioassemblies and aggregation process[17~20] and analytical applications in biochemical[21~23], and pharmaceuticals fields[24~26]. In our previous mini-review about the RLS technique theoretically and practically in 2003[27], we introduced the basic theory, a summary of applications from 2000 to 2002, and the main factors affecting the enhanced RLS signals[27]. The rapid development of new RLS techniques and newfound noble RLS probes has promoted the application of RLS technique in the last four years. Herein, we contribute a mini-review of the RLS technique and new applications since 2003.

1.3.2 Development of New RLS Techniques

RLS techniques have found wide applications in the detection of biomolecules for their simplicity and high sensitivity but suffer from flaws such as poor selectivity and stability. Therefore, improved RLS techniques such as the RLS imaging technique (RLSI)[28~31], wavelength-ratiometric RLS technique (WR-RLS)[32~26], backward light-scattering technique (BLS)[37~40], flow injection analysis-coupled RLS technique (FIA-RLS)[41~43], total internal reflected resonance light-scattering technique (TIRRLS)[44~50], and surface-enhanced light-scattering technique (SELS)[51] were established to solve these problems. Table 1 lists the newly derived RLS techniques and their applications in the last four years.

1.3.2.1 RLS Imaging Technique

The traditional RLS measurements reflect only average light-scattering signals of the aggregation species in bulk solution, failing to disclose more information such as the feature of the aggregation species and a single scatter. The RLS imaging technique, using a common microscope-coupled, charge-coupled device (CCD) camera and a laser beam, was established to observe light-scattering figures of the aggregation species[28]. Under laser excitation, a single aggregation species of $TPPS_4$ induced by proteins in bulk solution could be observed at a right angle to the excitation beam with a single CCD camera in situ. The RLS signals induced by a laser beam are more sensitive than the Newly derived RLS technique and their applications.

Table 1 Newly derived RLS technique and their applications

Methods	Analytes	Probes	Linear range	LOD (3σ)	Ref.
RLSI	BSA	$TPPS_4$	0.009–210 ng·mL^{-1}	8.6 pg·mL^{-1}	[28]
	HSA		0.010–210 ng·mL^{-1}	9.7 pg·mL^{-1}	
RLSI	ctDNA	TAPP	200–1100 ng·mL^{-1}	19.75 ng·mL^{-1}	[29]
	fsDNA		250–1100 ng·mL^{-1}	24.86 ng·mL^{-1}	
RLSI	Heparin	TAPP	0.02–0.6μg·mL^{-1}	1.3 ng·mL^{-1}	[30]
TIR-RLSI	fsDNA	CrHO	0.5–3.6 × 10^{-6}mol·L^{-1}	—	[31]
WR-RLS	Glucose	Con A	10–60 μmol·L^{-1}		[33]
		TAPP	0–4.0 ×10^{-7}mol·L^{-1}	—	
WR-RLS	Heparin	TMPyP-4	0–2.42×10^{-7}mol·L^{-1}		[34]
WR-RLS	Heparin	JGB	0.3–6000.0 ng·mL^{-1}	0.03 ng·mL^{-1}	[35]
WR-RLS	fsDNA	Hyamine 1622	5.0–3000.0 ng·mL^{-1}	0.50 ng·mL^{-1}	[36]
BLS	ctDNA	TPP	0.6–1200 ng·mL^{-1}	60 pg·mL^{-1}	[37]
	fsDNA		1.1–1200 ng·mL^{-1}	110 pg·mL^{-1}	
	HSA		1–1250 ng·mL^{-1}	75 pg·mL^{-1}	
BLS	BSA	Quercetin	2–1250 ng·mL^{-1}	180 pg·mL^{-1}	[38]
BLS	Cl^-	$AgNO_3$	0.02–4.26 μg·mL^{-1}	2.0 ng·mL^{-1}	[39]
BLS	Pb^{2+}	TPB	0.03–1.8 μg·mL^{-1}	2.6 ng·mL^{-1}	[40]
FIA-RLS	Proteins	Bromothymol blue	7–70 μg·mL^{-1}	3.75 μg·mL^{-1}	[41]
FIA-RLS	Heparin	Azure B	0.01–6.0 μg·mL^{-1}	6.4 ng·mL^{-1}	[42]
	HSA		0.005–18 μg·mL^{-1}	5.00 ng·mL^{-1}	
FIA-RLS	BSA	Biebrich scarlet	0.008–16 μg·mL^{-1}	7.80 ng·mL^{-1}	[43]
		SDBS	0.12–850 ng·mL^{-1}	12 pg·mL^{-1}	
TIR-RLS	Thiamine	SDS	0.20–850 ng·mL^{-1}	20 pg·mL^{-1}	[44]
		SLS	0.27–850 ng·mL^{-1}	27 pg·mL^{-1}	
TIR-RLS	Berberine	Fluorescein	3.2–3200×10^{-9} mol·L^{-1}	1.3 ng·mL^{-1}	[47]
	ctDNA		0.060–2.5 μg·mL^{-1}	6.0 ng·mL^{-1}	
TIR-RLS	fsDNA	CTAB	0.015–3.5 μg·mL^{-1}	1.5 ng·mL^{-1}	[45]
	yRNA		0.046–3.5 μg·mL^{-1}	4.6 ng·mL^{-1}	
	BP		0.10–1.0 ×10^{-6} mol·L^{-1}	3.48 ×10^{-8} mol·L^{-1}	
	OA		0.09–1.0 ×10^{-6} mol·L^{-1}	3.85 ×10^{-8} mol·L^{-1}	
TIR-RLS	AmP	Berberine	0.11–1.2 ×10^{-6} mol·L^{-1}	4.22×10^{-8} mol·L^{-1}	[48]

Continued

Methods	Analytes	Probes	Linear range	LOD (3*s*)	Ref.
	AmO		$0.12–1.2 \times 10^{-6}$ mol·L^{-1}	4.86×10^{-8} mol·L^{-1}	
	BP		$0.15–2.2 \times 10^{-6}$ mol·L^{-1}	4.87×10^{-8} mol·L^{-1}	
	OA		$0.10–2.0 \times 10^{-6}$ mol·L^{-1}	5.30×10^{-8} mol·L^{-1}	
TIR-RLS	AmP	CTMAB	$0.15–2.2 \times 10^{-6}$ mol·L^{-1}	5.84×10^{-8} mol·L^{-1}	([49]
	AmO		$0.20–2.2 \times 10^{-6}$ mol·L^{-1}	7.07×10^{-8} mol·L^{-1}	
TIR-RLS	ctDNA	Acrindine orange	0.0032–2.0 μg·mL^{-1}	0.32 ng·mL^{-1}	[46]
	fsDNA		0.0025–2.4 μg·mL^{-1}	0.25 ng·mL^{-1}	
	HSA		0.5–42.3 μg·mL^{-1}	0.198 ng·mL^{-1}	
TIR-RLS	BSA	Arsenazo-TB	0.5–41.0 μg·mL^{-1}	0.221 ng·mL^{-1}	[50]
SELS	*h*-IgG	Anti-*h*-IgG	0.1–10 μg·mL^{-1}	10 ng·mL^{-1}	[51]

Abbreviations: BSA, bovine serum albumin; HSA, human serum albumin; $TPPS_4$, *α*, *β*, *γ*, *δ*–tetrakis (p-sulfophenyl) porphyrin; TAPP, *α*, *β*, *γ*, *δ*-tetra(4-trimethylaminonium phenyl) porphine or *meso*-tetrakis [(trimethylammoniumyl) phenyl] porphyrin; fsDNA, fish sperm DNA; ctDNA, calf thymus DNA; yRNA, yeast RNA; CrHO, chromium(III) hydrolytic oligomers; Con A, concanavalin A; JGB, Janus green blue; TMPyP-4, *meso*-tetra (4-methylpyridy) porphyrin; TPP, tetraphenylporphyrin; TPB, sodium tetraphenylboron; SDBS, dodecylbenzene sulfonate; SDS, sodium dodecylsulfonate and; SLS, sodium lauryl sulfate; CTAB, cetyltrimethylammonium bromide; AmP, ampicillin; BP, benzyl penicillin; OA, oxacillin; AmO, amoxycillin; *h*-IgG, human immunoglobulin G.

RLS signals measured with a spectrofluorometer. The measured counts of aggregation species in these images are proportional to the concentrations of BSA and HSA in the range of nanogram with the limits of determination at picogram levels, indicating that the RLSI technique is much more sensitive and reliable[28]. The RLS imaging technique was also used to detect DNA and saccharide with high sensitivity in a similar manner[29,30].

However, the RLS imaging technique is limited by instability since the scatter in bulk solution is not static but in Brownian motion, making the light-scattering signals related to the scatter in the detection focus plane fluctuate. This flaw prompted a combination of the TIR-RLS technique, which can then provide an immobile platform at the liquid–liquid interface with the RLS imaging technique, allowing the scatter to be stably immobilized or controlled at the liquid–liquid interface for imaging[31]. In the performance of the TIR-RLS imaging technique, the feature of aggregation species of DNA biopolymer, which was selectively absorbed at the water–oil interface in the presence of triocyctyl phosphine oxide (TOPO), was observed by common microscope with high stability and sensitivity. It was also demonstrated that the large aggregations species at the interface have a stronger scattering ability than that in bulk solution, causing a strong lightscattering signal from H_2O–CCl_4 interface.

1.3.2.2 Backward Light Scattering (BLS)

These measurements of RLS method are commonly based on detecting the signals at the right angle of incident light. However, the scattered light both in forward and backward direction has been neglected. According to Rayleigh scattering law[52], the scattered light intensity from a spherical particle illuminated by a monochromatic light beam is angle dependent. The scattering light intensity from the backward direction of the incident light is two times greater than that from the right angle direction[40]. Therefore, backward light scattering is a good alternative if the apparatus is available. In fact, backward light-scattering spectroscopy has been used to provide structural and functional information of tissue in the fields of biomedical and biophysical sciences[53,54], acting as an optical probe technique to detect pre-cancerous and early cancerous changes in cellrich epithelia[55].

The basic theory and potential application of light scattering from backwards suggested the fabrication of the backward light-scattering technique. By coupling a homemade backward light-scattering optical assembly with a common spectrofluorometer, the BLS method was used to detect heavy metal ions[40] in environmental waters and chlorine ion[39] in human urine with higher sensitivity than the common RLS method. Backward RLS method was also performed on liquid–liquid interface to detect protein and nucleic with good selectivity, due to the extraction and separation process through the liquid–liquid interface[37,38]. With the development of the technique, we believe that the backward RLS technique, by combining a laser light source and a micro photomultiplier tube (PMT) detector, will become more sensitive and sufficiently general for various biochemical and environmental analysis.

1.3.2.3 Wavelength-Ratiometric RLS Technique

In the common RLS measurements, the data at the wavelength where maximum RLS intensity is available have been used to quantitatively detect aggregation species. Meanwhile, unavoidable changes of environmental conditions such as the fluctuation of temperature and voltage exerted on instruments will bring fluctuations to the measurement of RLS intensity at a single wavelength. From the advantages of fluorescence ratiometry, RLS ratiometry was developed to overcome the variation of the fluctuated RLS data. Lakowicz's group first reported the wavelength-ratiometric RLS technique by measuring the ratio of scattered intensities of gold colloid aggregation induced by avidin-biotin interactions at two incident wavelengths[32]. The advantages of the wavelength-ratiometric RLS measurements, briefly, are independent of the total concentration of analytical probesnot perturbed by excitation source instabilities or drifts[33]. The interaction between biopolymers with dual wavelength ratiometric was investigated and the RLS technique showed that compared with RLS at a single wavelength, dual wavelength ratiometric RLS techniques have more precise measurements with good repeatability and a wide linear range of analysis[34,35]. Furthermore, the data analysis method in the RLS ratiometry provided a good way to obtain more reliable information from the original signal, which could find wide applications in the field of biological, biomedical, and environmental analysis.

1.3.2.4 Flow Injection Analysis–Coupled RLS

Flow injection analysis (FIA), with the advantages of the perfect reproducibility and automation, is another way to overcome the poor stability of RLS technique. Ferna´ndez et al.[41] first combined the flow-injection analysis with Rayleigh light scattering to quantify the total protein in a real sample. The performance of integrated FIA-RLS technique on the analysis of heparin[42] and protein[43] indicated the good reproducibility and reliability of the new technique. In the detection of heparin sodium injection with the FIA-RLS technique, the recoveries are in agreement with the results given by the manufacturer at more than a 95% confidence level. The relative standard deviation (RSD) for the three samples ($n = 5$) was between 1.4% and 2.6%, and the within-day reproducibility and days reproducibility could be available with the RSD lower than 4%. Briefly, FIA-RLS technique is an improvement over conventional RLS in bulk and it overcomes shortcomings of the conventional RLS technique, such as poor reproducibility and laborious operation.

1.3.2.5 RLS at Liquid–Liquid Interface

Total internal reflected resonance light-scattering (TIR-RLS) technique established at the liquid–liquid interface has the following advantages[27]: (1) the selective absorption of analytes from bulk solution to liquid–liquid interface provides a good way of separation and pre-condensation of analytes from co-existing substances; (2) interaction between two immiscible substances can be studied at the oil–water interface by TIR-RLS; and (3) the interfacial region presents a good chance to study orientation of amphiphilic species. Recently, the combination of TIR-RLS technique with RLS imaging[31] and backward light scattering[37,38] also demonstrated the potential advantages of the liquid–liquid interface in the investigation of the interaction of organic small molecules (OSM) with bio-macromolecules.

1.3.2.6 Surface-Enhanced Light Scattering (SELS)

With the successful application of RLS at the liquid–liquid interface, we found that a solid interface (like a glass slide), which has similar properties to the liquid–liquid interface, is also a good substrate to investigate the interaction occurring at the interface. It has been found that the light scattering of an antigen-modified glass slide could be greatly enhanced by the binding of antibody. Then, an optical immuno-sensor based on measuring the surface-enhanced light-scattering (SELS) signals of glass slides was developed by simultaneously scanning the excitation and the emission monochromators of a common spectrofluorometer[51]. Under optimal experimental conditions, the sensor based on SELS has a high specificity with corresponding antigenother co-existing proteins, such as bovine serum albumin (BSA) and human serum albumin (HSA), do not show any interference effect. The system, besides the advantages of high sensitivity of RLS techniques and peculiar selectivity of immunoreactions, is label free, regenerative, simple, and rapid. It could be applicable to the determination of various proteins with antigen–antibody reactions due to the binding of large molecules on the solid interface.

1.3.3 New RLS Probes

1.3.3.1 Organic Small Molecule (OSM) Probes

Organic small molecules (OSM) are still used as common probes to detect biomolecules in the study of the interaction between dyes and protein and nucleic acids. New organic molecular probes, such as toluidine blue[56,57], imidacloprid[58], pyronine Y[59], bordeaux red[60], and solochrome cyanine R[61] were reported to successfully detect nucleic acids and proteins. For example, the near infrared cyanine dye, which possess high affinity for biological structures (especially DNA), produces enhancing RLS signals in near infrared region and was used to detect nucleic acid directly[62]. A near infrared RLS approach was developed combining the high sensitivity of RLS technique with the low interference of NIR measurement and could reduce possible spectral interference from some biological macromolecules occurred in visible region.

1.3.3.2 RLS Particles

Metal nanoparticles such as gold and silver nanoparticles (GNPs, SNPs) exhibit unique optical properties in the visible spectral range due to the excitation of the collective oscillations of conducting electrons known as plasmon resonances or surface plasmons[63]. The resonance frequency of surface plasmon strongly depends on the size, shape, and dielectric environment of nanoparticles, thus providing an effective way for tuning of their optical properties. Yguerabide et al. first reported that submicroscopic particles such as gold and silver nanoparticles with diameters between 40nm and 120 nm, which were discovered to generate colorful light-scattering signals, could be used as a novel fluorescent analogs in clinical and biological application[52,64]. Roll et al. reported a new approach to optical sensing using the light-scattering properties of colloidal gold[32]. Aslan et al. developed a glucose sensor by plasmon resonance–based light scattering of gold nanoparticles[33].

Recently, Li's group reported highly sensitive light-scattering assay for DNA hybridization in a homogeneous solution[65] by using gold nanoparticles as the label of oligo-nucleotide probes. The assay relies on the observation of greatly enhanced light scattering that originated from the aggregation of oligo-nucleotide–functionalized gold nanoparticles directed by the target DNA. The gold nanoparticles-based light-scattering strategy for target DNA detection has a detection limit (3σ, n=11) of 0.1 pmol·L^{-1}, which is much more sensitive than the previously reported homogeneous detection method. Furthermore, single-base mismatch in DNA targets could be easily discriminated using the light-scattering assay on a common spectrofluorometer without stringently controlling the temperature. The RLS immunoassay[66] is also reported to detect Apolipoprotein AI (ApoAI) and ApoB, using ApoAI and ApoB antibodies immobilized gold nanoparticles as a light-scattering probe. The results from the RLS immunoassay of 25 serum samples was reliable compared with immunoturbidimetry.

Silver nanoparticles is another suitable RLS probe with stronger light-scattering ability than gold nanoparticles. A simple light-scattering method to detect the Sudan dyes in food products based on the formation of silver nanoparticles was developed[67]. For the great light-scattering property of silver nanoparticles, the light-scattering signal of silver nanoparticles formed by the redox reaction of Sudan dyes and $AgNO_3$ can be visually detected with a simple laser pointer or light-emitting diode. The determination for real samples of cayenne oil and chili sauce demonstrated that this method was sensitive, effective, simple, reliable, and had the potential to be put into practice.

Other nanoparticles, such as ZnS, CdS, HgS, PbS, were used as a good RLS probe to detect proteins and nucleic acids[65~81]. Table 2 summarizes the analytical parameters of RLS measurement using nanoparticles as a probe in the last 4 years. We believe that the RLS technique will come up to a new development with the increasing application of nanoparticles.

Table 2 Analytical parameter of RLS technique using nanoparticles as a probe

Probes	Analytes	pH	λ_{max}	Linear range	LOD (3σ)	Ref.
Gold	DNA	7.0	315	0.7～119pmol·L^{-1}	0.1 pmol·L^{-1}	[65]
Gold	ApoAI	6.4	560	0.00833～0.3333 μg·mL^{-1}	2.04 ng·mL^{-1}	[66]
	ApoB			0.00197～0.1972 μg·mL^{-1}	0.96 ng·mL^{-1}	
Gold	Cysteine	5.0	556	0.01～0.25 μg·mL^{-1}	2.0 ng·mL^{-1}	[68]
Gold	Captopril	2.09	553	0.1～1.7 μg·mL^{-1}	32.0 ng·mL^{-1}	[69]
Gold	Thiamazole	5.2	555	0～1.05 μmol·L^{-1}	2.01 nmol·L^{-1}	[70]
Gold	Berberine	4.0	287	1.33～240 ng··mL^{-1}	0.40 ng/mL	[71]
Gold	Vitamin B1	4.0	368	0～2.8 ×10^{-7} mol·L^{-1}	0.9 ng·mL^{-1}	[72]
	BSA			0～0.8 μg·mL^{-1}	1.3 ng·mL^{-1}	
Silver	HAS	5.0	413	0～1.2 μg·mL^{-1}	10 ng·mL^{-1}	[73]
	γ-Globulin			0～2.5 μg·mL^{-1}	5.7 ng·mL^{-1}	
	Sudan I		452	0.2～2.4 μmol·L^{-1}	3.2 nmol·L^{-1}	
	Sudan II	Alkali		0.1～2.4 μmol·L^{-1}	3.0 nmol·L^{-1}	
Sliver	Sudan III	medium 452		0.1～2.4 μmol·L^{-1}	3.2 nmol·L^{-1}	[67]
	Sudan IV			0.2～3.0 μmol·L^{-1}	2.9 nmol·L^{-1}	
	HAS	3.95		0.1～15 μg·mL^{-1}	0.079 μg·mL^{-1}	
CdS/PAA	BSA		380	0.2～20 μg·mL^{-1}	0.078 μg·mL^{-1}	[74]
	γ-Globulin			0.1～50.0 μg·mL^{-1}	0.042 μg·mL^{-1}	
	Tobramycin			0.09～2.14 μmol·L^{-1}	68 nmol·L^{-1}	
Cds	Gentamicin	5.02	376	0.21～2.09 μmol·L^{-1}	84 nmol·L^{-1}	[75]
	Kanamycin			0.21～2.06 μmol·L^{-1}	190 nmol·L^{-1}	
HgS	γ-Globulin	5.03	362	10～140 ng·mL^{-1}	2.71 ng·mL^{-1}	[76]
PbS	γ-Globulin	7.0	385	10～500 ng·mL^{-1}	2.75 ng·mL^{-1}	[77]

Continued

Probes	Analytes	pH	λ_{max}	Linear range	LOD (3σ)	Ref.
	ctDNA			0.04～1.2 μg·mL^{-1}	19 ng·mL^{-1}	
ZnS	fsDNA	5.12	304.5	0.2～1.0 μg·mL^{-1}	23 ng·mL^{-1}	[78]
ZnS-Zn^{2+}	γ-Globulin	6.96	326	0.1～2.0 μg·mL^{-1}	0.0403 μg·mL^{-1}	[79]
CuS-Cu^{2+}	HSA		341	0.1～1.5 μg·mL^{-1}	0.0646 μg·mL^{-1}	
				0.02～4.0 μg·mL^{-1}	6.4 ng·mL^{-1}	
PVAK	BSA	3.0	380	0.02～3.5 μg·mL^{-1}	9.2 ng·mL^{-1}	[80]
	γ-Globulin			0.05～3.5 μg·mL^{-1}	12.5 ng·mL^{-1}	
	γ-Globulin			0.02～11.0 μg·mL^{-1}	6.0 ng·mL^{-1}	
PS-AA	BSA	6.9	342	0.04～10.0 μg·mL^{-1}	19.0 ng·mL^{-1}	[81]
	HSA			0.03～10.0 μg·mL^{-1}	15.0 ng·mL^{-1}	

Abbreviations: ApoAI, Apolipoprotein AI; ApoB, Apolipoprotein B; CdS/PAA, acrylic acid covered CdS; PVAK, polyvinyl alcohol keto-derivative nanoparticle; PS–AA, polystyrene–acrylic acid.

1.3.4 Applications of RLS Technique

1.3.4.1 Investigation on the Aggregation of Chromophores

Resonance light-scattering techniques, along with UV-vis absorption, fluorescence, and circular dichroism spectroscopy, are the main techniques used to measure the aggregation process of chromophores such as porphyrin. Here are some examples of reports in recent years[20,82～98]: (1) RLS technique was used to show the occurrence of acidity dependent structural rearrangements of J-aggregates porphyrin, formed by a zwitterionic diacid form of 5,10,15,20-tetrakis (4-sulfonatophenl) porphyrin ($H_2TPPS_4^{4-}$) under acidic conditions[97]. The combination of light-scattering techniques evidenced the occurrence of structural rearrangements of the clusters depending on the HCl concentration. (2) The aggregation of tetra(*p*-carboxyphenyl)porphyrin diacid (H_2TCPP^{2+}) in aqueous HCl and HNO_3 was identified with resonance light-scattering technique, fluorescence spectroscopy, and atomic force microscopy[82]. The results of the RLS showed the aggregation of H_2TCPP^{2+} formed in aqueous HNO_3 and HCl solutions with a pH less than 1 have different RLS signals at H and J aggregate absorption bands, which confirmed the existence of counterion-dependent aggregates of H_2TCPP^{2+}[20]. (3) Scolaro et al.[96] proposed a sensitive way to control the extent of porphyrin aggregation on a nucleic acid scaffold by exploiting competitive binding toward the biological scaffold between two chromophores that have different aggregating properties. The extent of aggregation could be monitored by the linearly changed RLS signals, which can be readily changed by varying the concentration of an added non-aggregating porphyrin and depend on the charge of the added species and the concentration of available binding site.

1.3.4.2 Quantitative Analysis

The RLS technique was used for quantitative analysis of analytes including nucleic acids[56～58,62,99～120], proteins[59～61,121～128], amino acids[68,129,130], pharmaceuticals[71～72,131,132], inorganic ions[39～40,133～137], surfactants[138～140], etc. It is worth noting that the successful application of the RLS technique on immunoassay[66] and DNA hybridization[65] could promote the application of RLS on clinical and biological chemistry. Tables 3 and 4 summarize the parameters of analytical systems using the RLS method to detect nucleic acids and protein assays since 2003.

1.3.4.3 Characterization of Nanostructure

The light-scattering properties of the gold nanoparticles[141], nanorods[142], and Au-Ag core-shell nanoparticles[143] with different shape, size, and concentration have been investigated and characterized using the RLS technique. It was found that the gold nanoparticles had maximum Rayleigh scattering peaks at 286 nm[141], and the intensity of Rayleigh scattering peaks have linear relationships with the diameters of gold nanoparticles. While gold nano-rods have two scattering peaks due to the transverse and longitudinal surface plasmon resonance[142].

Table 3 Determination of nucleic acids using RLS technique in the last four years

Analytes	Probes	pH	λ_{max} (nm)	Linear range ($ng \cdot mL^{-1}$)	LOD (3σ, $ng \cdot mL^{-1}$)	Ref.
ctDNA	Ru(phen)2 dppz^{2+}	2.3	336	40～4000	13.0	[99]
ctDNA	Ru(phen)2 dppx^{2+}	2.3	336	40～9000	4.2	[99]
ctDNA	Ru(bpy)2 dppz^{2+}	2.3	336	100～5000	51.5	[99]
ctDNA	Ru(bpy)2 dppx^{2+}	2.3	336	40～6000	3.0	[99]
ctDNA	Butyl rhodamine B	2	400	5.8～2688	5.8	[100]
ctDNA	Toluidine blue	11	350	0～900	6.75	[56]
ctDNA	Toluidine blue;	3.17	468	0～2800	31.7	[57]
ctDNA	Congo red	10.5	560	0.75～1000	0.89	[101]
ctDNA	Fluorescein	7.5	400	40～3100	16	[102]
ctDNA	Bromocresol green	11.0	336	50～800	16.2	[103]
ctDNA	Curcumin	4.3	392	3～1000	0.3	[104]
ctDNA	Xylenol orange-CTMAB	7.30	542	1000～3000	23.50	[105]
ctDNA	Near-infrared cyanine	7.55	823	0～400	3.5	[62]
ctDNA	Eu^{3+}-CTMAB	7.5	550	10～2000	1.7	[131]
ctDNA	Eu^{3+}-oxolinic acid	9.75	368	0.8～1000	0.011	[107]
ctDNA	Eu^{3+}-TTA-Phen	7.0	385.0	0.05～500	0.002	[108]
ctDNA	MnTSPc	11.60	346.2	400～1400	22.9	[109]
ctDNA	CuTSPc	10.50	383.6	200～1000	14.3	[110]
ctDNA	MnTSPc	11.60	346.2	400～1400	22.9	[111]
ctDNA	Pyronine B	7.4	377	0～1200	6.1	[112]
ctDNA	Imidacloprid	1.62	310	0～20000	12.8	[58]
ctDNA	Triadimenol	1.7	310	0～9000	24	[113]
ctDNA	Acetaiprid	1.68	313	100～1100	21	[114]
ctDNA	PDDA	7.3	300	30～2000	13	[115]
ctDNA	Lauryl betaine	9.30	388	20～3800	2.4	[116]
ctDNA	Cocamidopropyl hydroxysultaine	8.69	392	20～7300	1.5	[116]
ctDNA	La(phen) (o-phthalic acid)	6.75	400	23～1870	23	[117]
ctDNA	CetyIpyridinium bromide	10.4	363	200～1250	50	[118]
fsDNA	Alkali blue 6B	2.90	346	10～100.4	4.2	[119]
fsDNA	Violet-CTMAB	2.35	400	20～750	8.7	[120]
fsDNA	Toluidine blue	11	350	0～900	2.99	[56]
fsDNA	Toluidine blue	3.17	468	0～2200	22.7	[57]
fsDNA	Bromocresol green	11.0	336	50～800	15.3	[103]
fsDNA	Curcumin	4.3	392	1～1000	0.1	[104]
fsDNA	Xylenol orange-CTMAB	7.30	542	0～4750	21.13	[105]
fsDNA	Near-infrared cyanine	7.55	823	0～400	3.4	[62]

Continued

Analytes	Probes	pH	λ_{max} (nm)	Linear range (ng·mL^{-1})	LOD (3σ, ng·mL^{-1})	Ref.
fsDNA	Eu^{3+}-CTMAB	7.5	550	6～2000	0.36	[106]
fsDNA	Eu^{3+}-oxolinic acid	9.75	368	1～1000	20	[107]
fsDNA	Eu^{3+}-TTA-Phen	7.00	385.0	0.1～1000	0.03	[108]
fsDNA	MnTSPc	11.60	346.2	200～1400	14.4	[109]
fsDNA	CuTSPc	10.50	383.6	200～800	34.3	[110]
fsDNA	MnTSPc	11.60	346.2	200～1400	14.4	[111]
fsDNA	Pyronine B	7.4	377	0～800	11.2	[112]
fsDNA	Lauryl betaine	9.30	388	30～4200	3.0	[116]
fsDNA	Cocamidopropyl hydroxysultaine	8.69	392	10～8600	1.9	[116]
fsDNA	Cetylpyridinium bromide	10.4	363	200～2000	70	[118]
yRNA	Toluidine blue	3.17	468	0～500	5.1	[57]
yRNA	Congo red	10.5	560	0.75～2500	1.2	[101]
yRNA	Curcumin	4.3	392	1～1000	0.5	[104]
yRNA	Xylenol orange-CTMAB	7.30	542	0～3000	33.61	[105]
yDNA	Xylenol orange-CTMAB	7.30	542	500～3750	29.53	[105]
yDNA	Bromocresol green	11.0	336	50～900	12.7	[103]
yRNA	Violet-CTMAB	2.35	400	20～750	1.4	[120]
yRNA	Eu^{3+}-CTMAB	7.5	550	8～2000	0.21	[106]
yRNA	Eu^{3+}-oxolinic acid	9.75	368	1～1000	0.010	[107]
yRNA	Eu^{3+}-TTA-Phen	7.0	385.0	0.01～1000	0.006	[108]
yRNA	Pyronine B	7.4	377	40～1400	8.6	[112]
yRNA	Imidacloprid	1.62	310	4000～7000	35.5	[58]
yRNA	PDDA	7.3	300	100～4000	39	[115]
hsDNA	Congo red	10.5	560	1～1000	0.019	[101]
hsDNA	PDDA	7.3	300	30～3000	24	[115]
soRNA	Near-infrared cyanine	7.55	823	0～600	2.9	[62]
ssDNA	Imidacloprid	1.62	310	0～1460	29.5	[58]

Abbreviations: ctDNA, calf thymus DNA; fsDNA, fish sperm DNA; yDNA, yeast DNA; yRNA, yeast RNA; hsDNA, herring sperm DNA; soRNA, snake ovum RNA; ssDNA, salmon sperm DNA; CTMAB, cetyltrimethylammonium bromide; Eu^{3+}-TTA-Phen, europium(III)-2-thenoyltrifluoroacetne-1,10-phenanthroline; MnTSPc, manganese-tetrasulfonatophthalocyanine; CuTSPc, copper phthalocyanine tetrasulfonic acid; PDDA, poly(diallyldimethyl ammonium chloride); La(phen)(o-phthalic acid), lanthanum with ophenanthroline(phen) and o-phthalic acid.

Table 4 Determination of proteins using RLS technique in recent four years

Analytes	Probes	pH	λmax (nm)	Linear range (μg·mL^{-1})	LOD (3σ ng·mL^{-1})	Ref.
BSA	Fast Red VR	3.52	287	0.2～12.0	15.9	[121]
BSA	Bordeaux red	3.92	363	0.12～10.8	40	[60]
BSA	Congo red	2.7～3.0	360	0.05～8.0	14	[122]
BSA	Ponceau G	3.8	288	0.2～8.5	14.9	[123]
BSA	Solochrome	4.0	400	0～5.0	44.4	[61]
BSA	cyanine R	2.6	390	0.0075～15	1.8	[124]
BSA	SDBS SLS	2.6	390	0.020～10	12.8	[124]

Continued

Analytes	Probes	pH	λmax (nm)	Linear range (μg·mL^{-1})	LOD (3σ ng·mL^{-1})	Ref.
BSA	SLS	3.4	391	0.0025～1.2	1.3	[125]
BSA	CPB	10.93	460	0.005～2.5	3.0	[126]
BSA	CoTSPc	4.0	386	0.10～34.3	13.9	[127]
BSA	Fullerol	3.5	360	0.1～10.0	9.7	[128]
BSA	Pyronine Y	0.04 M H_2SO_4	400	0.15～3.6	21.0	[59]
HSA	Pyronine Y	0.04 M H_2SO_4	400	0.06～4.8	12.0	[59]
HSA	Fast Red VR	3.52	287	0.1～8.0	6.5	[121]
HSA	Bordeaux red	3.92	363	0.24～18.0	53	[60]
HSA	Congo red	2.7～3.0	360	0.001～6.0	0.28	[122]
HSA	Ponceau G	3.8	288	0.05～8.0	5.0	[123]
HSA	Solochrome cyanine R	4.0	400	0～4.5	45.4	[61]
HSA	SDBS	2.6	390	0.01～10	2.8	[124]
HSA	SLS	2.6	390	0.025～10	21.6	[124]
HSA	SLS	3.4	391	0.0075～0.9	0.8	[125]
HSA	CPB	10.93	460	0.025～3.5	10.0	[126]
HSA	CoTSPc	4.0	386	0.10～34.3	15.5	[127]
HSA	Fullerol	4.5	360	0.1～14.0	10.9	[128]
IgG	Fast Red VR	3.52	287	0.2～7.0	22.1	[121]
IgG	Ponceau G	3.8	288	0.2～5.0	24.0	[123]
IgG	Solochrome	4.0	400	0～4.0	60.6	[61]
IgG	cyanine R SLS	3.4	391	0.02～1.4	2.7	[125]
IgG	CoTSPc	4.0	386	0.10～34.3	15.6	[127]
Lysozyme	Fast Red VR	3.52	287	0.04～8.0	4.1	[121]
Lysozyme	Bordeaux red	3.92	363	0.12～5.4	64	[60]
Lysozyme	Solochrome cyanine R	4.0	400	0～4.0	65.5	[61]
Lysozyme	SLS	3.4	391	0.04～2.1	3.2	[125]
Lysozyme	CoTSPc	4.0	386	0.50～29.4	23.1	[127]
Lysozyme	Fullerol	5.0	360	0.5～14.0	57.4	[128]
Egg albumin	Bordeaux red	3.92	363	0.20～15.0	29	[60]
Egg albumin	Solochrome cyanine R	4.0	400	0～3.0	75.5	[61]
Egg albumin	SLS	3.4	391	0.02～0.8	3.9	[125]
Egg albumin	CoTSPc	4.0	386	0.20～29.4	17.9	[127]
Hemoglobin	Solochrome cyanine R	4.0	400	0～3.5	42.5	[61]
Hemoglobin	SLS	3.4	391	0.01～0.6	4.3	[125]
Hemoglobin	CoTSPc	4.0	386	0.10～34.3	25.3	[127]
α-chymo-sr]trypsin	Fast Red VR	3.52	287	0.2～7.0	18.0	[121]
Myoglobin	CoTSPc	4.0	386	0.10～37.2	11.8	[127]
Pepsin	Fullerol	3.0	360	0.5～18.0	8.5	[128]

Abbreviations: SDBS, sodium dodecyl benzene sulfonate; SLS, sodium lauroyl sarcosinate; CoTSPc, cobalt-tetrasulfonatophthalo-cyanine; CPB, utin–cetylpyridine bromide.

On the other hand, RLS techniques were first used to validate the micelle formation of proteins in aqueous solution. The critical micelle concentrations (CMC) of some proteins could be determinate by the light-scattering intensity of protein solution[144].

1.3.5 Future of RLS Technique

1.3.51 Highly Selective RLS Probes

RLS techniques have the advantages of sensitivity and simplicity but suffer from poor selectivity. Although a number of improved RLS methods have been established to overcome this problem, the RLS probe with high selectivity to analytes has become a choice, taking no account of modification of the common spectrofluorometer. New RLS probes that could induce enhanced light-scattering signals when selectively binded to an analyte are of great interest in the evolution of the RLS technique.

1.3.5.2 RLS Techniques Incorporated with Chromatographic Techniques

RLS techniques combined and used in chromatographic determination are of great interest. Detectors such as UV-Vis absorption, fluorescence, and diode array detection are the most important part of chromatographic analysis. However, it suffers problems such as low sensitivity. RLS techniques coupled with high-performance liquid chromatography (HPLC) or capillary electrophoresis (CE) are not only advantageous with the highly sensitive RLS signal but are also a complement to conventional chromatographic detectors.

1.3.5.3 RLS Particles in Cellular and Biological Imaging

Cellular imaging utilizing microscopy techniques and immunotargeted optical contrast agents provides anatomic details of cells and tissue architecture important for diagnosis of cancer and other disorders. The use of traditional fluorescent dyes such as malachite green and rhodamine-6G as contrast agents in biomedical imaging was limited due to their photo-bleaching[145]. While quantum dots with the advantage of unique size-dependent human toxicity and cytotoxicity of the semiconductor material. However, RLS particles such as gold nanoparticles are an alternative contrast agent due to their colorful scattering light under the excitation of white light and non-cytotoxicity as well as their non-susceptibility to photo-bleaching or chemical-thermal denaturation. The strong light scattering of gold nanoparticles has been exploited for real-time optical imaging of pre-cancer by using confocal reflectance microscopy[146]. El-Sayed et al. have demonstrated differentiation of cancerous cells from non-cancerous cells by dark-field light-scattering imaging of solid 40-mm gold nanospheres immunotargeted to epidermal growth factor receptor (EGFR) overexpressed on cancer cells[147]. We believe that the application based on the light-scattering signal of RLS particles in the field of cellular and biological imaging has a good future.

1.3.6 Conclusion

In this contribution, we briefly reviewed the development of RLS techniques since 2003. In the past four years, RLS techniques were theoretically and technically developed with the establishment of many newly derived RLS techniques to improve the performance or overcome the problems of the common RLS technique. RLS probes, not only organic small molecules but also polymers or nanomaterials, have been increasingly used in RLS measurements. With the wide application in biochemical analysis, immunoassay, pharmaceutical assay, and environmental analysis, we believe that RLS techniques still have great potential in analytical chemistry in the coming year.

Acknowledgements

All authors are grateful for the financial support of the National Natural Science Foundation of China (No. 20425517, No. 20675065, and No. 30570465) for this work.

References

[1] Bohren, C.F. and Huffman, D.R. (1998) Absorption and Scattering of Light by Small Particles; Wiley: New York.

[2] Yang, W.Z. (1992) Physical Chemistry Techniques; Peking University Press: Beijing.

[3] Pecora, R. (1985) Dynamic Light Scattering; Plenum Press: New York.

[4] Schure, M.R. and Palkar, S.A. (2002) Accuracy estimation of multiangle light scattering detectors utilized for polydisperse particle characterization with field-flow fractionation techniques: A simulation study. Analytical Chemistry, 74: 684～695.

[5] Magnuson, M.L., Lytle, D.A., Frietch, C.M., and Kelty, C.A. (2001) Characterization of submicrometer aqueous iron(III) colloids formed in the presence of phosphate by sedimentation field flow fractionation with multiangle laser light scattering detection. Analytical Chemistry, 73: 4815～4820.

[6] Pan, T. and Sevick Muraca, E.M. (2002) Volume of pharmaceutical powders probed by frequency-domain photon migration measurements of multiply scattered light. Analytical Chemistry, 74: 4228～4234.

[7] Lee, H., Williams, S.K.R., Allison, S.D., and Anchordoquy, T.J. (2001) Analysis of self-assembled cationic lipid-DNA gene carrier complexes using flow fieldflow fractionation and light scattering. Analytical Chemistry, 73: 837～843.

[8] Owens, P.K. and Johansson, J. (2000) Light-scattering studies of packed stationary phases for capillary electrochromatography. Analytical Chemistry, 72: 740～746.

[9] Szostek, B. and Koropchak, J.A. (1996) Condensation nucleation light scattering detection for capillary electrophoresis. Analytical Chemistry, 68: 2744～2752.

[10] Viebke, C. and Williams, P.A. (2000) The influence of temperature on the characterization of water-soluble polymers using asymmetric flow field-flow-fractionation coupled to multiangle laser light scattering. Analytical Chemistry, 72: 3896～3901.

[11] Takahashi, R., Al-Assaf, S., Williams, P.A., Kubota, K., Okamoto, A., and Nishinari, K. (2003) Asymmetrical-flow field-flow fractionation with on-line multiangle light scattering detection. 1. Application to wormlike chain analysis of weakly stiff polymer chains. Biomacromolecules, 4: 404～409.

[12] Fraunhofer, W., Winter, G., and Coester, C. (2004) Asymmetrical flow field-flow fractionation and multiangle light scattering for analysis of gelatin nanoparticle drug carrier systems. Analytical Chemistry, 76: 1909～1920.

[13] Risley, D.S. and Strege, M.A. (2000) Chiral separations of polar compounds by hydrophilic interaction chromatography with evaporative light scattering detection. Analytical Chemistry, 72: 1736～1739.

[14] Wei, Y. and Ding, M.-Y. (2000) Analysis of carbohydrates in drinks by high-performance liquid chromatography with a dynamically modified amino column and evaporative light scattering detection. Journal of Chromatography A, 904: 113 ～117.

[15] Pasternack, R.F., Bustamante, C., Collings, P.J., Giannetto, L.A., and Gibbs, E.J. (1993) Porphyrin assemblies on DNA as studied by a resonance light-scattering technique. Journal of the American Chemical Society, 115: 5393～5399.

[16] Pasternack, R.F. and Collings, P.J. (1995) Resonance light scattering: A new technique for studying chromophore aggregation. Science, 269: 935～939.

[17] Ribo´, J.M., Crusats, J., Sague´s, F., Claret, J., and Rubires, R. (2001) Chiral sign induction by vortices during the formation of mesophases in stirred solutions. Science, 292: 2063～2066.

[18] Kano, K., Fukuda, K., Wakami, H., Nishiyabu, R., and Pasternack, R.F. (2000) Factors influencing self-aggregation tendencies of cationic porphyrins in aqueous solution. Journal of the American Chemical Society, 122: 7494～7502.

[19] Micali, N., Mallamace, F., Romeo, A., Purrello, R., and Monsuscolaro, L. (2000) Mesoscopic structure of *meso*-tetrakis(4-sulfonatophenyl)porphine J-aggregates. Journal of Physical Chemistry B, 104: 5897～5904.

[20] Choi, M.Y., Pollard, J.A., Webb, M.A., and Mchale, J.L. (2003) Counteriondependent excitonic spectra of tetra (*p*-carboxyphenyl)porphyrin aggregates in acidic aqueous solution. Journal of the American Chemical Society, 125: 810～820.

[21] Huang, C.Z., Li, K.A., and Tong, S.Y. (1996) Determination of nucleic acids by a resonance light-scattering technique with α, β, γ, δ-tetrakis[4-(trimethylammoniumyl) phenyl]porphine. Analytical Chemistry, 68: 2259～2263.

[22] Huang, C.Z., Li, Y.F., and Liu, X.D. (1998) Determination of nucleic acids at nanogram levels with safranine T by a resonance light-scattering technique. Analytica Chimica Acta, 375: 89～97.

[23] Huang, C.Z., Li, Y.F., Mao, J.G., and Tan, D.G. (1998) Determination of protein concentration by enhancement of the preresonance light-scattering of α, β, γ, δ-tetrakis (5-sulfothienyl) porphine. Analyst, 123: 1401～1406.

[24] Liu, S., Luo, H., Li, N., Liu, Z., and Zheng, W. (2001) Resonance Rayleigh scattering study of the interaction of heparin with

some basic diphenyl naphthylmethane dyes. Analytical Chemistry, 73: 3907～3914.

[25] Feng, P., Shu, W.Q., Huang, C.Z., and Li, Y.F. (2001) Total internal reflected resonance light scattering determination of chlortetracycline in body fluid with the complex cation of chlortetracycline-europium-trioctyl phosphine oxide at the water/tetrachloromethane interface. Analytical Chemistry, 73: 4307～4312.

[26] Luo, H.Q., Liu, S.P., Li, N.B., and Liu, Z.F. (2002) Resonance Rayleigh scattering, frequency doubling scattering and second-order scattering spectra of the heparin–crystal violet system and their analytical application. Analytica Chimica Acta, 468: 275～286.

[27] Huang, C.Z. and Li, Y.F. (2003) Resonance light scattering technique used for biochemical and pharmaceutical analysis. Analytica Chimica Acta, 500: 105～117.

[28] Huang, C.Z., Liu, Y., Wang, Y.H., and Guo, H.P. (2003) Resonance light scattering imaging detection of proteins with α, β, γ, δ-tetrakis (*p*-sulfophenyl)porphyrin. Analytical Biochemistry, 321: 236～243.

[29] Liu, X.D., Huang, C.Z., Guo, H.P., and Huang, Y.M. (2006) Resonance light scattering imaging detection of single suprahelical species of DNA induced by α, β, γ, δ-tetrakis[4-(trimethylaminonium)phenyl]porphine. Chinese Journal of Chemistry, 24: 89～94.

[30] Guo, H.P., Huang, C.Z., and Ling, J. (2006) Resonance light scattering imaging determination of heparin. Chinese Chemical Letters, 17: 53～56.

[31] Ling, J., Huang, C.Z., and Li, Y.F. (2006) Directly light scattering imaging of the aggregations of biopolymer bound chromium(III) hydrolytic oligomers in aqueous phase and liquid/liquid interface. Analytica Chimica Acta, 567: 143～151.

[32] Roll, D., Malicka, J., Gryczynski, I., Gryczynski, Z., and Lakowicz, J.R. (2003) Metallic colloid wavelength-ratiometric scattering sensors. Analytical Chemistry, 75: 3440～3445.

[33] Aslan, K., Lakowicz, J.R., and Geddes, C.D. (2005) Nanogold plasmon resonance-based glucose sensing. 2. Wavelength-ratiometric resonance light scattering. Analytical Chemistry, 77: 2007～2014.

[34] Huang, C.Z., Pang, X.B., Li, Y.F., and Long, Y.J. (2006) A resonance light scattering ratiometry applied for binding study of organic small molecules with biopolymer. Talanta, 69: 180～186.

[35] Long, Y.J., Li, Y.F., and Huang, C.Z. (2005) A wide dynamic range detection of biopolymer medicines with resonance light scattering and absorption ratiometry. Analytica Chimica Acta, 552: 175～181.

[36] Dai, X.X., Li, Y.F., He, W., Long, Y.F., and Huang, C.Z. (2006) A dual-wavelength resonance light scattering ratiometry of biopolymer by its electrostatic interaction with surfactant. Talanta, 70: 578～583.

[37] Wang, Y.H., Guo, H.P., Tan, K.J., and Huang, C.Z. (2004) Backscattering light detection of nucleic acids with tetraphenylporphyrin-Al(III)-nucleic acids at liquid/liquid interface. Analytica Chimica Acta, 521: 109～115.

[38] Huang, C.Z., Wang, Y.H., Guo, H.P., and Li, Y.F. (2005) A backscattering light detection assembly for sensitive determination of analyte concentrated at the liquid/liquid interface using the interaction of quercetin with proteins as the model system. Analyst, 130: 200～205.

[39] Tan, K.J., Li, Y.F., Huang, C.Z., and Liu, X.L. (2006) Determination of chlorine in human urine by detecting backscattering signals with a new optical assembly. Chinese Chemical Letters, 17: 679～682.

[40] Tan, K.J., Huang, C.Z., and Huang, Y.M. (2006) Determination of lead in environmental water by a backward light scattering technique. Talanta, 70: 116～121.

[41] Vidal, E., Palomeque, M.E., Lista, A.G., and Fernańdez Band, B.S. (2003) Flow injection analysis: Rayleigh light scattering technique for total protein determination. Analytical and Bioanalytical Chemistry, 376: 38.

[42] Huang, C.Z., Pang, X.B., and Li, Y.F. (2005) Determination of heparin using azure B by flow injection analysis-resonance light scattering coupled technique. Analytical Letters, 38: 349～362.

[43] Tan, K.J., Li, Y.F., and Huang, C.Z. (2005) Flow injection resonance light scattering detection of proteins of nanogram. Luminescence, 20: 176～180.

[44] Lu, W., Huang, C.Z., and Li, Y.F. (2003) Novel assay of thiamine based on its enhancement of total internal reflected resonance light scattering signals of sodium dodecylbenzene sulfonate at the water/tetrachloromethane interface. Analytica Chimica Acta, 475: 151～161.

[45] Pang, X.B., Huang, C.Z., Li, Y.F., and Lu, W. (2003) Assay of nucleic acids at the water/tetrachloromethane interface with cetyltrimethylammonium bromide by total internal reflected resonance light scattering. Bulletin of the Chemical Society of Ja-

pan, 76: 1941～1946.

[46] Huang, C.Z., Lu, W., and Li, Y.F. (2003) Total internal reflected resonance light scattering detection of DNA at water/tetrachloromethane interface with acrindine orange and cetyltrimethylammonium bromide. Analytica Chimica Acta, 494: 11～19.

[47] Pang, X.B. and Huang, C.Z. (2004) A selective and sensitive assay of berberine using total internal reflected resonance light scattering technique with fluorescein at the water/1,2-dichloroethane interface. Journal of Pharmaceutical and Biomedical Analysis, 35: 185～191.

[48] Huang, C.Z., Feng, P., Li, Y.F., Tan, K.J., and Wang, H.Y. (2005) Adsorption of penicillin–berberine ion associates at a water/tetrachloromethane interface and determination of penicillin based on total internal-reflected resonance light scattering measurements. Analytica Chimica Acta, 538: 337～343.

[49] Huang, C.Z., Feng, P., Li, Y.F., and Tan, K.J. (2005) Pharmacokinetic detection of penicillin excreted in urine using a totally internally reflected resonance light scattering technique with cetyltrimethylammonium bromide. Analytical and Bioanalytical Chemistry, 382: 85～90.

[50] Dong, L., Chen, X., and Hu, Z. (2006) Total internal reflected resonance light scattering determination of protein in human blood serum at water/tetrachloromethane interface with arsenazo-TB and cetyltrimethylammonium bromide. Talanta, 71: 555～560.

[51] Zhao, H.W., Huang, C.Z., and Li, Y.F. (2006) A novel optical immunosensing system based on measuring surface enhanced light scattering signals of solid supports. Analytica Chimica Acta, 564: 166～172.

[52] Yguerabide, J. and Yguerabide, E.E. (1998) Light-scattering submicroscopic particles as highly fluorescent analogs and their use as tracer labels in clinical and biological applications: I Theory. Analytical Biochemistry, 262: 137～156.

[53] Perelman, L.T., Backman, V., Wallace, M., Zonios, G., Manoharan, R., Nusrat, A., Shields, S., Seiler, M., Lima, C., Hamano, T., Itzkan, I., Van Dam, J., Crawford, J.M., and Feld, M.S. (1998) Observation of periodic fine structure in reflectance from biological tissue: A new technique for measuring nuclear size distribution. Physical Review Letters, 80: 627.

[54] Gurjar, R.S., Backman, V., Perelman, L.T., Georgakoudi, I., Badizadegan, K., Itzkan, I., Dasari, R.R., and Feld, M.S. (2001) Imaging human epithelial properties with polarized light scattering spectroscopy. Nature Medicine, 7: 1245 ～1248.

[55] Backman, V., Wallace, M.B., Perelman, L.T., Arendt, J.T., Gurjar, R., Muller, M.G., Zhang, Q., Zonios, G., Kline, E., Mcgillican, T., and Shapshay, S. (2000) Detection of preinvasive cancer cells. Nature, 406: 35～36.

[56] Xiao, X.L., Wang, Y.S., Li, G.R., and Lv, C.G. (2004) Determination of deoxyribonucleic acids at nanograms levels with toluidine blue by a resonance light-scattering method. Spectrosc. Spect. Anal., 24: 190～193.

[57] Chen, L.-H., Nie, Y.-T., Liu, L.-Z., and Shen, H.-X. (2003) Determination of nucleic acids on the basis of enhancement effect of resonance light scattering of toluidine blue. Analytical Letters, 36: 107～122.

[58] Jia, G., Wang, P., Qiu, J., Sun, Y., Xiao, Y., and Zhou, Z. (2004) Determination of DNA with imidacloprid by a resonance light scattering technique at nanogram levels and its application. Analytical Letters, 37: 1339～1354.

[59] Feng, S., Pan, Z., and Fan, J. (2005) Determination of trace proteins with pyronine Y and SDS by resonance light scattering. Analytical and Bioanalytical Chemistry, 383: 255～260.

[60] Feng, S., Pan, Z., and Fan, J. (2006) Determination of proteins at nanogram levels with bordeaux red based on the enhancement of resonance light scattering. Spectrochimica Acta PartA, 64: 574～579.

[61] Feng, N.C., He, S.P., Zhang, J., and Liu, J.P. (2004) Resonance light scattering study on interaction of solochrome cyanine R with protein and light scattering determination of trace protein. Spectrosc. Spect. Anal., 24: 194～196.

[62] Fang, F., Zheng, H., Li, L., Wu, Y., Chen, J., Zhuo, S., and Zhu, C. (2006) Determination of nucleic acids with a near infrared cyanine dye using resonance light scattering technique. Spectrochimica Acta Part A, 64: 698～702.

[63] Kreibig, U. and Vollmer, M. (1995) Optical Properties of Metal Clusters; Springer-Verlag: Berlin.

[64] Yguerabide, J. and Yguerabide, E.E. (1998) Light-scattering submicroscopic particles as highly fluorescent analogs and their use as tracer labels in clinical and biological applications: II. Experimental characterization. Analytical Biochemistry, 262: 157～176.

[65] Du, B.-A., Li, Z.-P., and Liu, C.-H. (2006) One-step homogeneous detection of DNA hybridization with gold nanoparticle probes by using a linear light-scattering technique. Angewandte Chemie International Edition, 118: 8190～8193.

[66] Jiang, Z., Sun, S., Liang, A., Huang, W., and Qin, A. (2006) Gold-labeled nanoparticle-based immunoresonance scattering

spectral assay for trace apolipoprotein AI and apolipoprotein B. Clinical Chemistry, 52: 1389～1394.

[67] Wu, L.P., Li, Y.F., Huang, C.Z., and Zhang, Q. (2006) Visual detection of sudan dyes based on the plasmon resonance light scattering signals of silver nanoparticles. Analytical Chemistry, 78: 5570～5577.

[68] Li, Z.P., Duan, X.R., Liu, C.H., and Du, B.A. (2006) Selective determination of cysteine by resonance light scattering technique based on self-assembly of gold nanoparticles. Analytical Biochemistry, 351: 18～25.

[69] Liu, Z.D., Huang, C.Z., Li, Y.F., and Long, Y.F. (2006) Enhanced plasmon resonance light scattering signals of colloidal gold resulted from its interactions with organic small molecules using captopril as an example. Analytica Chimica Acta, 577: 244～249.

[70] Liu, X., Yuan, H., Pang, D., and Cai, R. (2004) Resonance light scattering spectroscopy study of interaction between gold colloid and thiamazole and its analytical application. Spectrochimica Acta Part A, 60: 385～389.

[71] Liu, S.P., Yang, Z., Liu, Z.F., Liu, J.T., and Shi, Y. (2006) Resonance Rayleigh scattering study on the interaction of gold nanoparticles with berberine hydrochloride and its analytical application. Analytica Chimica Acta, 572: 283～289.

[72] Liu, S.P., Chen, Y.H., Liu, Z.F., Hu, X.L., and Wang, F. (2006) A highly sensitive resonance Rayleigh scattering method for the determination of vitamin B1 with gold nanoparticles probe. Microchimica Acta, 154: 87～93.

[73] Fang, B., Gao, Y., Li, M., Wang, G., and Li, Y. (2004) Application of functionalized ag nanoparticles for the determination of proteins at nanogram levels using the resonance light scattering method. Microchimica Acta, 147: 81～86.

[74] Chen, H., Xu, F., Hong, S., and Wang, L. (2006) Quantitative determination of proteins at nanogram levels by the resonance light-scattering technique with composite nanoparticles of CdS/PAA. Spectrochimica Acta Part A, 65: 428 ～432.

[75] Liao, Q.G., Huang, C.Z., and Li, Y.F. (2006) A light scattering and fluorescence emission coupled ratiometry using the interaction of functional CdS quantum dots with aminoglycoside antibiotics as a model system. Talanta, 71: 567～572.

[76] Wang, L.-Y., Wang, L., Dong, L., Hu, Y.-L., Xia, T.-T., Chen, H.-Q., Li, L., and Zhu, C.-Q. (2004) Determination of γ-globulin at nanogram levels by its enhancement effect on the resonance light scattering of functionalized hgs nanoparticles. Talanta, 62: 237～240.

[77] Wang, L.Y., Chen, H.Q., Li, L., Dong, L., Xia, T.T., and Wang, L. (2004) Selective determination of nanogram g～globulin in human blood serum by resonance light scattering of functionalized nano-PbS. Chinese Chemical Letters, 15: 319～321.

[78] Li, Y., Chen, J., Zhuo, S., Wu, Y., Zhu, C., and Wang, L. (2004) Application of L-cysteine-capped ZnS nanoparticles in the determination of nucleic acids using the resonance light scattering method. Microchimica Acta, 146: 13～19.

[79] Wang, L., Xu, F., Zhou, Y., Wang, L., and Liu, Y. (2004) Preparation and application of MS-M^{2+} nanoparticles as a novel resonance light-scattering probe. Spectrochimica Acta Part A, 60: 2141～2145.

[80] Zhou, Y., She, S., Zhang, L., and Lu, Q. (2005) Determination of proteins at nanogram levels using the resonance light scattering technique with a novel PVAK nanoparticle. Microchimica Acta, 149: 151～156.

[81] Wang, L., Chen, H., Li, L., Xia, T., Dong, L., and Wang, L. (2004) Quantitative determination of proteins at nanogram levels by the resonance light-scattering technique with macromolecules nanoparticles of PS-AA. Spectrochimica Acta Part A, 60: 747～750.

[82] Doan, S.C., Shanmugham, S., Aston, E., and Mchale, J.L. (2005) Counterion dependent dye aggregates: Nanorods and nanorings of tetra(p-carboxyphenyl)-porphyrin. Journal of the American Chemical Society, 127: 5885～5892.

[83] Koti, A., Taneja, J., and Periasamy, N. (2003) Control of coherence length and aggregate size in the J-aggregate of porphyrin. Chemical Physics Letters, 375: 171～176.

[84] Mazzaglia, A., Angelini, N., Darcy, R., Donohue, R., Lombardo, D., Micali, N., Sciortino, M.T., Villari, V., and Scolaro, L.M. (2003) Novel heterotopic colloids of anionic porphyrins entangled in cationic amphiphilic cyclodextrins: Spectroscopic investigation and intracellular delivery. Chemistry–A European Journal, 9: 5762～5769.

[85] Chen, X.D. and Liu, M.H. (2003) Induced chirality of binary aggregates of oppositely charged water-soluble porphyrins on DNA matrix. Journal of Inorganic Biochemistry, 94: 106～113.

[86] Rosa, A., Ricciardi, G., Baerends, E.J., Romeo, A., and Scolaro, L.M. (2003) Effects of porphyrin core saddling, meso-phenyl twisting and counterions on the optical properties of meso-tetraphenylporphyrin diacids: The $[H_4TPP](X)_2$ (X=F, Cl, Br, I) series as a case study. Journal of Physical Chemistry A, 107: 11468～11482.

[87] Kuba´t, P., Lang, K., Procha´zkova´, K., and Anzenbacher, P., Jr. (2003) Self-aggregates of cationic meso-tetratolylporphyrins in aqueous solutions. Langmuir, 19: 422～428.

[88] Bordbar, A., Eslami, A., and Tangestaninejad, S. (2003) Solution properties of Cu(II) complex of a moderately hydrophobic water-soluble porphyrin and investigation of its interaction with human serum albumin. Polish Journal of Chemistry, 77: 283～293.

[89] Castriciano, M.A., Romeo, A., Villari, V., Micali, N., and Scolaro, L.M. (2004) Nanosized porphyrin J-aggregates in water/AOT/decane microemulsions. Journal of Physical Chemistry B, 108: 9054～9059.

[90] Genady, A.R., El-Zaria, M.E., and Gabel, D. (2004) Non-covalent assemblies of negatively charged boronated porphyrins with different cationic moieties. Journal of Organometallic Chemistry, 689: 3242～3250.

[91] Kano, K. (2004) Molecular complexes of water-soluble porphyrins. J. Porphyr. Phthalocya., 8: 148～155.

[92] Kuba´t, P., Lang, K., Zelinger, Z., and Kra´l, V. (2004) Aggregation and photophysical properties of water-soluble sapphyrins. Chemical Physics Letters, 395: 82～86.

[93] Maiya, B.G. (2004) New porphyrin architectures and host-guest chemistry. J. Porphyr. Phthalocya, 8: 1118～1128.

[94] Simplicio, F.I., Soares, R.R.D.S., Maionchi, F., Filho, O.S., and Hioka, N. (2004) Aggregation of a benzoporphyrin derivative in water/organic solvent mixtures: A mechanistic proposition. Journal of Physical Chemistry A, 108: 9384～9389.

[95] Li, X., Li, D., Han, M., Chen, Z., and Zou, G. (2005) Neutral porphyrin J-aggregates in premicellar sds solution. Colloids and Surfaces A, 256: 151～156.

[96] Scolaro, L.M., Romeo, A., and Pasternack, R.F. (2004) Tuning porphyrin/DNA supramolecular assemblies by competitive binding. Journal of the American Chemical Society, 126: 7178～7179.

[97] Castriciano, M.A., Romeo, A., Villari, V., Micali, N., and Scolaro, L.M. (2003) Structural rearrangements in 5,10,15,20-tetrakis(4-sulfonatophenyl)porphyrin J-aggregates under strongly acidic conditions. Journal of Physical Chemistry B, 107: 8765～8771.

[98] Togashi, D.M., Costa, S.M.B., Sobral, A.J.F.N., and Gonsalves, A.M. d'A.R. (2004) Self-aggregation of lipophilic porphyrins in reverse micelles of aerosol OT. Journal of Physical Chemistry B, 108: 11344～11356.

[99] Chen, F., Huang, J., Ai, X., and He, Z. (2003) Determination of DNA by Rayleigh light scattering enhancement of molecular light switches. Analyst,128: 1462～1466.

[100] Song, G.W., Cai, Z.X., and Li, L. (2004) Study of the interaction of butyl rodamine B with DNA and the determination of DNA based on resonance light scattering measurements. Indian Journal of Chemistry A, 43: 1099～1101.

[101] Wu, X., Wang, Y., Wang, M., Sun, S., Yang, J., and Luan, Y. (2005) Determination of nucleic acids at nanogram level using resonance light scattering technique with congo red. Spectrochimica Acta Part A, 61: 361～366.

[102] Cai, Z.X., Song, G.W., Li, L., and Liu, L.M. (2004) Determination of nucleic acid by a resonance light-scattering technique with fluorescein. Chinese Journal of Analytical Chemistry, 32: 647～650.

[103] Chen, X., Cai, C., Zeng, J., Liao, Y., and Luo, H. (2005) Study on bromocresol green-cetyltrimethylammonium- deoxyribonucleic acids system by resonance light scattering spectrum methods. Spectrochimica Acta Part A, 61: 1783～1788.

[104] Wang, F., Yang, J., Wu, X., Wang, F., and Ding, H. (2006) Investigation of the interaction between curcumin and nucleic acids in the presence of CTAB. Spectrochimica Acta Part A, in press.

[105] Chen, X., Cai, C., Luo, H., and Zhang, G. (2005) Study on the resonance light-scattering spectrum of anionic dye xylenol orange-cetyltrimethylammoniumnucleic acids system and determination of nucleic acids at nanogram levels. Spectrochimica Acta PartA, 61: 2215～2220.

[106] Ding, F., Zhao, H., Chen, S., Ouyang, J., and Jin, L. (2005) Study of the interaction of nucleic acid with europium(III) and CTMAB and determination of nucleic acids at nanogram levels by the second-order scattering. Analytica Chimica Acta, 536: 171～178.

[107] Wu, X., Sun, S., Yang, J., Wang, M., Liu, L., and Guo, C. (2005) Study on the interaction between nucleic acid and Eu^{3+}-oxolinic acid and the determination of nucleic acid using the resonance light scattering technique. Spectrochimica Acta Part A, 62: 896～901.

[108] Jia, Z., Yang, J., Wu, X., Sun, C., Liu, S., Wang, F., and Zhao, Z. (2006) The sensitive determination of nucleic acids using resonance light scattering quenching method. Spectrochimica Acta Part A, 64: 555～559.

[109] Li, Y., Zhu, C., and Wang, L. (2003) Determination of nucleic acid at nanogram levels with manganese-tetrasulfonatophthalocyanine sensitized by cetyltrimethylammonium bromide using a resonance light-scattering technique. Microchimica Acta, 142: 219～223.

[110] Li, Y., Wu, Y., Chen, J., Zhu, C., Wang, L., Zhuo, S., and Zhao, D. (2003) Simple and sensitive assay for nucleic acids by use of the resonance light-scattering technique with copper phthalocyanine tetrasulfonic acid in the presence of cetyltrimethylammonium bromide. Analytical and Bioanalytical Chemistry, 377: 675～680.

[111] Li, Y., Zhao, D., Zhu, C., and Wang, L. (2003) The sensitizing effect ofcetyltrimethylammonium bromide on the resonance light-scattering enhancementbetween the interaction of deoxyribonucleic acids and manganese-tetrasulfonatophthalocyanine. Chinese Journal of Analytical Chemistry, 31: 694～697.

[112] Gao, F., Li, Y.-X., Zhang, L., and Wang, L. (2004) Cetyltrimethylammonium bromide sensitized resonance light-scattering of nucleic acid–pyronine B and its analytical application. Spectrochimica Acta Part A, 60: 2505～2509.

[113] Jie, N., Hou, S., Du, F., Zhang, C., and Qin, G. (2004) The determination of deoxyribonucleic acids with triadimenol based on the enhancement of resonance light scattering. Nucleosides, Nucleotides & Nucleic Acids, 23: 725～734.

[114] Jie, N., Jia, G., Hou, S., Xiong, Y., and Dong, Y. (2004) Determination of deoxyribonucleic acids by a resonance light scattering technique and its application. Spectrochimica Acta PartA, 59: 3295～3301.

[115] Zhou, Y., Chang, W., and Li, Y. (2004) The resonance light scattering spectra caused by the interaction of poly (diallyldimethyl ammonium chloride) with nucleic acids and its analytical application. Chinese Journal of Analytical Chemistry, 32: 169–173.

[116] Chen, Z., Ding, W., Ren, F., Liu, J., and Yizeng (2005) A simple and sensitive assay of nucleic acids based on the enhanced resonance light scattering of zwitterionics. Analytica Chimica Acta, 550: 204～209.

[117] Song, G., Cai, Z., and Li, L. (2004) Determination of nucleic acid using the resonance light scattering technique with the mixed complex La(phen)(ophthalic acid). Microchimica Acta, 144: 23～27.

[118] Feng, S., Liu, X., and Fan, J. (2005) Resonance light scattering spectra of cetylpyridinium bromide and deoxyribonucleic acid system and its application to deoxyribonucleic acid assay. Chinese Journal of Analytical Chemistry, 33: 377～380.

[119] Long, Y.-F., Chen, X.-M., Wu, Q.-L., and Yang, W.-J. (2003) Determination of deoxyribonucleic acid with alkali blue 6B by resonance light scattering method. Spectrosc. Spect. Anal., 23: 458～460.

[120] Chen, Y., Yang, J., Wu, X., Cao, W., and Zhuang, H. (2003) Resonance light scattering of catechol violet-cetyltrimethylammonium bromide-nucleic acid system and its analytical application. Chinese Journal of Analytical Chemistry, 31: 1352～1355.

[121] Yang, C.X., Li, Y.F., and Huang, C.Z. (2003) Determination of proteins with fast red VR by a corrected resonance light-scattering technique. Analytical Sciences, 19: 211～215.

[122] Wu, X., Sun, S., Guo, C., Yang, J., Sun, C., Zhou, C., and Wu, T. (2006) Resonance light scattering technique for the determination of proteins with congo red and triton x-100. Luminescence, 21: 56～61.

[123] Huang, C.Z., Yang, C.X., and Li, Y.F. (2003) Determination of proteins with ponceau g by compensating for the molecular absorption decreased resonance light scattering signals. Analytical Letters, 36: 1557～1571.

[124] Liu, R., Yang, J., Sun, C., Wu, X., Li, L., and Li, Z. (2003) Resonance light-scattering method for the determination of BSA and HSA with sodium dodecyl benzene sulfonate or sodium lauryl sulfate. Analytical and Bioanalytical Chemistry, 377: 375～379.

[125] Chen, Z., Liu, J., Liang, Y., and Ren, F. (2006) Use of sodium lauroyl sarcosinate in a high-sensitivity protein assay by resonance light scattering technique. Journal of Biomolecular Screening, 11: 400～406.

[126] Liu, Y., Yang, J., Liu, S., Wu, X., Su, B., and Wu, T. (2005) Resonance light scattering technique for the determination of protein with rutin and cetylpyridine bromide system. Spectrochimica Acta Part A, 61: 641～646.

[127] Zhong, H., Wang, K., and Chen, H.-Y. (2004) Protein analysis with tetra-substituted sulfonated cobalt phthalocyanine by the technique of Rayleigh light scattering. Analytical Biochemistry, 330: 37～42.

[128] Zhao, G.-C., Zhang, P., Wei, X.-W., and Yang, Z.-S. (2004) Determination of proteins with fullerol by a resonance light scattering technique. Analytical Biochemistry, 334: 297～302.

[129] Chen, Z., Liu, J., Han, Y., and Zhu, L. (2006) A novel histidine assay using tetraphenylporphyrin manganese(III) chloride as a molecular recognition probe by resonance light scattering technique. Analytica Chimica Acta, 570: 109～115.

[130] Luo, H.Q., Li, N.B., and Liu, S.P. (2006) Resonance Rayleigh scattering study of interaction of hyaluronic acid with ethyl violet dye and its analytical application. Biosensors and Bioelectronics, 21: 1186～1194.

[131] Li, N.B., Luo, H.Q., and Liu, S.P. (2005) Resonance Rayleigh scattering study of the inclusion complexation of chloramphenicol with δ-cyclodextrin. Talanta, 66: 495～500.

[132] Liu, S.P., Luo, H.Q., Xu, H., and Li, N.B. (2005) Resonance Rayleigh scattering study of interaction of heparin with some cationic surfactants and their analytical application. Spectrochimica Acta Part A, 61: 861～867.

[133] Sun, S., Wu, X., Yang, J., Li, L., and Wang, Y. (2004) Determination of dysprosium by resonance light scattering technique in the presence of bpmphd. Spectrochimica Acta Part A, 60: 261～264.

[134] Jiang, Z.-L., Sun, S.-J., Kang, C.-Y., Lu, X., and Lan, J. (2005) A new and sensitive resonance-scattering method for determination of trace nitrite in water with rhodamine 6G. Analytical and Bioanalytical Chemistry, 381: 896～900.

[135] Jiang, Z.L., Zhou, S.M., Liang, A.H., Kang, C., and He, X. (2006) Resonance scattering effect of rhodamine dye association nanoparticles and its application to respective determination of trace ClO_2 and Cl_2. Environmental Science & Technology, 40: 4286～4291.

[136] Zhao, T., Zhang, J., Cheng, X., Chen, X., and Hu, Z. (2004) Sensitive determination of sulfate in drinks and vegetables digests by Rayleigh light scattering technique. Journal of Agricultural and Food Chemistry, 52: 3688～3692.

[137] Peng, J.D., Liu, S.P., Liu, Z.F., and Shi, Y. (2006) Resonance Rayleigh scattering spectrum for the chelate of lanthanum(III) with sodium tanshinon IIA silate and its analytical application. Science in China-Series B, 49: 423～429.

[138] Yang, C.X., Li, Y.F., and Huang, C.Z. (2002) Determination of cationic surfactants in water samples by their enhanced resonance light scattering with azoviolet. Analytical and Bioanalytical Chemistry, 374: 868～872.

[139] Liu, S.P., Shi, Y., Liu, Z.F., Luo, H.Q., and Kong, L. (2006) Resonance Rayleigh scattering method for the determination of cationic surfactants with chromium(VI)-iodide system. Analytical Sciences, 22: 769.

[140] Feng, S., Wang, J., and Fan, J. (2006) Determination of a cationic surfactant with naphthalene black 12B by the resonance light scattering technique. Annali di Chimica, 96: 293～300.

[141] He, Y.Q., Liu, S.P., Kong, L., and Liu, Z.F. (2005) A study on the sizes and concentrations of gold nanoparticles by spectra of absorption, resonance Rayleigh scattering and resonance non-linear scattering. Spectrochimica Acta Part A, 61: 2861～2866.

[142] Zhu, J., Huang, L., Zhao, J., Wang, Y., Zhao, Y., Hao, L., and Lu, Y. (2005) Shape dependent resonance light scattering properties of gold nanorods. Materials Science and Engineering B, 121: 199～203.

[143] Zhu, J., Wang, Y., Huang, L., and Lu, Y. (2004) Resonance light scattering characters of core–shell structure of Au–Ag nanoparticles. Physics Letters A, 323: 455～459.

[144] Zhao, H.W., Huang, C.Z., and Li, Y.F. (2006) Validation of micelle formation of proteins and determination of their critical micelle concentrations by measuring synchronous light scattering signals using a common spectrofluorometer. Chemistry Letters, 35: 418～419.

[145] Landsman, M.L., Kwant, G., Mook, G.A., and Zijlstra, W.G. (1976) Lightabsorbing properties, stability, and spectral stabilization of indocyanine green. Journal of Applied Physiology, 40: 575～583.

[146] Sokolov, K., Follen, M., Aaron, J., Pavlova, I., Malpica, A., Lotan, R., and Richards-Kortum, R. (2003) Real-time vital optical imaging of precancer using anti-epidermal growth factor receptor antibodies conjugated to gold nanoparticles1. CancerResearch, 63: 1999～2004.

[147] El-Sayed, I.H., Huang, X., and El-Sayed, M.A. (2005) Surface plasmon resonance scattering and absorption of anti-EGFR antibody conjugated gold nanoparticles in cancer diagnostics: Applications in oral cancer. Nano Letters, 5: 829～834.

(Jian Ling, Cheng Zhi Huang, Yuan Fang Li, Yun Fei Long, and Qie Gen Liao,
published in *Applied Spectroscopy Reviews*, 2007, 42:177～201.)

Chapter 2

Analytical Applications in DNA Detection of Light Scattering Technique

2.1 Determination of Nucleic Acids by a Resonance Light-scattering Technique with *α*, *β*, *γ*, *δ*-tetrakis [4-(trimethy-lammoniumyl) phenyl] Porphine

The resonance light-scattering technique, using a spectrofluorometer, was first developed as a sensitive instrumental analysis method. At pH 7.48 and ionic strength 0.004, the extent of light-scattering of *α*, *β*, *γ*, *δ*-tetrakis [4-(trimethylammoniumyl)phenyl]porphine (TAPP) is enhanced by nucleic acids near 432 nm. There are linear relationships between the enhanced extents of lightscattering and the concentrations of nucleic acids in the range of $1.8\times10^{-7}\sim10.8\times10^{-7}$ mol·L^{-1} for calf thymus and fish sperm DNA and in the range of $1.8\times10^{-7}\sim 1.8\times10^{-6}$ mol·L^{-1} for yeast RNA. The limit of determination (3 σ) is 4.1×10^{-8} mol·L^{-1} for calfthymus DNA, 4.6×10^{-8} mol·L^{-1} for fish sperm DNA, and 6.7×10^{-8} mol·L^{-1} for yeast RNA. Mechanism study indicates that nucleic acids react with the title porphyrin in two modes, depending on the concentrations of nucleic acids. When the molar ratio of nucleic acids to TAPP is smaller than 4:1, the hypochromicity and fluorescence quenching of TAPP by nucleic acids appear, and the enhancement of resonance light-scattering can be observed. When the molar ratio of nucleic acids to TAPP is larger than 4:1, a new fluorescent complex is formed.

The quantitative analysis of nucleic acids is very important since it is often used as a reference for measurements of other components in biological samples. There are two kinds of determination methods for nucleic acids: One is based on the reactions between the components of nucleic acids-phosphorus,[1] bases,[2] or sugar[3] and drugs such as diphenylamine,[3] indole,[4] *p*-nitrophenyl-hydrazine,[5] thiobarbituric acids,[6] etc. The other one is based on the reactions in which the double helix strands of DNA molecules are intercalated by or interact with drugs such as ethidium bromide,[7] diaminophenylindole (DAPI), and bisimidazole (Hoechst 33258).[8] Furthermore, the trivalent rare earth cations such as Tb(III),[9,10] Eu(III),[11] La(III),[12] and Y(III)[13] have been developed as fluorescence probes of the structure and function of nucleic acids in recent years. However, all of these methods are confined in spectrophotometry and fluorospectrometry.

A new determination method with high sensitivity for nucleic acids has been developed that uses resonance light-scattering in our laboratory. This assay is based on the interactions of *α*, *β*, *γ*, *δ*-tetrakis [4-(trimethylammoniumyl)phenyl] porphine (TAPP) with nucleic acids. At pH 7.48 and ionic strength 0.004, the extent of resonance light-scattering of TAPP can be enhanced by nucleic acids, and the extent of light-scattering enhancement is proportional to the concentrations of nucleic acids. Considering the fluorescence quenching effect of nucleic acids on the title porphyrin, the two methods were compared in terms of linear range and sensitivity.

2.1.1 Experimental Section

2.1.1.1 Apparatus

The resonance light-scattering spectrum, the extent ofresonance light-scattering, and the fluorescence intensity were measured with a Shimadzu RF-540 spectrofluorometer (Kyoto, Japan), equipped with a 150-W xenon lamp, a recorder, a dual monochromator, and a quartz cell (1×1 cm^2). The absorption spectrum was obtained with a Shimadzu UV-265 spectrophotometer. A WH-861 vortex mixer (Huangjing Instrumental Co., Jiang Su, China) was used to blend the solutions in volumetric flasks, and an 821 pH meter was used to measure the pH of the solution.

2.1.1.2 Reagents

Stock solutions of DNAs and RNA were prepared by dissolving commercial calf thymus DNA (Beitai Biochemical Co., Chinese Academy of Sciences, Beijing, China), fish sperm DNA, and yeast RNA (Shanghai Institute of Biochemistry, Chinese Academy of Sciences, Shanghai, China) in doubly deionized water. For DNAs, 24 h or more was needed at 4 ℃ , with gentle shaking occasionally. The concentrations of nucleic acids were calculated according to the absorbances at 260 nm by using ϵ_{DNA} (6600 $M^{-1}\cdot cm^{-1}$) and ϵ_{RNA} (7800 $M^{-1}\cdot cm^{-1}$),[14] respectively. The solutions of nucleic acids were prepared in the following concentration series ($\times10^{-5}$ $mol\cdot L^{-1}$): 0.3, 0.6, 0.9, 1.2, 1.5, 1.8, 2.1, 2.4, 2.7, 3.0, 3.3, 3.6, and 7.5.

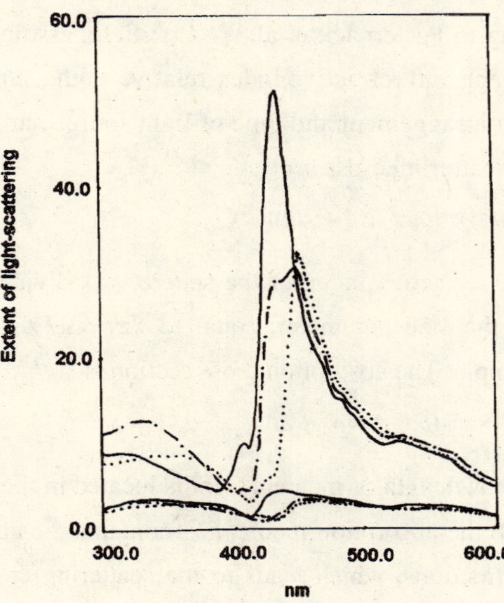

Fig. 1 Resonance light-scattering spectra at different pH values. Calf thymus DNA, 9.0×10^{-7} $mol\cdot L^{-1}$; TAPP, 1.2×10^{-6} $mol\cdot L^{-1}$. Symbols: (-) pH 7.48; (- · -), pH 3.79; (…) pH 2.02. Upper, DNA + TAPP; lower, TAPP.

The free base porphyrin, TAPP, synthesized in our laboratory and identified by ^{1}H NMR and IR, was dissolved in doubly deionized water. The concentration of the solution was determined according to its absorbance at 412.0 nm (the Soret maxima) by using $\epsilon=4.16\times10^5$ $M^{-1}\cdot cm^{-1}$ in pH 7.48 (I = 0.004).[15]

Tris-HCl buffer was prepared by dissolving 6.1 g of tris-(hydroxymethyl)aminomethane in 250 mL of water, adding 400 mL of 0.1 M HCl, and diluting to 1000 mL with water; the pH of the solution was 7.48.

All reagents were of analytical reagent grade without further purification. Water used throughout was doubly deionized.

2.1.1.3 Samples

According to the interferences of foreign substances, six synthetic samples were constructed.

2.1.1.4 Standard Procedure

In a dry 10-mL volumetric flask were added 0.60 mL of standard nucleic acid or sample solution and 0.60 mL of TAPP solution with different affluxes along the wall of volumetric flask. The mixture was vortexed, and 1.0 mL of Tris-HCl buffer solution was added. The mixture was diluted to 10 mL with water. The resonance light-scattering spectrum was obtained by scanning simultaneously the excitation and emission monochromators of the RF -540 spectrofluorometer from 300 to 600 nm. The spectrofluorometer was equipped with a 150-W xenon lamp which had been adjusted with constant geometry. The extent of light-scattering was measured at the maximum wavelength with slit width at 5.0 nm for the excitation and emission.

2.1.2 Results and Discussion

2.1.2.1 Resonance Light-Scattering Spectrum

Fig. 1 shows that the light-scattering of TAPP is very small, and near its Soret band (the Soret bands of TAPP at pH 7.48 and 2.02 are located at 412.0 and 432.0 nm, respectively[15]) the light-scattering becomes even smaller. However, enhanced light-scattering can be observed when TAPP coexists with nucleic acids near the Soret band, and before the enhancement region the light-scattering reaches a minimum. That is, the resonance light-scattering spectrum depends on the molecule's absorption. Shoulder peaks over the 530-580 nm region might be relative to Q absorption bands. According to Pasternack et al.,[16] a particle, assumed to be spherical, absorbs and scatters light depending on its size, shape and refractive index relative to the surrounding medium. When the instrumental conditions such as the exact arrangement and type of light source and detector are fixed, the extent of light-scattering is proportional to the scattering cross section:

$$c_{\text{sca}} = (\pi r^2)(8/3)X^4[(m^2-1)/(m^2+2)]^2$$

where r is the radius of spherical particle; m is the refractive index of the sphere, n_{sph}, divided by the refractive index of the surrounding medium, n_{med}; and x is the size parameter, equal to $2\pi r n_{\text{med}}/\lambda$. But the extent of light-scattering is reduced with absorption of the sample. The absorption cross section is

$$c_{\text{abs}} = (\pi r^2)4\times Im[(m^2-1)/(m^2+2)]$$

where I is the intensity of incident light. Since the wavelength of incident light is located in the visible region, and since, when the visible incident light passes through the absorption media, n_{sph} contains the absorption part,[17] m should be composed of scattering and absorption fractions, which leads to the scattering cross section being a stronger function of m than the absorption cross section. So, when the concentration is so low that the absorption of sample is low enough, enhanced scattering is observed.

Porphyrins can assemble on a biopolymer even without the requirement for aggregation of the template on which the biopolymer serves.[18] The driving force for the assembly formation is the tendency for porphyrins to form stacking-type aggregates. The hypochromicity of DNA on porphyrin (Fig. 2) reduced the absorption at the

Soret absorption band when DNA was added to porphyrin solution. The scattering experiments proved that the extent of scattering is very small and does not change with the concentrations of TAPP and DNA when they exist separately. However, when TAPP is mixed with DNA, TAPP molecules assemble on nucleic acids and form small particles, and then the enhanced scattering can be observed.

Fig. 3 shows that the enhancement of light-scattering changes only a little with pH in the range pH 4.49~9.26. The dependence of light-scattering on pH might be relevant to the form of TAPP. At pH<4.2, the free base form of TAPP is protonized, and this results in transfer of the Soret absorption band from 432.0 to 412.0 nm.[15] This also can be seen in Fig. 1.

2.1.2.2 Effects of the State of Nucleic Acids

Fig. 4 shows that the extent of scattering decreases with increasing ionic strength, but no change takes place in the pattern of the resonance lightscattering spectrum. That is ascribed to the change of the conformation of nucleic acidsthe template on which the TAPP assembles. As the concentration of NaCl increases, the flexible nucleic acid molecules become rigid, which inhibits the external (minor) groove binding or the intercalation of TAPP.[16] However, despite the strong dependence of the enhanced light-scattering of TAPP by nucleic acids on ionic strength, the extent of light scattering of TAPP is constant when ionic strength ranges from 0.004 to 0.40.

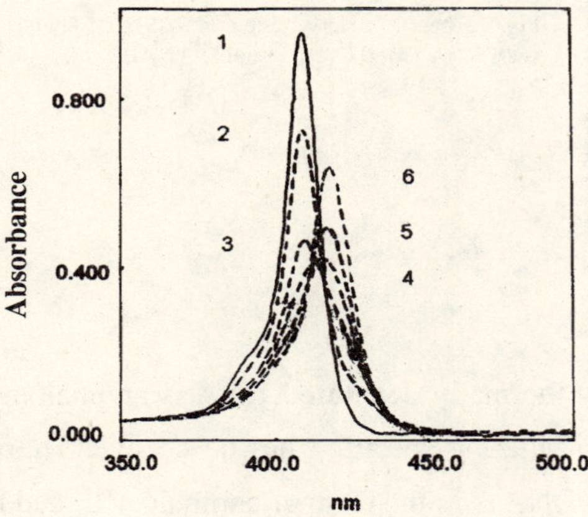

Fig. 2 UV spectra of the complex formed by calf thymus DNA and TAPP. Concentration of DNA: 1, 0.0; 2, 1.0×10^{-6} mol·L^{-1}; 3, 6.0×10^{-6} mol·L^{-1}; 4, 9.0×10^{-6} mol·L^{-1}; 5, 1.2×10^{-5} mol·L^{-1}; 6, 2.7×10^{-5} mol·L^{-1}. TAPP, 2.4×10^{-6} mol·L^{-1}. Similar spectra could be obtained for fish sperm DNA and yeast RNA.

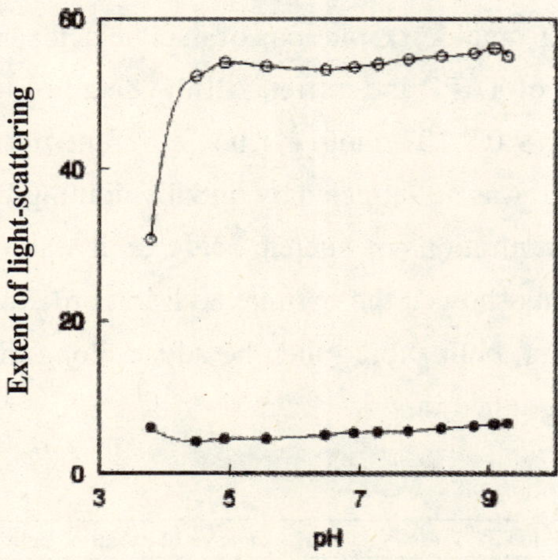

Fig. 3 Dependence of extent of RLS on pH. Symbols: (○) experimental data of DNA-TAPP complex; (●) experimental data of TAPP. Calf thymus DNA, 9.0×10^{-7} mol·L^{-1}; TAPP, 1.2×10^{-6} mol·L^{-1}; pH 7.48.

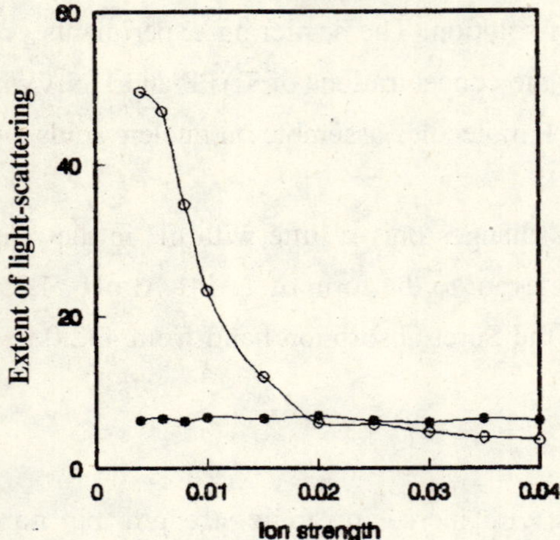

Fig. 4 Effect of ionic strength on RLS. Symbols: (○) experimental data of DNA-TAPP complex; (●) experimental data of TAPP. Calf thymus DNA, 9.0×10^{-7} mol·L^{-1}; TAPP, 1.2×10^{-6} mol·L^{-1}.

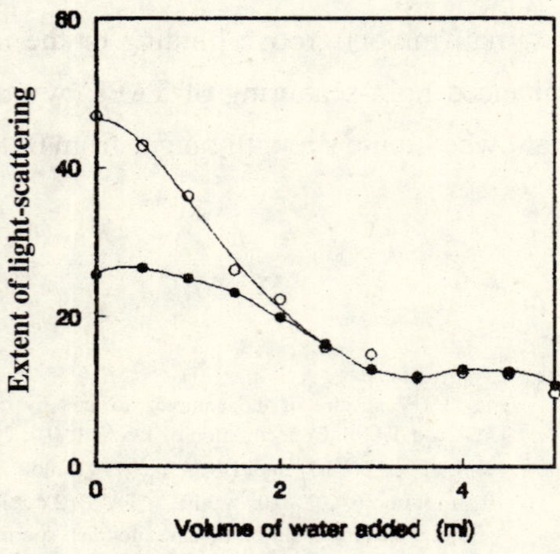

Fig. 5 Effect of water addition on RLS. Calf thymus DNA (○) and yeast RNA (●), 9.0×10^{-7} mol·L^{-1}; TAPP, 1.2×10^{-6} mol·L^{-1}; pH 7.48.

The enhancement of light-scattering of TAPP by thermally denatured DNA is anomalous and shows band reproducibility, but the pattern of the resonance light-scattering spectrum has no change. The reason maybe the change of conformation of DNA. Thermally denatured DNA is in the form of anomalous thread mat structure, and the assembly of TAPP on DNA is greatly different. It is noted that the enhanced extents of light-scattering by nucleic acids are different for different initial concentrations but same final concentrations of nucleic acids. Figure 5 gives the extent of light-scattering for 0.60 mL (1.5×10^{-5} mol·L^{-1}) solutions of nucleic acids into which different volumes of water had been added before the addition of TAPP and buffer. All the data in Fig. 5 were obtained with the same final concentrations of nucleic acids (9.0×10^{-7} mol·L^{-1}) but different initial concentrations. However, the fluorescence quenching of DNA on TAPP was not affected by initially diluting DNA. Changing the orders of addition of reagents can alter the initial concentrations of nucleic acids, so it was very important that the addition order of reagents be fixed. Our experiments showed the optimal addition order of reagents to be as follows: nucleic acids should be mixed with TAPP first, both should then be added along different affluxes of the wall of volumetric flask, and then the buffer can be added in.

Table 1 Tolerance of Foreign Substances

substances	concn coexisting ($\times10^{-7}$ mol·L^{-1})^a	change of extent of light-scattering(%)
protein, BSA	0.15	1.3
adenine	6.0	−7.8

Continued

substances	concn coexisting ($\times 10^{-7}$ mol·L^{-1})[a]	change of extent of light-scattering(%)
guanine	6.0	−2.9
cytosine	60.0	−3.1
thymine	6.0	−10.9
uracil	6.0	−3.0
$H_2PO_4^-$	6.0	4.6
Al(III) sulfate	0.12	−10.7
Zn(II) chloride	0.12	5.8
Ca(II) chloride	0.24	−0.1
Mg(II) chloride	0.24	−8.8
Co(II) nitrate	0.12	9.5
Cd(II) chloride	0.24	−7.8
Hg(II) nitrate	0.12	−0.1
Ni(II) nitrate	0.12	−0.8
Cu(II) nitrate	0.12	−4.7
Mn(II) nitrate	0.12	−7.4
Pb(II) nitrate	0.12	−6.6

[a] Calf thymus DNA, 9.0×10^{-7}mol·L^{-1}; TAPP, 1.2×10^{-6} mol·L^{-1}.

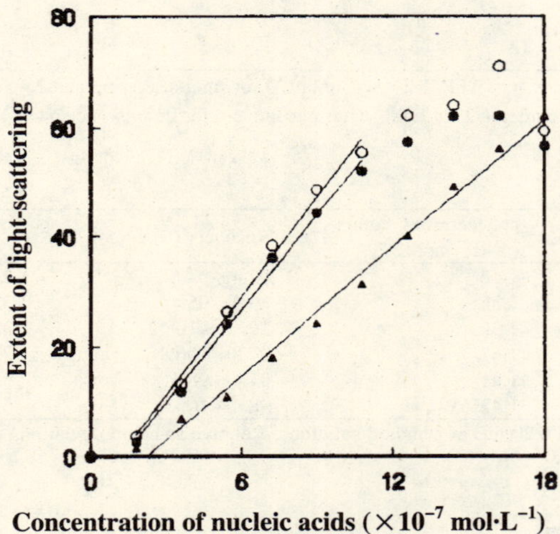

Fig. 6 Calibration curves for DNA and RNA. Calf thymus DNA (○); fish sperm DNA (●), yeast RNA (▲); TAPP, 1.2×10^{-6} mol·L^{-1}.

After the addition order of reagents and the volume of solution have been fixed, the experiments can be done at pH 7.48 and ionic strength 0.004. To achieve satisfactory reproducibility, the addition of reagents should follow different affluxes along the wall of volumetric flask. The standing time test showed that the system is stable for at least 6 h.

2.1.2.3 Tolerance of Foreign Coexisting Substances

Some interferences were tested, and the results are listed in Table 1. Considering the initial dilution of DNA by other reagents, a 0.60 mL solution of calf thymus DNA (1.5×10^{-5} mol·L^{-1}) containing the coexisting foreign materials was used to test the interferences.

2.1.2.4 Calibration Curves

According to the above standard procedures, 0.60 mL solutions of different concentrations of nucleic acids were used to construct the calibration curves (Fig. 6). The extents of light-scattering were obtained at 432.0 nm for DNA and at 436.0 nm for RNA. There are linear relationships between the extent of light-scattering and the concentrations of nucleic acids. All the analytical parameters are presented in Table 2. From Table 2 it can be seen that the resonance light-scattering technique (RLST) is much more sensitive than the fluorescence quenching method of nucleic acids on TAPP in terms of linear range and sensitivity (slope of linear regression equation). According to Table 2, the sensitivities of RLST and fluorescence quenching method have the same sequence: calf thymus DNA > fish sperm DNA > yeast RNA. It is unfortunate that the determination of nucleic acids is in the small linear range, but the limitation could be complemented by fluorescence quenching. According to Fig. 6, six synthetic samples constructed on the basis of the interferences of foreign substances (Table 1) were determined. As Table 3 shows, the results are satisfactory.

Table 2 Analytical Parameters for Determination by RLST and Fluorescence Quenching Method

nucleic acid	linear range ($\times 10^{-7}$ mol·L^{-1})	linear regression equation ($C\times 10^{-7}$ mol·L^{-1})[a]	limit of determination (3σ, $\times 10^{-8}$ mol·L^{-1})	r
calfthymus DNA	1.8～10.8	E_{sca}=-6.8 + 6.0C	4.1	0.9962
	15.0～90.0	F_{flu}=80.6 - 0.68C		0.9969
fish sperm DNA	1.8～10.8	E_{sca}=-6.8 + 5.9C	4.6	0.9962
	15.0～105.0	F_{flu}=81.1 - 0.61C		0.9960
yeast RNA	1.8～18.0	E_{sca}=-8.7 + 3.9C	6.7	0.9963
	15.0～105.0	F_{flu}=83.0 - 0.57C		0.9981

[a] E stands for extent of light-scattering, while F stands for fluorescence intensity. TAPP, 1.2×10^{-6} mol·L^{-1} for light-scattering and 2.4×10^{-6}mol·L^{-1} for fluorescence quenching method. Data were obtained by fixing the ordinate of recorder at 1 for light-scattering and at 4 for fluorescence quenching.

Table 3 Results of Synthetic Samples (n= 5)

nucleic acid (1.5×10^{-7}mol·L^{-1})	coexisting interferences	concentration Found ($\times 10^{-7}$mol·L^{-1})	Recovery (%, n=5)[a]	relative standard deviation(%)[b]
calf thymus DNA	BSA, Ca(II), Mg(II), Cd(II)	1.42	92.4～98.6	2.6
	A, G, C, T, U, $H2PO_4^-$	1.36	89.3～95.4	3.8
fish sperm DNA	BSA, Ca(II), Mg(II)	1.32	101.2～108.2	3.6
	A, G, C, T, U, $H2PO_4^-$	1.67	97.8～106.8	2.8
yeast RNA	BSA, Al(III), Hg(II)	1.41	91.4～98.6	5.1
	A, G, C, T, U, $H2PO_4^-$	1.42	98.4～109.8	5.1

a The recoveries were obtained by adding 0.40 mL of sample solution and 0.20 mL of standard solution, [b] Relative standard deviations were obtained for five measurements in the middle ofthe calibration curve.

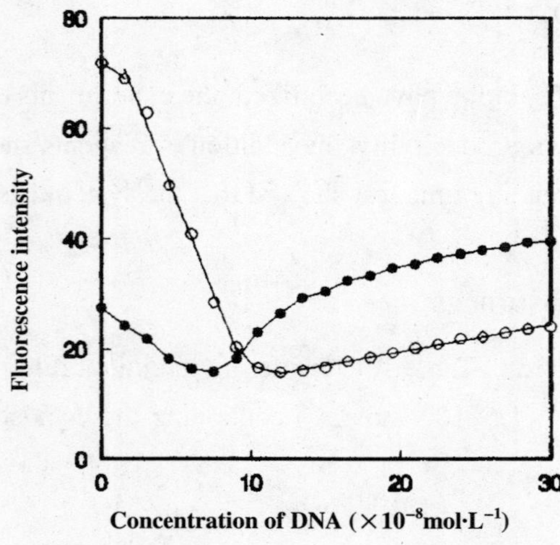

Fig. 7 Fluorescence reaction between calf thymus and TAPP. Fluorescence intensity (○) at 638.0 nm (excited at 413.0 nm) and (●) at 652.0 nm (excited at 422.0 nm). TAPP, 2.4×10^{-6} mol·L^{-1}.

2.1.2.5 Mechanism of the Reaction

It was found that, as the concentrations ofnucleic acids increase, the resonance wavelength shifts slightly forth and back (Table 4). As Figure 2 shows, calf thymus DNA decreases the absorption at 412.0 nm (hypochromicity), and a new peak at 420 nm appears when the molar ratio of DNA to TAPP is larger than 4:1. That indicates that a new complex is formed. The height of the new peak rises with increasing concentration ofnucleic acids. The new complex emits fluorescence with the emitted wavelength from 639.0 to 652.0 nm (Table 5). Fish sperm DNAand yeast RNAhave similar reactions.

Table 4 Wavelength Shifts of Light-Scattering (nm)[a]

	concentration of nucleic acids (10^{-7} mol·L^{-1})									
	1.8	3.6	5.4	7.2	9.0	10.8	12.6	14.4	16.2	18.0
calfthymus DNA	432.0	434.0	433.5	433.0	432.0	432.0	432.0	431.5	431.5	431.5
fish sperm DNA	432.0	433.0	434.0	432.5	432.0	432.0	432.0	432.0	431.0	431.5
yeast RNA	432.0	434.0	436.0	438.0	438.0	438.0	438.0	436.5	436.5	436.0

[a] Concentration of TAPP, 1.2×10^{-6} mol·L^{-1}.

Table 5 Wavelength Shifts of Fluorescence (nm)[a]

	concentration of nucleic acids ($\times10^{-6}$ mol·L^{-1})									
	0.0	3.0	6.0	9.0	12.0	15.0	18.0	21.0	24.0	27.0
calfthymus DNA										
excited	413	413	413	417	421	422	422	422	422	422
emitted	638	638	639	648	652	652	652	652	652	652
fish sperm DNA										
excited	413	413	414	415	422	423	423	423	423	423
emitted	638	639	640	648	652	652	652	652	652	652
yeast RNA										
excited	413	413	414	418	422	424	425	425	425	425
emitted	638	646	646	650	650	651	652	652	652	652

[a]Concentration of TAPP, 2.4×10^{-6} mol·L^{-1}.

As Fig. 2 and Fig. 7 depict, the new complex forms only when the molar ratio of DNA to TAPP is larger than 4:1. Thus, the reaction between nucleic acids and TAPP has two mechanisms, depending on the concentration of-nucleic acids: One characterizes the hypochromicity and fluorescence quenching effect of nucleic acids on TAPP when the molar ratio of nucleic acid to TAPP is smaller than 4:1, and at this time the enhancement of resonance light-scattering can be observed. The other characterizes a newly formed fluorescent complex when the molar ratio of nucleic acid to TAPP is larger than 4:1.

2.1.3 Conclusion

The resonance light-scattering technique is useful and sensitive in the determination of trace amounts of substances. All the experiments described here were done on a commonly used spectrofluorometer. Considering that the wavelength ofincidence equals the emitted wavelength, we think that RLST is related to Rayleigh scattering. Since the wavelength of incident light is located in the absorption region, the extent of light-scattering deviates by the -4 powers from the wavelength of the incident light. The deviation is ascribed to the change ofrefractive index.[17] That is, the major reason that enhanced light-scattering could be observed is the change of refractive index.

Acknowledgments

This project was supported by the National Natural Science Foundation of China (NNSFC), and all the authors express their deep thanks.

References

[1] Skidmore, W. D.; Duggan, E. L.; Donzales, L. J. Anal. Biochem. 1964, 9, 370-376. (b) Sheridan, R. E.; O'Donnell, C. M.; Pautler, E. R. Anal. Biochem. 1973, 52, 657～659.

[2] Huang, P. C.; Rosenbery, E. Anal. Biochem. 1966, 16, 107～113. (b) Marquet, R.; Houssier, C. Anal. Chem. 1989, 176, 265～268.

[3] Derallonne, J. R.; Weyns, J. C. Anal. Biochem. 1976, 74, 449. (b) Gendimenico, G. J.; Bouquin, P. L.; Tramposch, K. M. Anal. Biochem.19 8 8, 173, 45.

[4] Hubbard, R. W.; Matthew, W. T.; Moulton, D. W. Anal. Biochem. 1972, 46, 461～472.

[5] Martin, R. F.; Donohue, D. C. Anal. Biochem. 1972, 47, 562～574.

[6] Gold, D. V.; Shochat, D. Anal. Biochem. 1980, 105, 121～125.

[7] Strothkamp, K. G.; Strothkamp, R. E. J. Chem. Educ. 1994, 71, 77～79.

[8] Lankcker, M. V.; Gheyssens, L. C. Anal. Lett. 1986, 19, 615～623.

[9] Topal, M. D.; Fresco, J. R. Biochemistry 1980, 19, 5531～5537.

[10] Ci, Y. X.; Li, Y. Z.; Chang, W. B. Anal. Chim. Acta, 1991, 248: 589～594.

[11] Ci, Y. X.; Li, Y. Z.; Liu, X. J. Anal. Chem. 1995, 67, 1785～1788.

[12] Huang, C. Z.; Li, K. A.; Tong, S. Y. Anal. Lett., in press.

[13] Huang, C. Z.; Li, K. A.; Tong, S. Y. Mikrochim. Acta, submitted.

[14] Chen, Z.; Liu, J.; Luo, D. Biochemistry Experiments; Chinese University of Sciences and Technology Press: Hefei, PRC, 1994; p 111.

[15] (15) Zeng, Y. E.; Zhang, H. S.; Chen, Z. H. Handbook of Modern Chemical Reagents IV; Chemical Industry Press: Beijing, PRC, 1989; p 792.

[16] Pasternack, R. F.; Bustamante, C.; Collings, P. J.; Giannetto, A.; Gibbs, E. J. J. Am. Chem. Soc. 1993, 115, 5393-5399.

[17] Miller, G. A. J. Phys. Chem. 1978, 82, 616～618.

[18] Pasternack, F. F.; Gibbs, E. J. J. Inorg. Organomet. Polym. 1993, 3, 77～88.

(Cheng Zhi Huang, Ke An Li, and Shen Yang Tong, published in *Analytical Chemistry*, 1996, 68,2259～2263.)

2.2 Hybridization Detection of DNA by Measuring Organic Small Molecule Amplified Resonance Light Scattering Signals

The interaction of organic small molecules (OSMs) with a biological molecule is very important. In this contribution, quinone-imine dyes including Acridine Yellow (AY), Neutral Red (NR), Acridine Orange (AO), Brilliant Cresyl Blue (BCB), Thionin (TN), Azur A(AA), Azur B(AB), and Methylene Blue (MB) respectively with double strand DNA (dsDNA) and single strand DNA (ssDNA) were investigated based on the measurements of enhanced resonance light scattering (RLS) and TEM. Mechanism investigations have shown that groove binding occurs between dsDNA and these OSMs, which depends on G-C sequences of dsDNA and the volumes of OSMs. With the amplified RLS signals resulting from the interactions of OSMs with DNA, a new technique has been proposed to detect the hybridization and mismatch of DNA labeling neither the target nor the probe DNA. The results have suggested that the extent of the amplified RLS signals of dsDNA by AY is the maximum among these eight OSMs, and therefore, it has been selected as a typical model system for further discussions.

2.2.1 Introduction

Hybridization detection of DNA has been a significant topic for its application in the diagnosis of pathogenic and genetic diseases.[1,2] So far, hybridization detections have been involved in chip-based microarrays technique,[3] molecular beacons,[4] surface plasmon resonance,[5] molecular spectrophotometry,[6] reflective interferometry,[7,8] chemiluminescence,[9] radioactive measurements,[10] and so on. Most of them, however, require a special label with the drawbacks of a time-consuming and complicated process. To overcome these disadvantages, labelfree hybridization detections binding through base pairing have been reported based on optical,[11~14] electrochemical,[15] piezoelectric,[16] and nanomechanical techniques.[17]

By coupling and scanning the excitation and the emission monochromators of a common spectrofluorometer simultaneously, Pasternack found that it was easy to get enhanced resonance light scattering (RLS) signals when assembly species were excited by a light beam with a wavelength close to the region of their absorption bands.[18] Subsequently, wide applications have been found with RLS spectroscopy in detecting biosamples.[19–21] To improve the sensitivity, selectivity, and automation, techniques like total internally reflected RLS,[22] RLS imaging,[23] flow-injection RLS,[24] and microarray RLS techniques[25] have been developed. Of these studies, the most interesting one is the microarray RLS technique, which has been used to detect DNA hybridization with high sensitivity, but the target DNA must be labeled. Herein we propose a RLS signalamplified technique, in which neither the target nor the probe DNA needs labeling to detect the hybridization and sequence specificity of DNA by the groove binding property with organic small molecules (OSMs) using Acridine Yellow (AY) as an example.

2.2.2 Experimental Section

2.2.2.1 Apparatus

RLS and fluorescence spectra were measured with a Hitachi F-4500 spectrofluorometer (Tokyo, Japan) with use of a 200-μL microquartz fluorescence cell. Absorption spectra were measured by a Hitachi U-3010 spectrophotometer (Tokyo, Japan), and TEM observations were carried out on a TecNai 10 electron microscope (FEA, USA.). A pHS-3C digital pH meter (Leici, China) was used to detect the pH values.

2.2.2.2 Reagents

Oligonucleotide sequences were synthesized by Beijing Sunbio-technology Co. (Beijing, China), and used without further purification. The used oligonucleotide probes (P) and targets (T) respectively include P1, 5'-GAA CGA AAC CAT TAT ACG AT-3', its complementary sequences T1, 5'-ATC GTA TAA TGG TTT CGT TC-3', and its two-basemismatched sequences MT1, 5'-ATT TTA TAA TGG TTT CGT TC-3'; P2, 5'-ATA ATT TAT T-3', and its complementary T2, 5'-AAT AAA TTA T-3' ; and P3, 5'-CGC GCC CGC C-3', and its complementary T3, 5'-GGC GGG CCG C-3'. Thermally denatured fish sperm DNA (fsDNA) was used for comparison, which was obtained by incubating fsDNA in a boiling water bath for 10 min and cooling immediately in ice water.

All chemicals were analytical reagents and were used without further purification. Milli-Q purified water (18.2 MΩ) was used for all sample preparations. The concentration of fsDNA was determined according to the absorbance values at 260.0 nm by using ϵ_{DNA} 6600 $mol \cdot L^{-1}$ cm^{-1}.[26] The 0.1 $mmol \cdot L^{-1}$ stock solutions of eight OSMs, including Acridine Yellow (AY), Neutral Red (NR), Acridine Orange (AO), Brilliant Cresyl Blue (BCB), Thionin (TN), Azur A(AA), Azur B(AB), and Methylene Blue (MB) (Shanghai Chemical Reagents Co. Shanghai, China) were prepared by dissolving the commercial products in water in 250 mL volumetric flash. Hybridization buffer was Tris-HCl (pH 7.2) containing 10 $mmol \cdot L^{-1}$ Tris, 140 $mmol \cdot L^{-1}$ NaCl, and 80 $mmol \cdot L^{-1}$ $MgCl_2$.

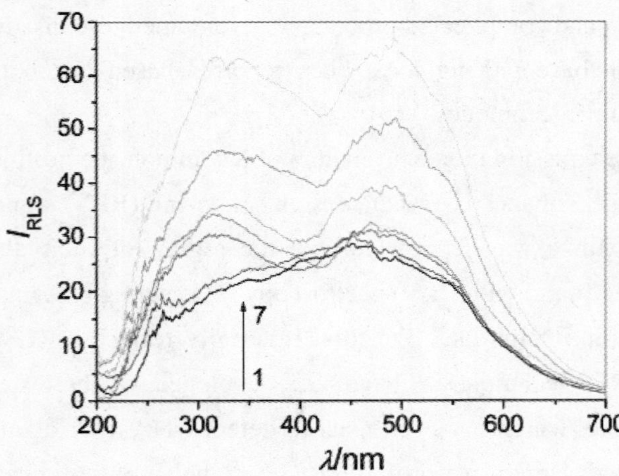

Fig. 1 RLS spectra of bindings of P1 and P1≈T1 with AY: (1) P1 (black); (2) P1≈T1 (red); (3) AY (blue); (4) P1-AY (aubergine); (5-7) P1≈T1-AY. c_{AY} = 2.0 × 10^{-5} $mol \cdot L^{-1}$; c_{P1} = 1.0 × 10^{-7} $mol \cdot L^{-1}$. c_{T1} (× 10^{-7} $mol \cdot L^{-1}$) = 0.3 (curve 5, green blue), 0.7 (curve 6, green), and 1.0 (curve 7, yellow). pH 7.2.

2.2.2.3 Experimental Procedure

A 20.0μL probe (P) solution, 40.0 μL of hybridization buffer solution, and an appropriate volume of target DNA (T) solution according to the desired concentration were added to a 1.5-mL microtube. After the mixture was incubated for 30 min for hybridization at 37℃, 20.0 μL of a 0.1 m $mol \cdot L^{-1}$ OSMs solution was added. The mixture was diluted to 100.0 μL with water, and then vortex-mixed thoroughly before the RLS measurements. All RLS spectra were obtained by scanning the excitation and emission monochnoromators simultaneously (namely $\triangle\lambda = 0$ nm) from 200.0 to 700.0 nm. The RLS intensity was measured at 494.4 nm with a slit width at 5.0 nm for the excitation and emission.

TEM specimens were prepared by dropping the solution onto copper grids covered with a self-prepared film, subsiding for 5~8 min, and using acetate uranium (1%) negative staining for 5 min.

2.2.3 Results and Discussion

2.2.3.1 RLS Spectral Properties and the Application

The RLS spectral properties of P1 (a kind of ssDNA), P1≈T1 (the hybridization complexes formed from P1 and T1, a kind of dsDNA, herein we use "≈" to indicate a double strand), OSMs (including AY, NR, AO, BCB, TN, AA, AB, and MB), P1-OSMs (the mixture of P1 and OSMs), and P1≈T1-OSMs (the mixture of P1≈T1 and OSMs) were studied. Figure 1 shows the typical one involving in the interactions of AY with P1≈T1 and P1. It can be seen that the RLS signals of AY, P1-AY, P1, and P1≈T1 are weak over the range of 200.0 to 700.0 nm. AY has two weak and wide RLS peaks at 315.6 and 470.0 nm, which are related to the molecular absorption of AY at 264.0 and 434.0 nm (Fig. 2 in the Supporting Information), according to the RLS theory.[27~29] The RLS signals of P1 and P1≈T1 are almost identical (curves 1 and 2 in Fig. 1), and when AY solution was added to P1 or T1 solution, negligible enhanced RLS signals could be observed. If AY was added to the solution of P1≈T1, however, greatly enhanced RLS signals could be observed with RLS peaks characterized at 315.6 and 494.4 nm, respectively. Therefore, it is apparent that AY could amplify the RLS signals of P1≈T1.[16,17] Furthermore, the amplified extent ($\triangle I_{RLS}$) of P1≈T1 at 494.4 nm is in good proportion to the concentration of T1 at a given amount of P1, and the dependence of $\triangle I_{RLS}$ on the concentration of T1 follows a linear function of $\triangle I_{RLS} = -3.0 + 372.0c$ ($r = 0.994$, $n = 4$) over the range of 0.01 to 0.1 μmol·L^{-1} at 1.0×10^{-7} mol·L^{-1} P1.

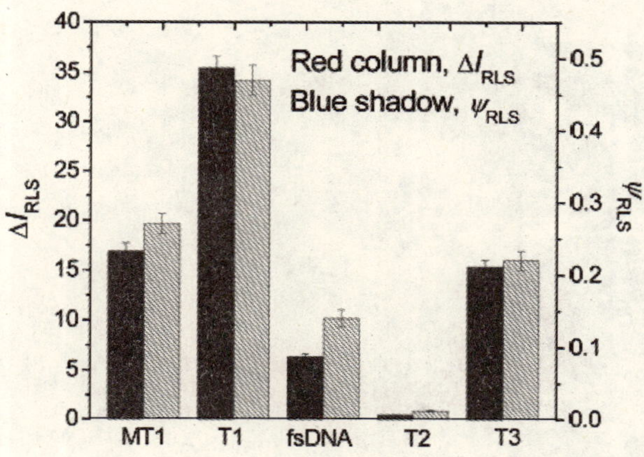

Fig. 2 RLS efficiency and sequence selectivity detection. From left to right, P1 and AY used for detection of MT1, T1, and fsDNA; P2 and AY are used for T2; and P3 and AY are used for T3. $c_{AY}=2.0 \times 10^{-5}$ mol·L^{-1}. All oligonucleotides are 1.0×10^{-7} mol·L^{-1}. pH 7.2.

By using the amplified RLS signals by AY, different $\triangle I_{RLS}$ signals at 494.4 nm could be detected when equivalent contents of T1, MT1, and fsDNA were incubated with P1, respectively. As shown in Figure 2 (and Figure S3 in the Supporting Information), the $\triangle I_{RLS}$ produced by T1 is approximately 5-fold and 2-fold stronger than that by fsDNA and MT1, which indicates that P1 has the ability to selectively bind with the complementary DNA sequences.

As for the interactions of other quinone-imine dyes, the results (Figure S4 in the Supporting Information) show that AA and AY display the same properties, which can clearly amplify the RLS signals of P1≈T1, but hardly amplify those of P1, while AO amplifies the RLS signals of neither $P1 \approx T1$ nor P1; and others amplify the RLS signals ofboth $P1 \approx T1$ and P1 without obvious differences. Since the extent of the amplified RLS signals of $P1 \approx T1$ by AY is the maximum among these eight OSMs, AY has been selected as an example for further discussions.

2.2.3.2 RLS Efficiency Definition and Detection

To show the efficiency of RLS, a term of RLS efficiency is introduced and defined in eq 1(seen in the Supporting Information)[30,31]

$$\varphi_{\mathrm{RLS}} = \frac{C_{\mathrm{sca}}}{C_{\mathrm{ext}}} = \frac{C_{\mathrm{sca}}}{C_{\mathrm{abs}} + C_{\mathrm{sca}}} = \frac{(2.63\times10^{20})C_{\mathrm{sca}}}{\epsilon} \qquad (1)$$

where C_{sca}, C_{ext}, and C_{abs} are the light scattering cross section, the extinction cross section, and the absorption cross section, respectively; ϵ is the molar extinction coefficient (M^{-1} cm^{-1}). By using polystyrene latex particles as a standard ($\varphi_{\mathrm{RLS}}^{\mathrm{PS}}(\lambda) = 1$), the RLS efficiency of a sample($\varphi_{\mathrm{RLS}}^{\mathrm{X}}(\lambda)$) could be calculated by eq 2 (seen in the Supporting Information)

$$\varphi_{\mathrm{RLS}}^{X}(\lambda) = \frac{A_{\mathrm{PS}}(\lambda)}{A_{\mathrm{X}}(\lambda)} \cdot \frac{I_{\mathrm{X}}(\lambda)}{I_{\mathrm{PS}}(\lambda)} \qquad (2)$$

where $A_{\mathrm{PS}}(\lambda)$ and $A_{\mathrm{X}}(\lambda)$ are the absorbance of polystyrene latex particles and sample, and $I_{\mathrm{PS}}(\lambda)$ and $I_{\mathrm{X}}(\lambda)$ are the RLS intensities of polystyrene latex particles and sample. According to eq. 2, we measured the RLS efficiency ($\varphi_{\mathrm{RLS}}^{\mathrm{X}}(\lambda)$) of the mixture of the hybridization complex and AY (Fig. 2). The results have showed that different hybridization complexes in the presence of AY have different RLS efficiencies, and the full complementary hybridization complex with G-C sequences in the presence of AY has the highest RLS efficiency. Thus, we could use the RLS efficiency to detect the interaction between different kinds of DNAs and OSMs.

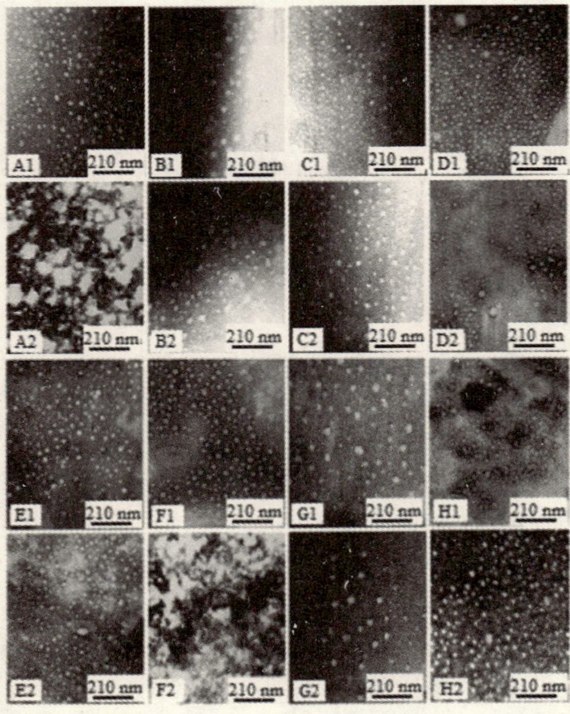

Fig. 3 TEM images of P1-OSMs and $P1 \approx T1$-OSMs (A1, A2: AY; B1, B2: NR; C1, C2: AO; D1, D2: BCB; E1, E2: NT; F1, F2: AA;G1, G2: AB; H1, H2: MB); c_{OSMs}= 2.0×10^{-5}mol·L^{-1}; c_{P1} and c_{T1} = 1.0×10^{-7}mol·L^{-1}. pH 7.2.

2.2.3.3 The Essential Need for Amplified RLS Signals

According to the RLS theory, the intensity of RLS signals observed from the vertical direction of the incident light for a spherical scattering particle with absorbance could be calculated as follows[27~29]

$$I = \frac{24A^2\pi^2 N v^2}{\lambda^4}\left(\frac{m^2-1}{m^2+2}\right)^2 \qquad (3)$$

where I is the incident light wavelength in the medium, A is the amplitude of the incident light, N is the number of the scattering particles per unit volume, V is the volume of one particle, and m is the relative refractive index of the particle versus its surrounding medium. When the conditions of the instrument and the solvent remain constant, the RLS intensity of the detection system may increase with the increased v, or N or both v and N for the other parameters are invariable. To understand the factors that result in the amplified RLS signals of P1≈T1 by AY or AA, we analyzed the TEM of the system.

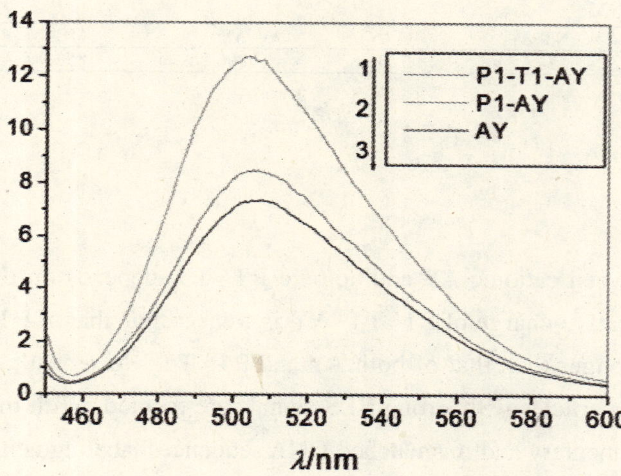

Fig. 4 The fluorescence spectra of the interactions: (1) P1≈T1-AY (blue); (2) P1≈AY (red); (3) AY (black). c_{AY} = 2.0 × 10^{-5}mol·L^{-1}. c_{P1} and c_{T1} = 1.0 × 10^{-7}mol·L^{-1}. pH 7.2.

AA is 98 nm, larger than the 19 nm of P1-AA, indicating that the interactions of AY or AA with P1≈T1are different from those of P1. In addition, A2 in Figure 3 displays that there are small assemblies similar to P1-AY around P1≈T1-AY, indicating that equilibrium exists among T1-AY, P1-AY, and P1≈T1-AY. Similar equilibrium also exists among T1-AA, P1-AA, and P1≈T1-AA (F2 in Fig. 3). It is for these equilibria that we chose ten big particles for roughly evaluating the sizes of P1≈T1-AY and P1≈T1-AA aggregations. By comparing these RLS measurement results of the interactions of eight OSMs with P1 and P1 ≈T1, we can infer that the main essential of amplified P1 ≈T 1 RLS signals by AY or AA is the formation of the large particles, which is consistent with eq 3.

To learn the nature of the amplified RLS signals of P1≈T1 by AY further, we also studied the fluorescence properties. The fluorescence emission of AY at 504 nm when excited at 445 nm (Fig. 4) could be strongly enhanced by P1≈T1, but slightly enhanced by P1 or T1. Thus, the interactions between AY and P1≈T1 mainly involve in intercalative, or groove, or both, which could also be identified by the enhanced fluorescence polarization with the increased concentration of P1≈T1 (Table S2 in the Supporting Information).[32,33] Considering the fact that the$\triangle I_{RLS}$) is relative to the dsDNA and it is very difficult to observe the enhanced RLS signals for the intercalative interaction,[34,35] we could infer that the interactions between cationic AY and anionic T1≈P1 might involve the groove binding, which is the only interaction mode between OSMs and dsDNA except for the intercalative. The groove binding compound ($P1 \approx T1$-AY) has a weaker negative charge than $P1 \approx T1$, and has a stronger hydrophobic property than that of both AY and $P1 \approx T1$, which induces the assembly of $P1 \approx T1$-AY (Fig. 3 B) and leads to the formation of large particles with strong RLS signals.[36]

To understand the groove binding nature further, we measured RLS spectra of the mixtures of AY and different DNAs including P2, T2, $P2 \approx T2$, P3, T3, and $P3 \approx T3$. Results have showed that the RLS signals of $P3 \approx T3$ amplified by AY are easily observed (Fig. 2), while those of P2, T2, $P2 \approx T2$, P3, and T3 are hardly observed, indicating that AY prefers to bind with G-C sequences in the groove of dsDNA, which has a similar property to Thioflavin T.[37]

To learn why only AY and AA show the amplified RLS signals of $P1 \approx T1$, we have calculated the molecular volumes of eight OSMs with the calculation software of HyperChem 7 Professional, showing that AY has the volume 742.64 Å[3], very close to 753.28 Å[3] of AA (Table 1), which be fit for the groove space of $P1 \approx T1$. Certainly, other properties of OSMs may also influence the amplified RLS signals of $P1 \approx T1$.

Table 1 The Calculated Volume (Å[3]) of Typical OSMs[a]

AY	NR	AO	BCB	NT	AA	AB	MB
742.64	785.66	844.45	861.50	654.65	753.28	806.84	852.90

[a]The calculation was made through software of HyperChem 7 Professional.

2.2.4 Conclusion

In summary, the groove binding property between cationic AY and anionic $P1 \approx T1$ depends on the G-C sequences of DNA and the volume of AY. The negative charge of $P1 \approx T1$-AY is weaker than that of $P1 \approx T1$, and the hydrophobic property of $P1 \approx T1$-AY is stronger than that of both AY and $P1 \approx T1$. As a result, the assemblies of AY-$P1 \approx T1$ are induced, and the large particles with strong RLS signals are formed. With the RLS measurements, it is very easy to detect the complementary and mismatched DNA sequences labeling neither the target nor the probe DNA.

Acknowledgments.

This work has received support from the Ministry of Science and Technology of the People's Republic of China (No. 2006CB933100) and the National Natural Science Foundation of China (NSFC, No. 20425517).

Supporting Information Available

Molecular structure of quinone-imine dyes, optimal condition of the interaction of P1 and T1, absorption spectra of AY, spectra of sequence selectivity detertion, RLS spectra of the interaction of P1 and $P1 \approx T1$ with quinone-imine dyes, RLS efficiency definition, and fluorescence polarization and anisotropy values. This material is available free of charge via the Internet at http://pubs.acs.org.

References

[1] Wood, K.; Little, C. S.; Little, R. R.; Hammond, P. T. Angew. Chem., Int. Ed. 2005, 44, 6704.

[2] Behr, J. P. Acc. Chem. Res. 1993, 26, 274.

[3] Sterrenburg, E.; Turk, R.; Boer, J. M.; van Ommen, G. B.; den Dunnen, J. T. Nucleic Acids Res. 2002, 21, e116.

[4] Wang, L.; Yang, C. J.; Medley, C. D.; Benner, S. A.; Tan, W. H. J. Am. Chem. Soc. 2005, 127, 15664.

[5] Hutter, E.; Pileni, M. P. J. Phys. Chem. B 2003, 107, 6497.

[6] Elghanian, R.; Storhoff, J. J.; Mucic, R. C.; letsinger, R. L.; Mirkin, C. A. Science 1997, 277, 1078.

[7] Lin, V. S. Y.; Moteshareі, K.; Dancil, K. P. S.; Sailor, M. J.; Ghadiri, M. R. Science 1997, 278, 840.

[8] Pan, S.; Rothberg, L. J. Nano Lett. 2003, 3, 811.

[9] Miao, W. J.; Bard, A. J. Anal. Chem. 2004, 76, 5379.

[10] Kuhnast, B.; Dolle, F.; Terrazzino, S.; Rousseau, B.; Loch, C.; Vaufrey, F.; Hinnen, F.; Doignon, I.; Pillon, F.; David, C.; Crouzel, C.; Tavitian, B. Bioconj. Chem. 2000, 11, 627.

[11] Yu, F.; Yao, D.; Knoll, W. Nucleic Acids Res. 2004, 32, e75.

[12] Peterson, A. W.; Wolf, L. K.; Georgiadis, R. M. J. Am. Chem. Soc. 2002, 124, 14601.

[13] Watts, H. J.; Yeung, D.; Parkes, H. Anal. Chem. 1995, 67, 4283.

[14] Li, H. X.; Rothberg, L. J. Proc. Natl. Acad. Sci. U.S.A. 2004, 101, 14036.

[15] Wang, J. Anal. Chim. Acta 2002, 469, 63.

[16] Hook, F.; Ray, A.; Norden, B.; Kasemo, B. Langmuir 2001, 17, 8305.

[17] Fritz, J.; Baller, M. K.; Lang, H. P.; Rothuizen, H.; Vettiger, P.; Meyer, E.; Guntherod, H. J.; Gerber, C.; Gimzewski, J. K. Science 2000, 288, 316.

[18] Pasternack, R. F.; Bustamante, C.; Collings, P. J.; Giannetteo, A.; Gibbs, E. J. J. Am. Chem. Soc. 1993, 115, 5393.

[19] Huang, C. Z.; Li, K. A.; Tong, S. Y. Anal. Chem. 1996, 68, 2259.

[20] Huang, C. Z.; Li, K. A.; Tong, S. Y. Anal. Chem. 1997, 69, 514.

[21] Aslan, K.; Lakowicz, J. R.; Geddes, C. D. Anal. Chem. 2005, 77, 2007

[22] Feng, P.; Shu, W. Q.; Huang, C. Z.; Li, Y. F. Anal. Chem. 2001, 73, 4307.

[23] Huang, C. Z.; Liu, Y.; Wang, Y. H. Anal. Biochem. 2003, 376, 38.

[24] Tang, K. J.; Li, Y. F.; Huang, C. Z. Luminescence 2005, 20, 176.

[25] Bao, P.; Frutos, A. G.; Greef, C.; Lahiri, J.; Muller, U.; Peterson, T. C.; Wardern, L.; Xie, X. Anal. Chem. 2002, 74, 1792.

[26] Karlsson, H. J.; Eriksson, M.; Perzon, E.; Akerman, B.; Lincoln, P.; Westman, G. Nucleic Acids Res. 2003, 31, 6227.

[27] Fu, X. C.; Shen, W. X.; Yao, T. T. Physical Chemistry; High Education Press: Beijing, China 1993; p 1008.

[28] Akins, D. L.; Zhu, H. R.; Guo, C. J. Phys. Chem. 1994, 98, 3612.

[29] Miller, G. A. J. Phys. Chem. 1978, 82, 616.

[30] Yguerabide, J.; Yguerabide, E. E. Anal. Biochem. 1998, 262, 137.

[31] Yguerabide, J.; Yguerabide, E. E. Anal. Biochem. 1998, 262, 157.

[32] Yoshio, Q.; Kuniharu, I.; Yukihiro, M. Langmuir 1993, 9, 19.

[33] Li, W. Y.; Xu, J. G.; Guo, X. Q.; Zhu, Q. Z.; Zhao, Y. B. Spectrochim. Acta, Part A 1997, 53, 781.

[34] Pasternack, R. F.; Collings, P. J. Science 1995, 269, 935.

[35] Huang, C. Z.; Li, Y. F.; Liu, X. D. Anal. Chim. Acta 1998, 375, 89.

[36] Berlepsch, H. V.; Böttcher, C.; Ouart, A.; Burger, C.; Dähne, S.; Kirstein, S. J. Phys. Chem. B 2000, 104, 5255.

[37] Ilanchelian, M.; Ramaraj, R. J. Photochem. Photobiol. A 2004, 162, 129.

(Yun Fei Long, Cheng Zhi Huang, and Yuan Fang Li, published in *Journal of Physical Chemistry B*, 2007, 111, 4535~4538)

2.3 Determination of Nanograms of Nucleic Acids by Their Enhancement Effect on the Resonance Light Scattering of the Cobalt(II)/4-[(5-chloro -2-pyridyl) azo]-1,3-diaminobenzene Complex

Using a common spectrofluorometer to measure the intensity of resonance light-scattering, a method for determination of nucleic acids in the nanogram range has been developed. In the pH range 11.5～12.0, the resonance light-scattering of the binary comlpex of cobalt(II)/ 4-[(5-chloro-2-pyridyl) azo]-1, 3-diaminobenzene(5-Cl-PADAB) is greatly enhanced by nucleic acids, with the maximum scattering peak located at 547.0 nm. The enhanced intensity of resonance light-scattering is in proportion to the concentration ofcalfthymus DNA in the range 0～400 $ng{\cdot}mL^{-1}$ and to that of fish sperm DNA and yeast RNA in the range 0～300 $ng{\cdot}mL^{-1}$. The limits of detection are 1.4 $ng{\cdot}mL^{-1}$ for calf thymus DNA, 0.8 $ng{\cdot}mL^{-1}$ for fish sperm DNA, and 1.3 $ng{\cdot}mL^{-1}$ for yeast RNA. Precision at 200 $ng{\cdot}mL^{-1}$ for the three nucleic acids is 1.9 %, 2.0 %, and 0.8 %, respectively. Six synthetic samples were determined satisfactorily. Mechanism studies showed that the nature of the reaction is that the binary complex of Co(II)/5-Cl-PADAB reacts with single-stranded nucleic acid, and the enhancement effect of nucleic acids on the resonance light scattering ofthe binary complex is due to the stacking ofthe binary complex on nucleic acids, which act as a template.

The quantitative analysis of nucleic acids is very important because it can be used as a reference for measurements of other components in biological fluids and genetic diagnosis. The most sensitive quantitation of nucleic acids at present is generally according to their fluorescence enhancement effect on organic dyes such as ethidium bromide (EB) and its homo- or heterodimer,[1,2] diaminophenylindole (DAPI),[3] and bisimidazole (Hoechst 33258).[4] By using laser facilities and the fluorescence enhancement effect of nucleic acids on the organic dyes with double functional groups, single DNA molecules and the growth of DNA in PCR can be detected.[5,6]

Scattering light is highly applicable to the polymer sciences, and particularly dynamic Rayleigh scattering is an important tool for the study oftranslational and rotational motions ofmolecules in solutions.[7] The technique, however, suffers the disadvantages of low signal levels and lack of sensitivity unless laser facilities are employed. Recently, Pasternack et al.[8～11] developed a technique to detect the intensity ofscattering light by using a common spectrofluorometer. We think the technique is useful in analytical chemistry because of the simplicity and sensitivty. With this technique, we have established a sensitive method for studying trace amounts of-biological substances.[12] In this paper, we present a new method for determination of nucleic acids with high sensitivity and discuss the reaction mechanism according to the resonance light-scattering data. The basis for the method is the enhancement effect ofnucleic acids on the scattering light ofthe binary complex of Co(II)/4-[(5-chloro -2-pyridyl)azo]-1,3- diaminobenzene (5-Cl-PADAB).

The intensity of Rayleigh light scattering by transparent isotropic media is in proportion to λ^{-4}, where is the wavelength of incident light in free space. The intensity deviates from the dependence of λ^{-4}, and it is possible that the intensity become quite large when the incident wavelength is near the absorption band of the analyte molecules. This phenomenon is known as resonance-enhanced Rayleigh scattering and is predicted by the same theory that predicts resonance-enhanced Raman scattering.[13] According to macroscopic fluctuation theory and Mie theory, Miller[14] had made theoretical studies. Further theoretical and practical studies had been made by Anglister and Steinberg,[15] Stanton and Pecora,[13] and Pasternack et al.[8~11] In general, the intensity oflight scattering depends on the volume ofthe species, the wavelength of incident light, and the real and imaginary parts of the scatterer's polarizability. So strong light-scattering bands are expected for large aggregates at the wavelength where the molar absorptivity of the aggregate is large, but very weak or no light-scattering signals can be detected for those species whose volume are small, even ifthe incident wavelength is close to their strong absorption bands. With resonance light-scattering spectroscopy, the self-aggregation of chlorophyll α and sulfotophenylporphyrins[10] and the interaction ofthe metallointercalator cationic complex (2,2':6',2"-terpyridine)methylplatinum(II) with DNA[11] have been studied.

5-Cl-PADAB is a commercial organic reagent and has extensive applications in the sensitive determination of metal ions.[16] As we previously reported,[17] the interaction of the binary complex of Co(III)/ 5 -PADAB with nucleic acids occurs in such a way that each nucleotide residue can bind two molecules of the binary complex. That mimics the stacking of the binary complex on nucleic acids, which act as a template.[18] Since the stacking species have high absorptivity (for example, ε(ctDNA/Co(III)/ 5-Cl-PADAB) = $5.1 \times 10^{-4} M^{-1} \cdot cm^{-1}$ [19]) and possibly large volume, it is expected that the resonance light scattering of the binary complex can be enhanced by nucleic acids.

2.3.1 Experimental Section

2.3.1.1 Apparatus

The resonance light-scattering spectrum and the intensity of resonance light scattering were measured with a Shimadzu RF-540 spectrofluorometer (Kyoto, Japan). A WH-861 vortex mixer (Huangjin Instrumental Co., Jiangsu, China) was used to blend the solution.

2.3.1.2 Reagents

Stock solutions of nucleic acids were prepared by directly dissolving commercial calfthymus DNA(Beitai Biochemical Co., Chinese Academy of Sciences, Beijing, China), fish sperm DNA, and yeast RNA (Shanghai Institute of Biochemistry, Chinese Academy of Sciences, Shanghai, China) in doubly deionized water at 0-4℃. Twenty -four hours or more was needed for complete dissolution of DNAs, even if occasional gentle shaking was done. The concentrations of DNAs were calculated according to the absorbance at 260.0 nm. All the working concentrations of nucleic acids were 2.5 $\mu g \cdot mL^{-1}$.

The stock solution of Co(II) was prepared by dissolving cobalt metal (99.99%) in nitric acid, and the working solution of Co(II) was obtained by diluting the stock solution to $1.0 \times 10^{-4} mol \cdot L^{-1}$ with water. The stock solution of 5-Cl-PADAB was prepared by dissolving 61.92 mg of the crystallized 5-Cl-PADAB (Merck, Germany) in thermal dehydrated alcohol, and after the solution had been cooled, dehydrated alcohol was added to 500 mL. The working solution of 5-Cl-PADAB was made 1.0×10^{-4} $mol \cdot L^{-1}$ (containing 40%(v/v) ethanol) by diluting the stock solution with water. In addition, 0.01 and 0.30 $mol \cdot L^{-1}$ NaOH solutions were used.

All reagents were of analytical grade without further purification. Water used throughout was doubly deionized.

2.3.1.3 Preparation of Synthetic Samples

According to the tolerances offoreign substances, interfering components were added in an appropriate volume ofstandard solution to make up synthetic samples. To test the practicability of the method, six samples were constructed.

2.3.1.4 Standard Procedure

In a dry 10 mL volumetric flask were added 0.50 mL of Co(II) solution, 0.50 mL of 5-Cl-PADAB solution, 0.25 mL of dehydrated alcohol, and 1.0 mL of 0.3 $mol \cdot L^{-1}$ NaOH. The mixture was vortexed, and then nucleic acid standard solution or sample solution was added, and the mixture was vortexed again. Before the addition of nucleic acids, it was necessary to add an appropriate volume of water to keep the total initial volume of the mixture at 3.40 mL. Fifteen minutes later, the mixture was diluted to 10 mL with doubly deionized water and mixed thoroughly. The resonance light-scattering spectrum and the intensity of scattering were measured against the binary complex as a reference during the period of 20~100 min after the last mix.

The resonance light-scattering spectrum was obtained by scanning simultaneously the excitation and emission monochromators ofthe RF -540 spectrofluorometer from 400 to 700 nm (namely, $\Delta\lambda = 0$ nm). The intensity of light scattering was measured at the wavelength where the maximum scattering peak is located. Both the intensity measurement and the spectrum scanning ofthe resonance light scattering were made by keeping the slit-width of the excitation and the emission of the spectrofluorometer at 5.0 nm.

2.3.2 Results and Discussion

2.3.2.1 Spectral Characteristics

Fig. 1 displays the resonance light-scattering spectrum of the binary complex of Co(II)/ 5-Cl-PADAB and its enhanced resonance light-scattering spectra by nucleic acids. In the wavelength range 400~650 nm, the resonance light scattering of the binary complex is rather weak; even so, the resonance light scattering in the 540~600 nm wavelength range is stronger than that in the 480~510 nm range because of the molecular absorption of the binary complex (see below). In the wavelength range 400~700 nm, the resonance light scattering of the binary complex is enhanced by nucleic acids, with the maximum scattering peak located at 547.0 nm. Shoulder peaks in the range 480~510 nm can be observed. In addition, the enhanced extent ofthe light scattering differs for different nucleic acids. Fig. 1 shows the enhanced order for different nucleic acids as follows: fish sperm DNA > yeast RNA > calf thymus DNA (on the basis of $ng \cdot mL^{-1}$). As a matter offact, the comparison for the enhanced order should be based on the molecular mass or the length of nucleic acids. By using ε_{DNA}=6600 $M^{-1} \cdot cm^{-1}$ and ε_{RNA}=7800 $M^{-1} \cdot cm^{-1}$,[20] we find that the enhanced order yeast RNA > fish sperm DNA > calfthymus DNA (on the basis of $mol \cdot L^{-1}$) is followed.

The features of those spectra can be elucidated by the theory of resonance depolarized Rayleigh scattering. When the incident light passes through a transparent isotropic medium, the intensity of light scattering is proportional to λ^{-4}, but if λ is near an absorption band of the molecules and if there are aggregates in the system, the scattering cross section of the system, $C_{sca,}$ the ratio of the rate of energy scattering out of the incident beam (in all directions) to the intensity of the incident beam, can be expressed as[8,9,13~15]

$$c_{sca} = (k_m{}^4)|\alpha|^2/(6\pi) = (k_m{}^4)(\alpha_r{}^2 + \alpha_i{}^2)/(6\pi) \quad (1)$$

where k_m is the wave vector of light in the solvent, $k_m=2\pi/\lambda_m$, and α_r and α_i are the real and imaginary parts of the polarizability of the aggregates. The absorption cross section of the system, c_{abs}, the ratio of the rate of energy absorption from the incident beam to the intensity of the incident beam, depends on α_i only,

$$c_{abs} = k_m\alpha_i \quad (2)$$

and the absorbance A of a sample of thickness L is

$$A = 2.3^{-1}(N/V)c_{\text{abs}}L \qquad (3)$$

where N/V is the number of aggregates per unit volume. From the C_{abs} equation, the absorption depends on the first power of the polarizability, which in turn depends linearly on the volume of the aggregate. Thus, a solution with a fixed concentration of the aggregating component will exhibit no change in A as aggregation occurs, because the product of N/V and α_i stays constant. However, the intensity of scattering depends on the square of the volume of the aggregate, and thus it increases as a result of aggregation; resonance light scattering is, therefore, extremely sensitive to even low concentrations of extended aggregates.

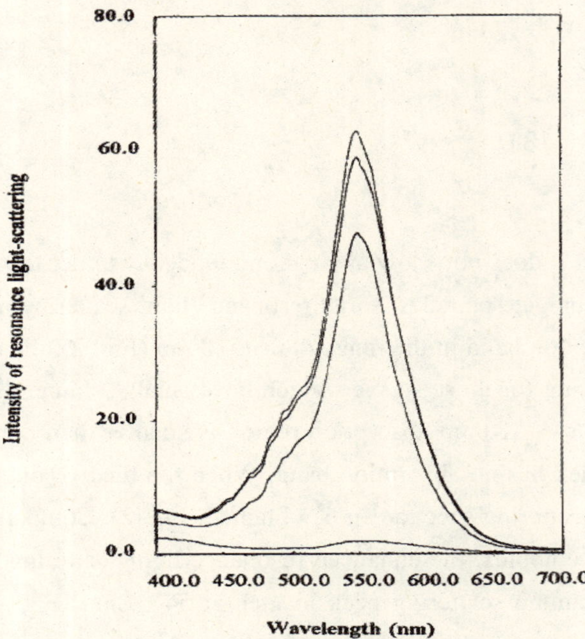

Fig. 1 Resonance light-scattering spectra. From top to bottom, ternary systems of fish sperm DNA, yeast RNA, calf thymus DNA, and the binary complex of Co(II)/5-Cl-PADAB. Concentrations: calf thymus DNA, 200.0 ng·mL^{-1}; $c_{\text{Co(II)}}$ = $0.5c_{\text{5-Cl-PADAB}}$ = 5.0 ×10^{-6} mol·L^{-1}; ethanol, 12.9% (v/v) in period 1.

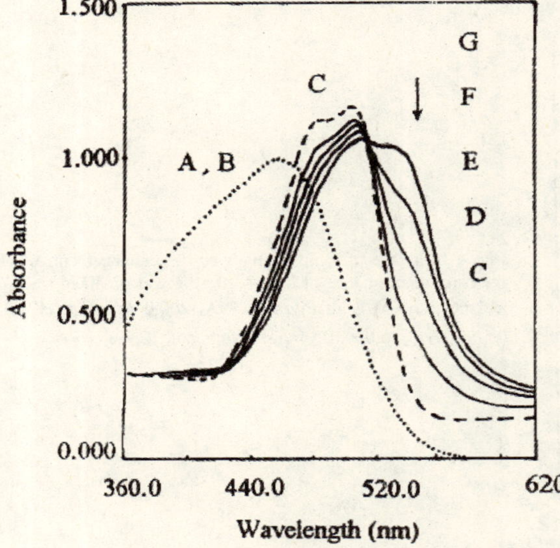

Fig. 2 Absorption spectra of 5-Cl-PADAB(A), DNA + 5-Cl-PADAB(B), Co(II) + 5-Cl-PADAB(C), and Co(II) + 5-Cl-PADAB + DNA(D-G). Concentrations: $c_{\text{Co(II)}} = 0.5c_{\text{5-Cl-PADAB}}$ = 2.0× 10^{-5} mol·L^{-1}; calf thymus DNA, D 1.0, E 2.0, F 3.0, G 4.0 g·mL^{-1}; ethanol, 20.7% (v/v) in period 1.

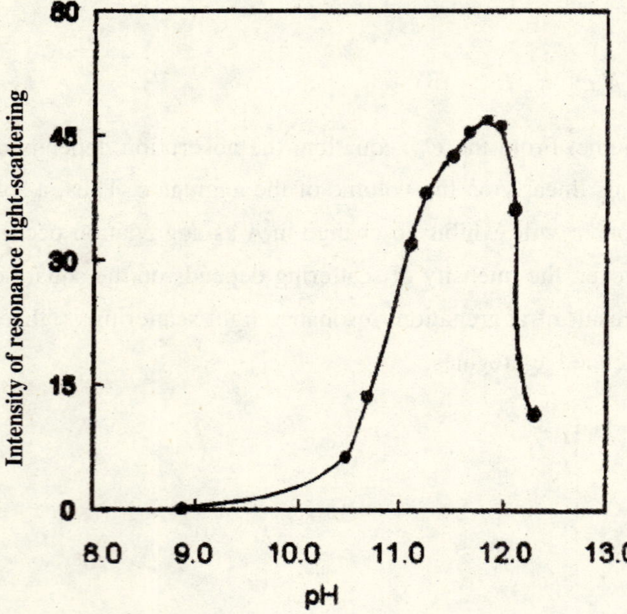

Fig. 3 Dependence of the enhancement of RLS on pH. Concentrations: calf thymus DNA, 200 ng·mL^{-1}; $c_{Co(II)}$ $=0.5c_{5\text{-Cl-PADAB}} = 5.0\times10^{-6}$ mol·L^{-1}; ethanol, 12.9% (v/v).

The binary complex has high absorptivity,[16] but it does not show aggregating tendency under the experimental case and has small volume compared with aggregate particles, so its resonance light scattering is rather weak. Even so, since the binary complex has an absorption band in the range 480～510 nm (Fig. 2), the absorption band usually reducing the resonance light scattering for those species which have small volume, the resonance light scattering of the binary complex in the 480～510 nm absorption region is smaller than that in the range 540～600 nm (Fig. 1), where the binary complex has no absorption band. When the binary complex interacts with nucleic acids, enhanced resonance light-scattering spectra can be obtained (Fig. 2). Compared with the resonance light-scattering spectrum of the binary complex, the enhanced resonance light-scattering spectra have strong resonance light scattering, with the maximum scattering peak located at 547.0 nm (Fig. 1). The maximum scattering peak is almost the same as the maximum absorption wavelength of the ternary system near 545.0 nm (Fig. 2).

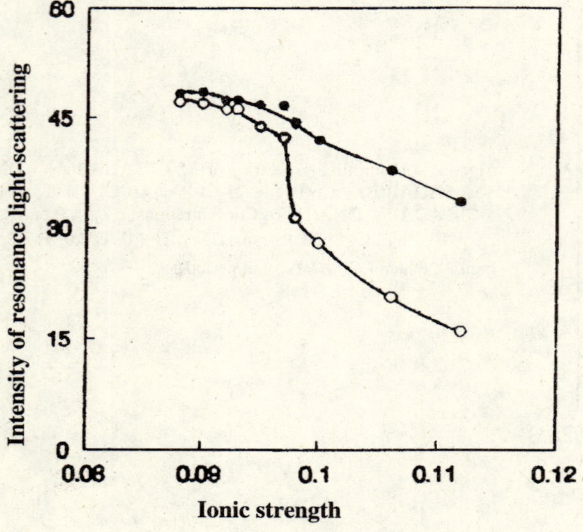

Fig. 4 Influence of ionic strength on the enhancement of RLS. Intensity of resonance of light-scattering was obtained at 20 (O) and 60 min (●). Calf thymus DNA, 200.0 ng·mL^{-1}; cCo(II) = $0.5c_{5\text{-Cl-PADAB}} = 5.0\times10^{-6}$ mol·L^{-1}; ethanol, 12.9% (v/v).

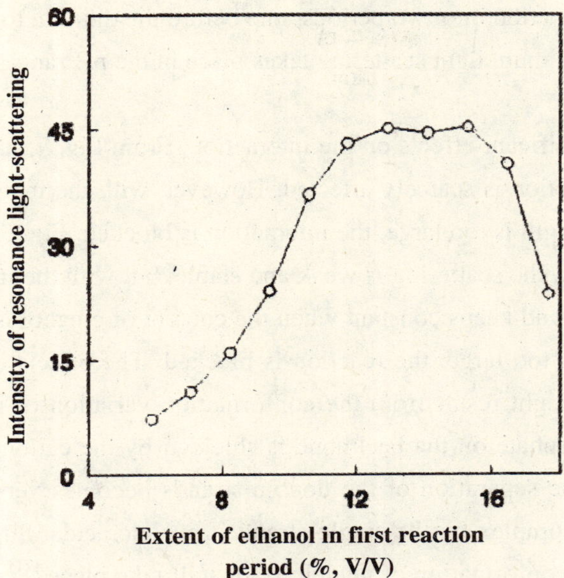

Fig. 5 Effect of the content of ethanol. Concentrations: calf thymus DNA, 200.0 ng·mL^{-1}; $c_{Co(II)} = 0.5c_{5\text{-Cl-PADAB}} = 5.0 \times 10^{-6}$ mol·L^{-1}.

As we previously reported,[17] the interaction mechanism of the binary complex with nucleic acids mimics the stacking of the binary complex on the nucleic acids, which act as a template, so the enhanced resonance light scattering, with its maximum scattering peak located at 547.0 nm, results from the enhancement effect of Rayleigh lightscattering of the binary complex by nucleic acids. The shoulder peaks, observed in the range 480～510 nm, which may disclose the absorption of the binary complex in the ternary system, support the stacking mechanism ofthe binary complex on nucleic acids.

2.3.2.2 Optimization of the General Procedure.

By using 200.0 ng·mL^{-1} calf thymus DNA, 5.0×10^{-6} mol·L^{-1}Co(II), and 1.0×10^{-5} mol·L^{-1} 5-Cl-PADAB (the choice of the concentration of Co(II) and 5-Cl-PADAB will be explained later), the optimal conditions were tested.

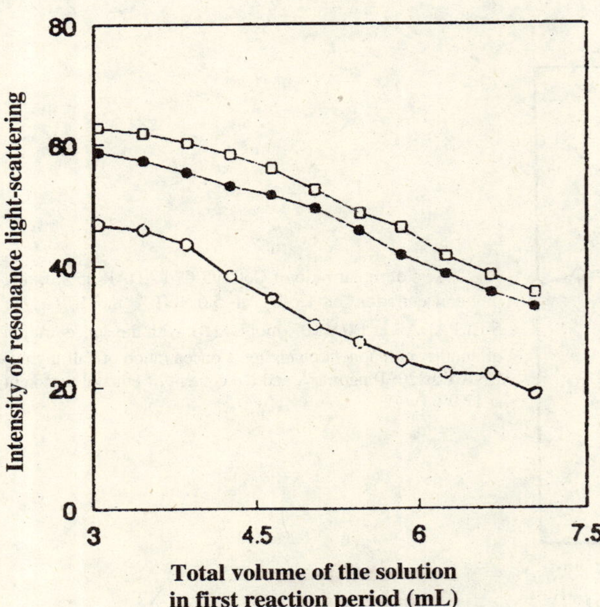

Fig. 6 Choice of the volume of the mixture in period 1. The total volume of ethanol coming from 5-Cl-PADAB and extra addition is 0.45 mL, and the content of ethanol can be calculated from the total volume of ethanol (0.45 mL) and the total volume of the mixture in the period 1. Concentration of nucleic acids, 200.0 ng·mL^{-1}; $c_{Co(II)} = 0.5c_{5\text{-Cl-PADAB}}) = 5.0 \times 10^{-6}$ mol·L^{-1}. From top to bottom, fish sperm DNA, yeast RNA, and calf thymus DNA.

To understand the reaction better, we divided the reaction into two periods, one before the dilution to 10 mL and the other after the dilution. Fig. 3 shows that the maximum light scattering takes place in the pH range 11.5～12.0 in period 1.

Ionic strength and the content of ethanol have significant effects on the interaction. From Fig. 4, it can be seen that, when ionic strength is low ($I<0.1$), the reaction is scarcely affected. However, with the increase of ionic strength, the reaction slows down. If the ionic strength is too large, the interaction is blocked. Fig. 5 shows the effect of ethanol. When the content of ethanol is low, the scattering is weak and stable, but with the increase of the content of ethanol, the scattering becomes strong and keeps constant when the content of ethanol is in the range 11.8%～15.3% (v/v). If the content of ethanol is too large, the reaction is blocked. The effects of both ionic strength and ethanol content on the interaction might result from the conformation variation of nucleic acids. With increasing ionic strength, the anion of phosphate on the backbone is shielded by the cation ion of the ionic strength controller (Na^+, for instance), and the separation of the double strands becomes very difficult,[21] i.e., unfavorable to the stacking of the binary complex on the single-stranded nucleic acids. Similarly, with increasing the content of ethanol, variation of the conformation of nucleic acids will take place,[21] so it is difficult for the binary complex to stack on the single-stranded nucleic acids.

Fig. 6 depicts the influence of the volume of the mixture in the first reaction period. It shows that, the larger the volume of the solution mixture in period 1, the smaller the intensity of resonance light scattering is. So, the division of the reaction into two periods is of benefit to the sensitivity. According to Fig. 6, we can calculate the optimal content of ethanol ranging from 14.8% to 11.7% (v/v), which parallels the finding of Fig. 5. In addition, we found that the reaction time of period 1 plays a very important role, and the suitable reaction time of period 1 is 12～20 min. Since alkaline denaturation of nucleic acids should take place at pH>11.3,[21] it is possible that, in period 1, the interaction of the binary complex with nucleic acids involves the separation of the double strands of nucleic acids. The use of thermally and alkalinously denatured nucleic to speed up the interaction[17] supports the interaction process. As for period 2, the intensity of scattering can reach its maximum in 20 min after the last dilution, and there would be a slight increase, but it is admittable with the allowed intensity error of 5% if the determination is finished in 100 min.

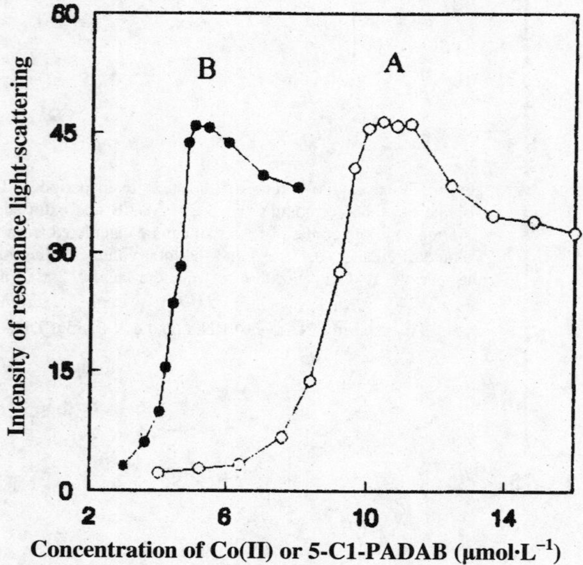

Fig. 7 Test of molar ratio of Co(II)/5-Cl-PADAB upon fixing the concentration of Co(II) at 5.0×10^{-6} mol·L^{-1}(A) or 5-Cl-PADAB at 1.0×10^{-5} mol·L^{-1}(B), with the concentration of another component changing. Concentration of calf thymus DNA was 200.0 ng·mL^{-1}, and the content of ethanol was kept at 12.9% (v/v).

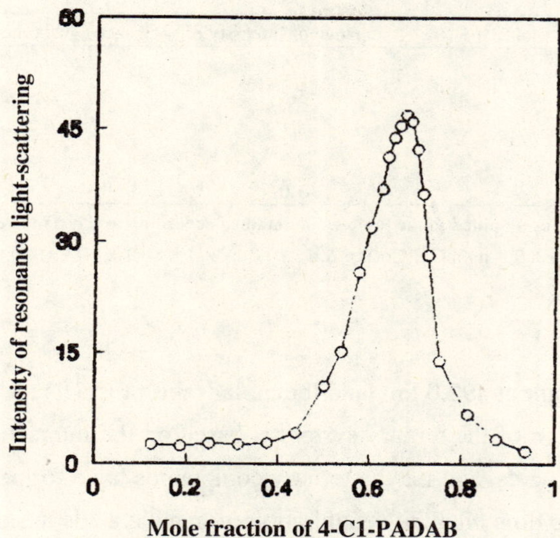

Fig. 8 Test of molar ratio of Co(II)/5-Cl-PADAB upon keeping the total concentration of Co(II) and 5-Cl-PADAB at 1.6×10^{-5} mol·L^{-1} with the concentrations of the two components changing simultaneously. Concentrations of DNA and content of ethanol are the same as in Fig.5.

2.3.2.3 Molar Ratio of Co(II)/5-Cl-PADAB in the Ternary System

By spectrophotometry,[17] we have obtained that the molar ratio of Co(II) to 5-Cl-PADAB of the ternary system is 1:2, which is in agreement with the molar ratio of Co(II) to 5-Cl-PADAB of the binary complex.[16] The identical result can be obtained with the resonance light-scattering method also.

Under the experimental conditions, by keeping the concentration of nucleic acids constant, the molar ratio of Co(II) to 5-Cl-PADAB of the ternary system can be measured by two methods. One method is that the concentration of one of the two components (Co(II) and 5-Cl-PADAB) is kept constant and that of the other component is changed. Fig. 7 shows that, whether the concentration of Co(II) or 5-Cl-PADAB changes with the other component being kept constant, the molar ratio of Co(II) to 5-Cl-PADAB is 1:2. The other method is to hold the total concentration of Co(II) and 5-Cl-PADAB at 1.6×10^{-5} mol·L^{-1} while the concentrations of the two components are changed simultaneously. Figure 8 shows that, when the molar fraction of 5-Cl-PADAB is 0.675, namely the molar ratio of Co(II) to 5-Cl-PADAB is 1:2, the intensity of light-scattering reaches maximum.

Table 1 Interferences of Foreign Coexisting Substances

substance	concentration coexisting ($\times 10^{-6}$ mol·L^{-1})	change of intensity of resonance light scattering (%)
protein, BSA	240.0*	6.4
protein, HSA	240.0*	9.0
protein, γ-IgG	240.0*	7.4
base, A	18.0	-7.7
base, G	0.36	-3.4
base, C	18.0	-8.7
base, T	5.0	-2.4
base, U	15.0	-2.4
$PO4^{3-}$Na(I)	18.0	-7.4
Al(III), SO_4^{2-}	1.0	-9.8
Ca(II), Cl^-	3.6	-10.0
Cd(II), SO_4^{2-}	0.6	-5.6
Cr(III), Cl^-	1.8	-0.1
Cu(II), Cl^-	1.8	-7.7
Hg(II), NO_3^-	0.04	-0.2

Continued

substance	concentration coexisting ($\times 10^{-6}$ mol·L^{-1})	change of intensity of resonance light scattering (%)
Mg(II), Cl^-	1.0	-9.5
Mn(II), NO_3^-	0.5	-6.8
Ni(II), NO_3^-	0.5	-8.1
Pb(II), NO_3^-	1.8	-2.3
Zn(II), Cl^-	3.6	-5.0

[a]Concentrations of proteins are represented as ng·mL^{-1}. All the values obtained in the table were obtained according to the standard procedure, and the concentrations of reagents are as follows: calf thymus DNA, 200.0 ng·mL^{-1}; Co(II), 5.0×10^{-6} mol·L^{-1}; 5-Cl-PADAB, 10.0×10^{-6} mol·L^{-1}; ethanol (first reaction period), 12.9%(v/ v).

2.3.2.3 Nature of the Reaction

According to Fig. 2, which has an isobestic point at 492.0 nm, and the molar ratio of Co(II) to 5-Cl-PADAB of the ternary system, it is apparent that the formation of the ternary system is based on the interaction of the binary complex of Co(II)/ 5-Cl-PADAB with nucleic acids, and maybe ternary compounds have formed. As the reaction takes place in the pH range 11.5~12.0, at the time alkaline denaturation of nucleic acids has occurred, and both the alkaline and thermal denaturation of DNA speeds up the reaction,[17] the nature of the interaction is based on the binary complex and the single-stranded nucleic acids. In addition, by spectrophotometry we found that each nucleotide residue can bind two binary complex molecules,[17] so the enhancement effect of nucleic acids on the resonance light-scattering of the binary complex is due to the stacking of binary complex on nucleic acids, which act as a template. Therefore, when the ionic strength is large, the double strands of nucleic acids are difficult to separate because of the shielding effect of Na^+, and the reaction is blocked.

2.3.2.4 Interferences of Coexisting Foreign Substances

The influences offoreign coexisting substances such as proteins,bases, and metal ions were tested. The results are presented in Table 1. Of the tested metal ions, Ca(II), Cr(III), Cu(II), Mg(II), Pb(III), and Zn(II) ions can be allowed with relatively higher concentration (the allowed maximum concentration can reach 1.8×10^{-6} mol·L^{-1}), but Hg(II) ion can be allowed with very low concentration ($<4.0\times10^{-8}$mol·L^{-1}). However, the allowed concentration of those interference ions is still larger than that in biological fluids.

2.3.2.5 Characteristics of the Resonances Light-Scattering Method

As stated above, resonance light-scattering spectra were obtained by scanning simultaneously the excitation and emission monochromators. So, resonance light-scattering spectra are synchronous ones. In addition, scattering light stems from the aggregate when it is excited by a light beam with the emission in all directions, and the emission wavelength is equal to the scattering light wavelength, which means the aggregate is a new luminophor that remits light with the same wavelength as the incident light. Thus, the resonance light scattering belongs to synchronous luminescence, with its particularities of $\Delta\lambda=0$ nm and no electronic excitation after light absorption. According to the equation of synchronous luminescence,[22]

$$I_s = kcdE_{ex}(\lambda_{ex})E_{em}(\lambda_{ex}+\Delta\lambda) \qquad (4)$$

where E_{ex} is the excitation function at the given excitation wavelength $\lambda_{ex}=\lambda_{em}-\Delta\lambda$, E_{em} is the normal emission function at the corresponding emission wavelength $\lambda_{em}=\lambda_{ex}+\Delta\lambda$, c is the analyte concentration, d is the thickness of the sample cell, and K is the characteristic constant comprising the "instrumental geometry factor" and related parameters. When $\Delta\lambda=0$, we can get

$$I_s = kcdE_{ex}(\lambda_{ex})E_{em}(\lambda_{ex}) \qquad (5)$$

where I_s is the intensity of synchronous luminescence at $\Delta\lambda=0$.

As the resonance light scattering is a particular synchronous luminescence, the relationship between the intensity of resonance light scattering (I_{RLS}) and the concentration of the aggregate should follow eq 5. Since the nature of the interaction of the binary complex with nucleic acids is the stacking of the binary complex of the single-stranded nucleic acids, in the case the binary complex is excessive, the concentration of aggregate is equal to the concentration of nucleic acids. The correlation between I_{RLS} and the concentration of nucleic acids can be seen from Table 2. All the regression equations in Table 2 have small intercepts in I_{RLS}, so I_{RLS} is in direct proportion to the concentration of nucleic acids. Those equations, along with limits of detection and precision, were obtained according to the general procedure. The proportional correlation of the enhanced intensity of light scattering with the concentration of calf thymus DNA is in the range 0~400 ng·mL^{-1}, with those of fish sperm DNA and yeast RNA in the range 0~300 ng·mL^{-1}. Table 2 presents the parameters involved in the analytical applications of the enhancement effect of nucleic acids on the resonance light scattering of Co(II)/ 5-Cl-PADAB. Table 3 gives the results of determination for six synthetic samples which were based on the tolerance of foreign coexisting substances presented in Table 1. From Table 3, it can be seen that the values found for the six synthetic samples are identical with the expected ones, and the recovery and relative standard deviation are very satisfactory. Therefore, the resonance light-scattering method ofnucleic acids is applicable. Both Tables 2 and 3 show that, by using the resonance light-scattering technique, nucleic acids in nanogram quantities can be determined with high reproducibility, sensitivity, and simplicity.

Table 2 Analytical Parameters of the Determination

nucleic acids	linear regression equation (c, ng·mL^{-1})^a	limit of determination (3 , ng·mL^{-1})	r^b	precision at 200.0 ng·mL^{-1}(%)
calfthymus DNA	I= 0.1+0.238C	1.4	0.9994	1.9
fish sperm DNA	I= -1.0+0.293 C	0.8	0.9996	2.0
yeast RNA	I= -0.1+0.277C	1.3	0.9996	0.8

[a] I is the enhanced intensity of resonance light scattering. [b] r is the correlation coefficient.

Table 3 Results and Determination for Synthetic Samples

nucleic acids contained in samples (amount μg·mL^{-1})	main interferences	amount found (μg·mL^{-1}, n= 5)	recovery (%, n) 5)^a	RSD (%)^b
calfthymus, DNA 3.00	BSA, Ca(II), Mg(II)	2.97	95.6~100.4	0.9
calfthymus DNA2.00	A, G, C, T, $H_2PO_4^-$	2.06	97.6~106.4	1.2
fish sperm DNA 2.50	HSA, Zn(II), Cd(II), Cu(II)	2.58	94.6~102.6	2.7
fish sperm DNA 2.00	A, G, C, T, $H_2PO_4^-$	2.14	92.0~100.8	2.9
yeast RNA 3.00	-IgG, Mn(II), Ni(II), Pb(II)	3.15	90.0~107.6	3.44
yeast RNA 2.50	A, G, C, T, $H_2PO_4^-$	2.45	90.8~101.2	2.9

[a] The recoveries were obtained by adding 0.40 mL of sample solution and 0.40 mL of 2.5 μg·mL^{-1} standard solution of nucleic acids. [b] RSD is relative standard deviation for five measurements of samples.

Based on the fluorescence resonance energy transfer (FRET), fluorometric methods are sensitive for the determination of DNA and RNA[1~6], but the organic dyes are carcinogenic and difficult for a common lab to obtain. Still more, the limit of detection, for example, that of EB being 10 ng·mL^{-1}, is higher than that ofour method. Of course, laser-induced fluorescence methods are highly sensitive, but we are not sure; if laser facilities are used, the resonance light scattering technique should be much more sensitive.

2.3.3 Conclusion

The enhancement of Rayleigh scattering resulting from the absorption of aggregates is a very common phenomenon and, therefore, may provide important applications in a wide range of areas. Besides the sensitive determination of nucleic acids, we have proved that, with the light-scattering technique, proteins in nanogram quantities can be determined[19].In addition, the technique can be used to study the mechanism of interactions of porphyrins with nucleic acids or proteins to monitor the formation of the suprahelical helix of nucleic acids[23]. Although the resonance light-scattering technique is in its infancy, it has many potential applications. For example, the experimental approach can be expanded to time-resolved measurements in the way of time-resolved fluorescence and to the study on the scattering light probe of inhomogeneous systems, particularly biological macro molecular interacting systems. Sensitive determination of antigens in immunochemistry is very crucial. Considering its high sensitivity, the resonance light-scattering technique may have applications in immunochemistry if unlabeled antigen can form a large species with antibody but labeled antigen cannot or if labeled antigen can form a large species with antibody but unlabeled antigen cannot. The formation of the suprahelical helix of nucleic acids in the scattering signals being observed, suggests to us that the resonance light-scattering technique may have applications in genetic diagnosis and PCR for the in vitro exponential amplification of specific nucleic acid sequence. We believe that the resonance light-scattering technique, if equipped with laser facilities, will be highly applicable to analytical chemistry and analytical biochemistry.

Acknowledgments

This project is supported by the National Natural Science Foundation of China (NNSFC), and all authors here express their deep thanks.

References

[1] (a) Pandey, P. C.; Weetall, H. H. Anal. Chem. 1995, 67, 787～792. (b) Harriman, W. O.; Wabl, M. Anal. Biochem. 1995, 228, 336～342. (c) Strothkamp, K. G.; Strothkamp, R. E. J. Chem. Educ. 1994, 71, 77～79. (d) Sari, M. A.; Battioni, J. P.; Duppre, D.; Mansuy, D.; Le Peck, J. B. Biochemistry 1990, 29, 4205～4215. (e) Markovits, J.; Roques, B. P.; Le Pecq, J. B. Anal. Biochem. 1979, 94, 259～264.

[2] (a) Piuno, P. A. E.; Krull, U. J. Anal. Chem.1995, 67, 2635～643. (b) Piuno, P. A. E.; Krull, U. J.; Hudson, R. H. E.; Damha, M. J.; Cohen, H. Anal. Chim. Acta 1994, 288, 205～214.

[3] (a) Daxhelet, G. A.; Kohnen, M. M.; Coene, M. M.; Hoet, P. P. Anal. Biochem. 1990,190, 116～119. (b) Daxhelet, G. A.; Coene, M. M.; Hoet, P. P.; Cocito, C. G. Anal. Biochem. 1989, 179, 401～403.

[4] (a) Rao, J.; Otto, W. R. Anal. Biochem. 1992, 207, 186-192. (b) Rago, R.; Mitchen, J.; Wilding, G. Anal. Biochem. 1990, 191, 31～34. (c) Lipman, J. M. Anal. Biochem. 1989, 176, 128～131

[5] (a) Benson, S. C.; Zeng, Z. X.; Glazer, A. N. Anal. Biochem. 1995, 231, 247～255; 256-260. (b) Rye, H. S.; Drees, B. L.; Nelson, H. C. M.; Glazer, A. N. J. Biol. Chem. 1993, 268, 25229～25238. (c) Glazer, A. N.; Rye, H. S. Nature (London) 1992, 359, 589～561. (d) Petty, J. T.; Johnson, M. E.; Goodwin, P. M.; Martin, J. C.; Jett, J. H.; Keller, R. A. Anal. Chem. 1995, 67, 1755～1761. (e) Haab, B. B.; Mathies, R. A. Anal. Chem. 1995, 67, 3253～3260. (f) Zhu, H. P.; Clark, S. M.; Benson, S. C.; Rye, H. S.; Glazer, A. N.; Mathies, R. A. Anal. Chem. 1994, 66, 1941～1948.

[6] (a) Skogerboe, K. J. Anal. Chem. 1995, 67, 499R～4554R. (b) Perez-Howard, G. M.; Weil, P. A.; Beenchem, J. M. Biochemistry 1995, 34, 8005～8017. (c) Devlin, R.; Studholme, R. M.; Dandliker, W. B.; Fahy, E.; Blumeyer, K.; Ghosh, S. S. Clin. Chem. 1993, 65, 2352～2359.

[7] Zuo, J. The Principles and Applications of Laser Light Scattering in Polymer Science; Henan Science and Technology Press:

Zhengzhou, 1994; pp 1～180.

[8] Pasternack, R. F.; Collings, P. J. Science 1995, 269, 935～939.

[9] Pasternack, R. F.; Bustamante, C.; Collings, P. J.; Giannetto, A.; Gibbs, E. J. J. Am. Chem. Soc. 1993, 115, 5393～5399.

[10] (a) Paula, J. C.; Robblee, J. H.; Pasternack, R. F. Biophys. J. 1995, 68, 335～341. (b) Pasternack, R. F.; Schaefer, K. F. Inorg. Chem. 1994, 433, 2062～2065.

[11] Arena, G.; Scolaro, L. M.; Pasternack, R. F.; Romeo, R. Inorg. Chem. 1995, 34, 2994～3002.

[12] Huang, C. Z.; Li, K. A.; Tong, S. Y. Anal. Chem. 1996, 68, 2259～2263.

[13] Stanton, S. G.; Pecora, P. J. Phys. Chem. 1981, 75, 5615～5626.

[14] Miller, G. A. J. Phys. Chem. 1978, 82, 616～618.

[15] (a) Anglister, J.; Steinberg, I. Z. Chem. Phys. Lett. 1979, 65, 50-54. (b) Anglister, J.; Steinberg, I. Z. J. Chem. Phys. 1983, 78, 5358～5368.

[16] Cheng, K. L.; Ueno, K.; Imamura, T. CRC Handbook of Organic Analytical Reagents (Chinese Version); Geology Press: Beijing, 1982; pp 142～143.

[17] Huang, C. Z.; Li, K. A.; Tong, S. Y. Anal. Chim. Acta, in press.

[18] Pasternack, R. F.; Gibbs, E. J. J. Inorg. Organomet. Polym. 1993, 3, 77～88.

[19] Huang, C. Z. Ph.D. Dissertation, Peking University, Beijing, 1996; p 35.

[20] Chen, Z.; Liu, J.; Luo, D. Biochemistry Experiments; Chinese University ofSciences and Technology Press: Hefei, PRC, 1994; p 111.

[21] Sun, L. E.; Sun, D. X.; Zhu, D. X. Molecular Genetics; Nanjing University Press: Nanjing, 1995; pp 6～28.

[22] Rubio, S.; Gomez-Hens, A.; Vaalcarce, M. Talanta 1986, 33, 633～640.

[23] Huang, C. Z.; Li, K. A.; Tong, S. Y. Bull. Chem. Soc. Jpn., submitted

(Cheng Zhi Huang, Ke An Li, and Shen Yang Tong, Published in *Analytical Chemistry*, 1997, 69, 514～520)

2.4 Interactions of Janus Green B with Double Stranded DNA and the Determination of DNA Based on the Measurement of Enhanced Resonance Light Scattering

Abstract: A novel assay of DNA with a sensitivity at the nanogram level is proposed based on the measurement of enhanced resonance light scattering (RLS) signals resulting from the interaction of Janus Green B (JGB) with DNA. At pH 6.37 and ionic strength <0.20, the RLS signals of JGB were greatly enhanced by DNA in the region of 300～650 nm characterized by three peaks at 416.0, 452.0 and 469.2 nm. The binding properties were examined using a Scatchard plot based on the measurement of the enhanced RLS data at 416.0 nm at a high JGB: DNA molar ratio ($R>2.22$), and an aggregation mechanism of JGB in the presence of DNA at the nanogram level is proposed. Linear relationships can be established between the enhanced RLS intensity and DNA concentration in the range 0～3.5 $\mu g \cdot mL^{-1}$ for both calf thymus DNA (ctDNA) and fish sperm DNA (fsDNA) if 2.0×10^{-5} $mol \cdot L^{-1}$ JGB is employed. The limits of determination were 8.7 $ng \cdot mL^{-1}$ for ctDNA and 9.9 $ng \cdot mL^{-1}$ for fsDNA, respectively. Synthetic samples were analysed satisfactorily.

2.4.1 Introduction

In the development of methods for mutation detection, elucidation of complex biological problems, molecular diagnosis and prognosis of disease and assessment of treatment,[1,2] one important topic is the resonance energy transfer from organic dyes to nucleic acids. Owing to the fluorescence enhancement resulting from the resonance energy transfer, binding studies of organic dyes with nucleic acids have found wide applications in the design of new luminescent chromophores,[3] immunoassays[4] and DNA chips.[5] If laser facilities are employed, the fluorescence enhancement effect of DNA on organic dyes with double functional groups can be applied to the detection of single DNA molecules and the growth of DNA in a PCR test.[6,7]

Recently, a promising tool concerning enhanced resonance light scattering (RLS) has attracted strong interest from chemists and biochemists since it is highly sensitive to the characterization of the binding properties of organic dyes with nucleic acids.[8,10] An RLS spectrum can be easily obtained by simultaneously scanning the excitation and emission monochromators of a common spectrofluorimeter with $\Delta\lambda = 0$ nm.[8,9] The principle of RLS is based on refractive index fluctuation near the absorption band in an aqueous medium, in which particles of nanometer size are formed.[11] In a transparent isotropic medium, the light scattering for molecular particles with the particle size 20-fold smaller than the wavelength of the incident beam follows the Rayleigh scattering law because the imaginary part of the refractive index originating from the molecular absorption can be neglected.[8] If the wavelength of the incident beam is close to the absorption band of the molecular particles whose size is at the nanometer level, however, enhanced RLS can be expected since the fluctuation of the imaginary part of the refractive index is significant and may be comparable to that of the real part of the refractive index.[8] By using a common spectrofluorimeter to measure the RLS signals, Pasternack *et al.*[8,9] studied the aggregation of porphyrins. Later, we discovered that by employing the enhanced RLS signals of quinonimine dyes,[10] free base porphyrins[12,13] or metal complex dyes,[14] trace amounts of nucleic acids[10,12,14] and proteins[13] in synthetic[10,12,14] and practical[13] samples can be sensitively determined. The formation of the suprahelical helixes of nucleic acids[15] and the aggregation of porphyrins in the presence of proteins[16] can also be investigated. Here by employing the RLS technique, we studied the interaction of Janus Green B (JGB) with double stranded DNA.

DNA has long been recognized as an important target for photoactive dyes, which have proved to photosensitize biological damage. In living systems, these dyes are possibly photocytotoxic and can cause photoinduced mutagenic effects if cell killing is incomplete.[17] In this study, it was found that the binding of JGB with DNA involves the long range assembly of JGB on the molecular surface of double stranded DNA in a neutral aqueous medium. With the enhanced RLS signals of the long-range assembly process, nanogram levels of DNA can be determined.

2.4.2 Experimental

2.4.2.1 Apparatus

RLS spectra and intensities were measured with a Shimadzu (Kyoto, Japan) RF-540 spectrofluorimeter and the absorption spectrum was scanned with a Hitachi (Tokyo, Japan) U-3400 spectrophotometer. An S-10A digital pH meter (Xiaoshan Scientific Instruments Plant, Zhejiang, China) was used to measure the pH values of aqueous solutions and an MVS-1 vortex mixer (Beide Scientific Instrumental, Beijing, China) was used to mix solutions in calibrated flasks.

2.4.2.2 Reagents

Stock standard solutions of DNA were prepared by dissolving calf thymus DNA (ctDNA) (Beitai Biochemical, Chinese Academy of Sciences, Beijing, China) and fish sperm DNA (fsDNA) (Shanghai Institute of Biochemistry, Chinese Academy of Sciences, Shanghai, China) in doubly distilled water. A period of 24 h or more was needed and occasionally gentle shaking was necessary for dissolution at 4 °C. Concentrations of DNA were determined according to the absorbances at 260 nm after establishing that the absorbance ratio A_{260}/A_{280} was in the range 1.80～1.90. The molarities of DNA, where necessary, were calculated by using the molar absorptivity of double stranded DNA at 260 nm: [18] $\varepsilon_{DNA} = 6600\ \text{L}\cdot\text{mol}^{-1}\cdot\text{cm}^{-1}$. A working standard solution of DNA of 25.0 $\mu\text{g}\cdot\text{mL}^{-1}$ ($7.5\times10^{-1}\ \text{mol}\cdot\text{L}^{-1}$) was prepared.

A stock standard solution of JGB (for the molecular structure, see Fig. 1) was prepared by dissolving the crystalline product (Merck, Darmstadt, Germany) in doubly distilled water. A working standard solution of $2.0\times10^{-4}\ \text{mol}\cdot\text{L}^{-1}$ was prepared.

Britton–Robinson buffer solution was used to control the acidity of the interacting system and 0.1, 1.0 and 4.0 $\text{mol}\cdot\text{L}^{-1}$ NaCl solutions were used to adjust the ionic strength of the aqueous solutions. All other reagents were of analytical-reagent grade and used without further purification. Doubly distilled water was used throughout.

2.4.2.3 General procedures

In a 10 mL calibrated flask were placed 1.00 mL of JGB solution, 1.0 mL of buffer solution and an appropriate volume of DNA solution or a sample solution containing DNA. The mixture was vortex mixed after each addition of the interacting additives, then diluted to 10 mL using doubly distilled water. The mixture was well mixed manually after the flask piston had been fitted. All of the absorption and RLS measurements were obtained against parallel blank solutions treated in the same way but without DNA.

2.4.3 Results and discussion

2.4.3.1 Features of resonance light scattering spectra

Fig. 2 shows the RLS spectral features of JGB, DNA and JGB– DNA. Both JGB and DNA have weak RLS signals over the wavelength range 300～650 nm (lines 1 and 2 in Fig. 2). DNA has a very weak RLS signal at pH 6.37 even if its concentration reaches 30.0 $\mu g \cdot mL^{-1}$(line 1 in Fig. 2). However, a wide, strong RLS band in the range 300～650 nm can be observed for the mixture of JGB and DNA, which indicates that interaction of JGB with DNA has occurred. As can be seen in Fig. 2, the wide, strong RLS spectrum of JGB –DNA was overloaded with three peaks at 416.0, 452.0 and 469.2, with two overshoot shoulder peaks at 350 and 572 nm. It was found that these enhanced RLS signals increased with increasing DNA concentration in the $R>$ 1.67 range ($R = c_{JGB}/c_{DNA}$) (Fig. 2). Similar RLS signals could be obtained for the interaction of JGB with fsDNA.

According to the macroscopic fluctuation theory,[8,9] scattering light originates from the fluctuation of the refractive index of a solution.[8,9] If the wavelength of the incident beam is close to the absorption band of molecular particles, the refractive index of the solution varies strongly, which leads to both the real and imaginary parts of the refractive index making contributions to the scattering light, resulting in enhanced RLS signals.[8,9] Hence the RLS features in Fig. 2 are undoubtedly associated with the absorption properties of the interacting systems, and in such a case it is necessary to consider the absorption features of the interacting components.

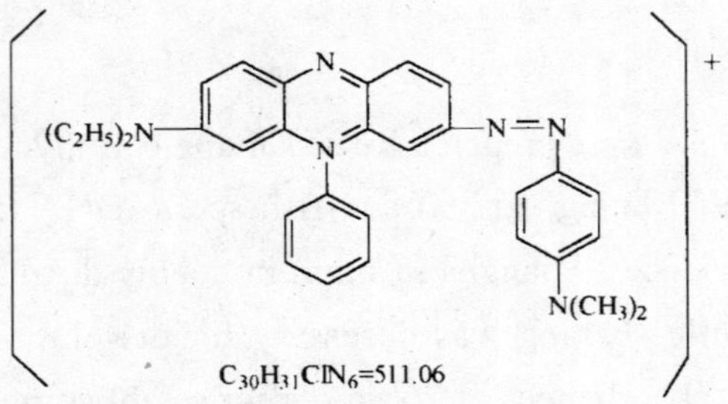

$C_{30}H_{31}ClN_6$=511.06

Fig. 1 Molecular structure of Janus Green B (JGB).

In the visible region, DNA has no absorption band, whereas JGB has two characteristic absorption bands located at 396 nm (λ_1) and 603 nm (λ_2) (Fig. 3). When interaction of JGB with DNA occurs, the two absorption bands display different features depending on the R values. If $R>1.67$, a hypochromic effect can be observed for the λ_2 band with the maximum wavelength shifting towards the blue to 584.6 nm, while a hyperchromic effect can be observed for the λ_1 band with a slight wavelength shift. With further addition of DNA to keep $0.22<R<1.67$, although the blue shift of the λ_2 band continues to 569.0 nm, a hyperchromic effect of the λ_2 band is obtained. An isosbestic point at 500.0 nm can be observed in this R range. If more DNA was added to keep $R<0.22$, the blue-shifted λ_2 band at 569.0 nm shifts bathochromically with a slight hyperchromic effect. If DNA is in a 30-fold excess, the λ_2 band could reach 616.0 nm. These absorption features indicate that the interaction of JGB with DNA involves different interaction processes depending on the R values, *i.e.*, at $R>1.67$, $0.22<R<1.67$ and $R<0.22$.

2.4.3.2 Assignment of JGB aggregation by absorption and RLS spectra

It was found that the JGB absorption has an aggregation tendency in aqueous solution with increasing concentration or ionic strength of the medium. At pH 6.37 and ionic strength 0.006, although the λ_1 band displayed hardly any wavelength shift with increasing JGB concentration, the λ_2 band showed a hypsochromic effect. If the JGB concentration is $>1.0\times10^{-4}$ mol·L^{-1}, the λ_2 band can reach 592.3 nm from 603.0 nm. Furthermore, it was found that the λ_2 absorption band begins to deviate from Beer's law if the JGB concentration is $>6.0\times10^{-5}$ mol·L^{-1}.

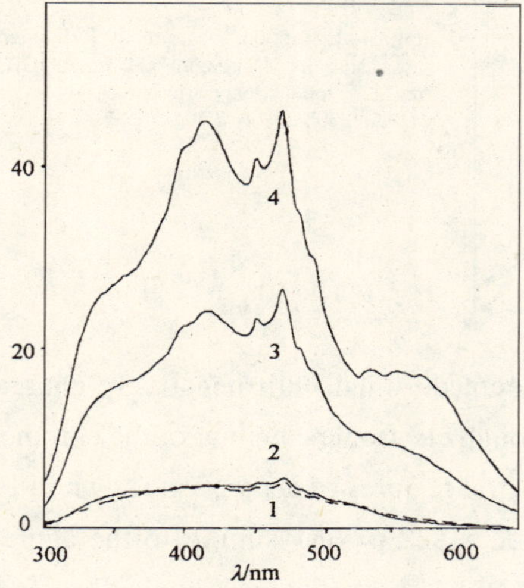

Fig. 2 RLS spectrum of JGB (line 1), ctDNA (line 2) and JGB–ctDNA (lines 3 and 4). pH, 6.37; ionic strength, 0.006. Concentrations: JGB, 2.0×10^{-5} mol·L^{-1} but line 1 without any JGB; ctDNA (μg·mL^{-1}): 1, 30.0; 2, 0.0; 3, 1.0; 4, 2.0.

With increasing ionic strength of the medium, the λ2 band decreases and shifts towards the blue to 566.0 nm, whereas the λ_1 band decreases slightly without a significant wavelength shift (Fig. 4). A clear isosbestic point at 551.0 nm can be observed in Fig. 4, which indicates that H-aggregation of JGB has occurred.[19] The H-aggregate species is responsible for the 566.0 nm band, the corresponding RLS signals of which are located in the 570 nm region (Fig. 5). At an ionic strength of 0.006, 2.0×10^{-5} mol·L^{-1} JGB solution shows very weak RLS signals. With increase in ionic strength, however, the weak RLS signals increase, and three characteristic RLS peaks occur at 415.0, 452.0 and 468.0 nm (Fig. 5). A shoulder RLS peak is also present in the 345 nm region, which is probably associated with the λ_1 absorption band. Hence, it is reasonable that JGB displays an aggregation tendency with increasing ionic strength of the aqueous medium, resulting in H-aggregate species.

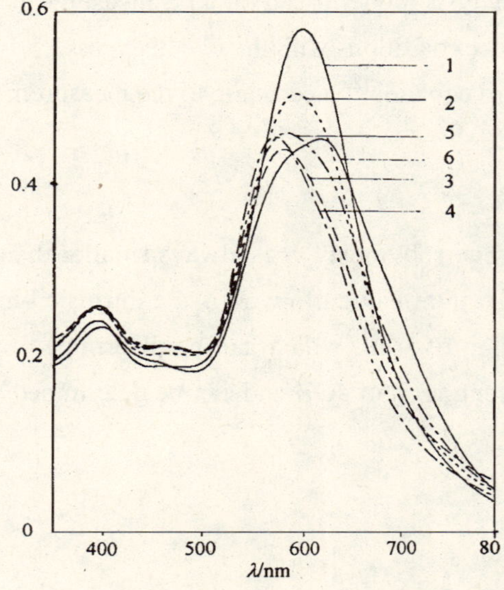

Fig. 3 Absorption spectra of the interacting system of JGB with ctDNA. pH, 6.37; ionic strength, 0.003. Concentrations: JGB, 2.0×10^{-5} mol·L^{-1}; ctDNA (μg·mL^{-1}): 1, 0; 2, 2.0 (R = 3.33); 3, 4.0 (R = 1.67); 4, 30.0 (R = 0.22); 5, 100.0 (R = 0.067); 6, 150.0 (R = 0.027).

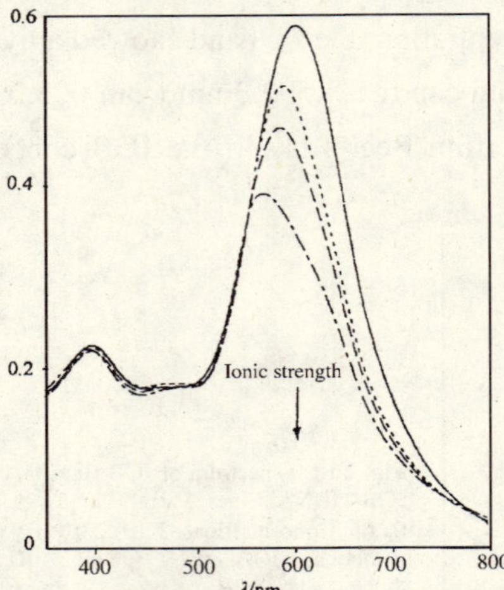

Fig. 4 Absorption spectrum of JGB aggregation with increasing ionic strength. pH, 6.37; JGB, 2.0×10^{-5} $mol \cdot L^{-1}$; ionic strength (in decreasing order at 600 nm): 0.006; 0.206; 0.806; 2.506.

As a positively charged molecule, JGB can undoubtedly bind with negatively charged DNA polyanion through electrostatic attraction, and this is possible through electronic coupling of the chromophore between JGB and the base of DNA molecules. By comparing the spectral features of absorption shown in Fig. 3 and Fig. 4, the interaction of JGB with DNA in the molar ratio range $R > 0.22$ is very similar to the aggregation of JGB that occurs in a high ionic strength medium. Both Figs. 3 and 4 show a hypochromic effect and a blue shift for the λ_2 absorption band. In terms of the RLS spectra in Figs. 2 and 5, they both show three similar weak over-loaded RLS peaks in the 415～470 nm range and two shoulder peaks in 345 and 470 nm regions. Hence the binding mechanism of JGB with DNA at $R > 0.22$ is the same as the aggregation of JGB that occurs in a neutral medium of high ionic strength. In other words, the aggregation of JGB could occur in the presence of double stranded DNA when $R > 0.22$.

2.4.3.3 Equilibrium of the interaction between JGB and DNA

In the investigation of interactions of organic dyes with macromolecules, a Scatchard plot is commonly used to discuss the binding properties in terms of measuring the binding number and binding constant. The data for Scatchard analysis are usually used based on measurements of absorbance or fluorescence intensity of the interacting system.[16] We have established a Scatchard analysis model based on RLS measure- ments and to investigate the interaction of safraine T with nucleic acids under conditions with the dye in excess.[10]

In this work, we established the following Scatchard equation[20] according to the measurement of RLS data:

$$\frac{m}{[\mathrm{JGB}]} = n\,K - m\,K \qquad (1)$$

where m is the molar ratio of bound JGB to DNA base pair (obviously m is always smaller than R, which is the molar ratio of added JGB to added DNA), n is the maximum value of m, K is the intrinsic binding constant of JGB to DNA and [JGB] is the equilibrium concentration of JGB, which can be determined by using [JGB] = c_{JGB}-[JGB·DNA], where [JGB·DNA] is the bound concentration of JGB and can be determined as described in a previous paper.[10]

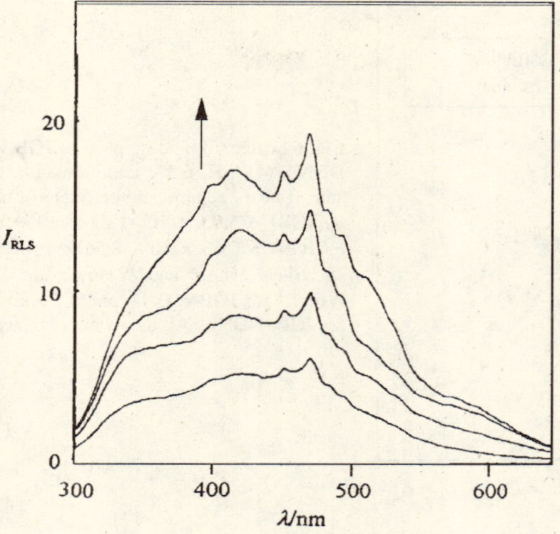

Fig. 5 RLS spectrum of JGB aggregation with increasing ionic strength. Conditions as in Fig. 4. Ionic strength (in increasing order at 400 nm): 0.006; 0.206; 0.806; 2.506.

Fig. 6 displays the results of the Scatchard plot concerning the interaction equilibrium of JGB with ctDNA and fsDNA. The linear regression equations for the interactions of JGB with ctDNA and fsDNA are $m/[JGB] = 5.93 \times 10^6 - 1.25 \times 10^6 m$ $(r=-0.9939)$ and $m/[JGB]=3.63 \times 10^6 - 8.56 \times 10^5 m$ $(r=-0.9495)$, respectively. Hence we can obtain the values of n and K for the interactions of JGB with ctDNA as 4.7 and 1.25×10^6 L·mol^{-1} and those with fsDNA as 4.2 and 8.56×10^5 L·mol^{-1}, respectively.

2.4.3.4 Nature of the interaction of JGB with DNA

By comparing Figs. 2 and Fig. 5 and Fig. 3 and Fig. 4, we conclude that the interaction of JGB with DNA in the range $R>0.22$ is very similar to the aggregation of JGB that occurs in a neutral medium of high ionic strength. There is a possibility that DNA plays the role of supplying negative charges to neutralize the positive charges of JGB molecules, and then encourages the ***H***-aggregation of JGB. The aggregate of JGB deposits on the backbone of DNA molecules on which many negatively charged phosphate ions exists, in agreement with the results of Scatchard analysis, which indicate that one nucleotide residue can bind about four JGB molecules. Hence the interaction of JGB with DNA is ascribed to the electrostatic attraction between the positively charged JGB and the negatively charged DNA molecules. As can be seen in Fig. 6, at high binding molar ratios the Scatchard plots cannot return to the abscissa but curve upwards, indicative of cooperative binding,[17] namely the long- range assembly of the organic dye molecules on the molecular surface of DNA.[9,10] Experiments showed that enhanced RLS occurs in the range $R>1.67$ with increasing DNA concentra- tion. Hence the strongly enhanced RLS signals at $R>1.67$ indicate that the interaction of JGB with DNA involves the long-range assembly of JGB on the DNA molecular surface. It was found that if $R<1.67$, the RLS signals begin to decrease with increasing DNA concentration, which means that the binding mode of long-range assembly begins to change. At $R<0.22$, the RLS signals are hardly detected. The bathchromic effect and strong hypochroism from the free JGB in this R range (Fig. 2) suggest a strong interaction between the electronic states of the intercalating chromophore and that of the DNA base[21]. Hence it is possible that the intercalative of JGB with DNA involves the intercalative binding of JGB into the DNA base pairs in the presence of large amounts of DNA. In such a case, the binding spectra at $0.22<R<1.67$ possibly indicate an equilibrium between the long-range assembly species and the intercalative species.

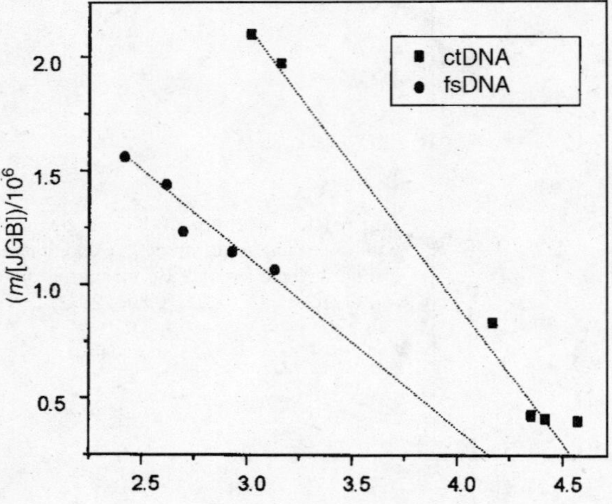

Fig. 6 Scatchard binding plots of JGB with ctDNA (-) and fsDNA (4). pH, 6.37; ionic strength, 0.006. The regression linear equations for ctDNA and fsDNA were $m/[JGB] = 5.93 \times 10^6 - 1.25 \times 10^6 m$ (r = 20.9939) and $m/[JGB] = 3.63 \times 10^6 - 8.56 \times 10^5 m$ (r = 20.9495), respectively. The n and K values are 4.7 and 1.25×10^6 $L \cdot mol^{-1}$ for JGB–ctDNA and 4.2 and 8.56×10^5 $L \cdot mol^{-1}$ for JGB–fsDNA. All data were obtained at 20 °C at 416.0 nm.

2.4.3.5 Optimization of the general procedures

The RLS signals reflect the binding properties between JGB and DNA at high R values, so it can supply reference information on the long-range assembly of JGB on the DNA molecular surface. Since the interaction products depend on the interacting components, the RLS signals reveal the change of state of the two interacting components. In addition to the molar ratio, the H-aggregation of JGB in the presence of DNA depends on pH and ionic strength. Fig. 7 shows that the RLS intensity remains constant in the pH range 5.7～6.8, and a reduced RLS intensity is obtained at any pH value outside this range. It is possible that the decrease in RLS can be ascribed to the change of state of DNA at pH$<$5.7, where an indirect proton–phosphate interaction *via* water and the protonation of nitrogen atoms of bases could occur. As other reports have shown, protonation of cytosine N-3 (pKa = 4.24) and adenine N-1 sites (pKa = 3.20) occurs at pH 5.3, while guanine N-7 (pKa = 2.30) will be protonated at pH$<$3.[22] Hence the dependence of RLS intensity on the pH of the medium can characterize the state of DNA.

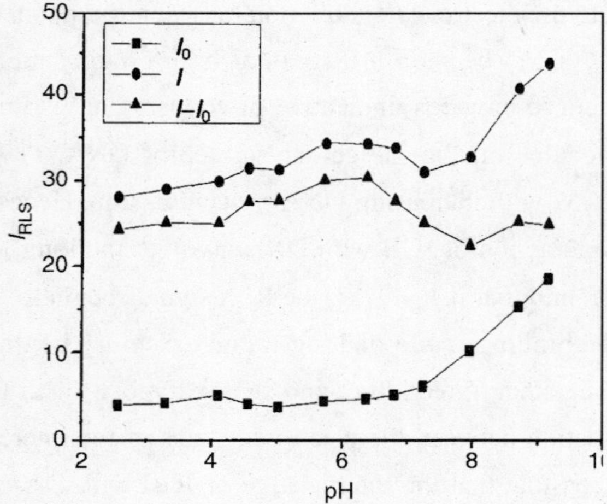

Fig. 7 pH effect on the RLS signals of JGB (■, I_0), and JGB–ctDNA (●, I). The enhanced RLS intensity was defined as $\Delta I_{RLS} = I - I_0$. ctDNA, 2.0 $\mu g \cdot mL^{-1}$; JBG, 2.0×10^{-5} $mol \cdot L^{-1}$. All the data were obtained with the ionic strength maintained at 0.010 and the data were collected up at 416.0 nm.

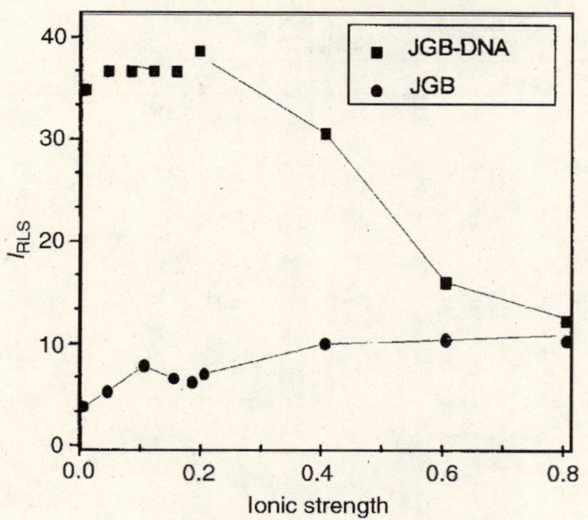

Fig. 8 Effect of ionic strength on JGB (●, I_0), and JGB–ctDNA (■, I). ctDNA, 2.0 μg·mL^{-1}; JGB, 2.0 × 10^{-5} mol·L^{-1}. pH, 6.37. All the data were obtained at 416.0 nm.

Similarly, as can be seen in Fig. 8, the RLS intensity remains constant if the ionic strength of the solution is <0.2, indicating strong binding properties of JGB with double stranded DNA and in agreement with the results of Scatchard analysis. Hence the electrostatic interaction of JGB with DNA and the electronic coupling of the chromophore between JGB and the base of DNA molecules are very strong.

2.4.2.6 Tolerance of the method to foreign substances

In addition to the state of the interacting components, foreign substances, including various ions, sugars, surfactants and nucleotides, have proved to exert effects on the interaction of JGB with ctDNA. As Table 1 shows, Mg^{2+}, Na^{+}, K^{+}, Ca^{2+} can be tolerated at high concentration levels. The reason is possibly that they are hard ions and could tend to bind almost exclusively to the phosphate groups of DNA, stabilizing the Watson–Crick double stranded helix. In contrast, soft ions, such as Hg^{2+}, which appear to bind exclusively with the base moiety of DNA to form internal chelates, interstrand complexes or cross-links,[22] can be tolerated at low concentration levels. Surfactants, such as sodium dodecyl sulfate (SDS), cetyltrimethylammonium bromide (CTMAB), gelatin, Triton X-100, β-cyclodextrin and sugars, can be tolerated at higher levels. Proteins can also be tolerated at higher concentration levels, which provides this assay with the possibility of determining the content of DNA in practical samples.

Table 1 Tolerance of the method to foreign substances[a]

Substance	Concentration (10^{-6} mol·L^{-1})	Change of I_{RLS} (%)
Al(III), SO_4^{2-}	18.0	−5.6
Ca(II), Cl-	2500.0	−9.0
Cd(II), Cl^-	1.00	−3.2
Co(II), Cl^-	0. 1	−11.8
Cr(III), Cl^-	2.0	−5.2
Hg(II), SO_4^{2-}	0.05	−8.5
K(I), Cl^-	5000.0	−5.6
Mg(II), Cl^-	1000.0	−2.1
Mn(II), SO_4^{2-}	0.5	−7.9
Na^+, Cl^-	5000.0	−6.2
NH_4^+, Cl^-	6700.0	+7.7
Pb^{2+}, Cl^-	0.02	−2.7
Zn^{2+}, Cl^-	4.0	−5.2
Glucose	1.0	−3.5
Lactose	1.0	+10.1

Continued

Substance	Concentration (10^{-6} mol·L^{-1})	Change of I_{RLS} (%)
Maltose	1.0	−7.2
Sucrose	5.0	+5.0
b-Cyclodextrin (b-CD)	300.0	−2.5
Gelatin	0.5^b	+0.5
Triton X-100	0.4^c	+7.2
CTMAB	2.5	+1.9
SDS	0.5	−5.8
Protein, BSA	1.0^b	+7.2
Protein, HSA	1.0^b	−3.2
5^A-AMP	1.0	−9.5
5^A-GMP	1.0	−11.3
5^A-CMP	1.0	−6.2
5^A-UMP	1.0	+5. 1

^{a} Concentrations: JGB, 2.0 × 10^{-5} mol·L^{-1}; ctDNA, 2.0 μg·mL^{-1}. pH 6.37; ionic strength 0.006. All data were obtained at 416.0 nm·μg·mL^{-1}. ^{c} %.

2.4.2.7 Calibration curves and analysis of synthetic samples

Under optimum conditions according to the optimum proce- dures, calibration curves for ctDNA and fsDNA were con- structed with different concentrations of JGB with increasing ctDNA and fsDNA concentrations. There are linear relation- ships between the enhanced RLS intensity ($\Delta I_{RLS} = I - I_0$) and DNA concentration for an appropriate JGB solution. All of the analytical parameters were regressed and are presented in Table 2. It was found that JGB concentration affects the linear range and the sensitivity of the determination method. As Table 2 shows, with increasing JGB concentration, the linear range is extended, but the sensitivity decreases. It is worth noting that although enhanced RLS signals can be obtained in the range $1.67 < R < 2.22$, no linear relationships can be obtained and the R value at the upper limit of the linear range is about 2.2.

To test the method, four synthetic samples, which were constructed based on the tolerance levels of foreign substances (Table 1), were analysed according to the results given in Table 2. As Table 3 shows, the results are reproducible and reliable.

2.4.3 Conclusion

In a neutral aqueous solution of ionic strength <0.2, the interaction of JGB with double stranded DNA involves two interaction mechanisms depending on the molar ratio of the two interacting components, namely long-range assembly and intercalative binding. Long-range assembly occurs when $R > 1.67$, resulting in strongly enhanced RLS signals. Through Scatchard analysis with the enhanced RLS data, the binding constant is found to be at the 10^6level, and the binding number is about 4 in the long-range assembly process. Intercalative binding occurs at $R < 0.22$, and there is an equilibrium of the long-range assembly and the interactive binding in the range $0.22 < R < 1.67$. It was found that the enhanced RLS intensity of RLS in the long-range assembly in proportional to the concentration of ctDNA and fsDNA, and on this basis determination method of DNA at nanogam level can be established.

Table 2 Analytical parameters of the determination[a]

DNA	Concentration of JGB/10^{-5} mol·L^{-1}	Linear range (μg·mL^{-1})	R range	Linear regression equation (c/μg·mL^{-1})	LOD^b (3σ)/ μg·mL^{-1}	Correlation coefficient (r)
ctDNA	1.0	0～1.5	≥2.22	$\Delta I_{RLS} = 0.6 + 18.9c$	7.5	0.9982 (n =4)
	2.0	0～3.5	≥2.22	$\Delta I_{RLS} = -0.1 + 17.3c$	8.7	0.9966 (n =8)
	3.0	0～5.0	≥2.0	$\Delta I_{RLS} = 0.5 + 13.7c$	10.3	0.9944 (n =11)

Continued

DNA	Concentration of JGB/10^{-5} mol·L^{-1}	Linear range (μg·mL^{-1})	R range	Linear regression equation (c/μg·mL^{-1})	LOD[b] (3σ)/ μg·mL^{-1}	Correlation coefficient (r)
fsDNA	1.0	0～1.5	≥2.22	ΔI_{RLS} = -0.4 + 20.1c	7.5	0.9970 (n =4)
	2.0	0～3.5	≥2.22	ΔI_{RLS} = -0.3 + 15.2c	9.9	0.9937 (n =8)
	3.0	0～4.0	≥2.50	ΔI_{RLS} = 1.8 + 11.4c	13.2	0.9941(n =9)

[a] pH 6.37; ionic strength, 0.006. All the data were obtained at 416.0 nm. [b] Limit of determination.

Table 3 Results for analysis of synthetic samplesa

DNA in sample/μg·mL^{-1}	Main additives[b]	Found value/μg·mL^{-1} (n = 5)	Recovery range (%) (n =5)	RSD (%) (n = 5)
ctDNA 25.0	Mg(II), Ca(III), Co(II), K(I)	24.8	94.9～103.0	2.0
ctDNA 15.0	β-CD, SDS, BSA	15.4	97.3～107.0	2.5
fsDNA 20.0	Mg(II), Ca(III), Cr(III), β-CD	19.6	92.1～-104.9	2.7
fsDNA 10.0	5^-AMP, 5^-GMP, 5^-CMP	10.5	95.2～103.2	1.4

[a] pH 6.37; ionic strength 0.006. All the data were obtained at 416.0 nm. [b] Concentrations of additives: BSA, 0.05 μg·mL^{-1}; nucleotide: 6.0 × 10^{-7} mol·L^{-1} β-CD, 1.2 × 10^{-6} mol·L^{-1}; Ca^{2+}, 8.0 × 10^{-6} mol·L^{-1}; Cr^{3+}, 4.0 × 10^{-9} mol·L^{-1}; Mg^{2+}, 8.0 × 10^{-7} mol·L^{-1}; K^{+}, 8.0 × 10^{-6} mol·L^{-1}; Co^{2+}, 2.4 × 10^{-9} mol·L^{-1}; SDS, 2.0 × 10^{-8} mol·L^{-1}. JGB, 4.0 × 10^{-5} mol·L^{-1}.

Acknowlegment

This program is supported by the National Natural Science Foundation of China (NSFC, No. 29875019), to whom the authors express their gratitude.

References

[1] F. S. Collins, A. Patrinos, E. Jordan, A. Chakravti, R. Gesteland and L. Walters, Science, 1998, 282, 682.
[2] T. K. Christopoulos, Anal. Chem., 1999, 71, 425R.
[3] M. Schena, D. Shalon, R. Heller, A. Chai, P. O. Brown and R. W. Davis, Proc. Natl. Acad. Sci. USA, 1996, 93, 10614.
[4] M. Hall, I. Kazakova and Y. M. Yao, Anal. Biochem,, 1999, 272, 165.
[5] Marshall and J. Hodgson, Nature Biotechnol., 1998, 16, 27.
[6] N. Glazer and H. S. Rye, Nature (London), 1992, 359, 589.
[7] C. Benson, Z. X. Zeng and A. N. Glazer, Anal. Biochem., 1995, 231, 247.
[8] R. F. Pasternack and P. J. Collings, Science, 1995, 269, 935.
[9] R. F. Pasternack, C. Bustamante, P. J. Colings, A. Giannetto and E. J. Gibbs, J. Am. Chem. Soc., 1993, 115, 5393.
[10] Z. Huang, Y. F. Li and X. D. Liu, Anal. Chim. Acta, 1998, 375, 89.
[11] Z. P. Li, K. A. Li and S. Y. Tong, Analyst, 1999, 124, 907.
[12] Z. Huang, K. A. Li and S. Y. Tong, Anal. Chem., 1996, 68, 2259.
[13] C. Z. Huang, Y. F. Li, J. G. Mao and D. G. Tan, Analyst, 1998, 123, 1401.
[14] C. Z. Huang, K. A. Li and S. Y. Tong, Anal. Chem., 1997, 69, 514.
[15] C. Z. Huang, K. A. Li and S. Y. Tong, Bull. Chem. Soc. Jpn., 1997, 70, 1843.
[16] C. Z. Huang, Y. F. Li, N. Li, K. A. Li and S. Y. Tong, Bull. Chem. Soc. Jpn., 1998, 71, 1791.
[17] Tuite and J. M. Kelly, Biopolymers, 1995, 35, 419.
[18] Y. E. Zeng, H. S. Zhang and Z. H. Chen, Handbook of Modern Chemical Reagents, Chemical Industry Press, Beijing, 1989, vol. 4.
[19] D. L. Arkins, H. R. Zhu and C. Guo, J. Phys. Chem., 1994, 98, 3612.
[20] K. G. Strothkamp and R. E. Strothkamp, J. Chem. Educ., 1994, 71, 77.
[21] C. V. Kumar and E. H. Asuncion, J. Am. Chem. Soc., 1993, 115, 8547.
[22] K. B. Jacobson and J. E. Turner, Toxicology, 1980, 16, 1.

(Cheng Zhi Huang, Yuan Fang Li, Xin Hua Huang and Ming Li,
published in *The Analyst,* 2000, 125, 1267～1271)

2.5 A Sensitive and Selective Assay of Nucleic Acids by Measuring Enhanced Total Internal Reflected Resonance Light Scattering Signals Deriving from the Evanescent Field at the Water/Tetrachloromethane Interface

A total internal reflected resonance light scattering (TIR-RLS) technique, the coupling of resonance light scattering (RLS) technique with total internal reflected light at the interface of two immiscible liquids, where the steep change of the refractive indexes occurs to result in an evanescent field, is proposed with the characteristics of separation and enrichment properties of analytes and direct use of oil-soluble reagents free from surfactants. At pH 8.69 and ion strength 0.008, ternary amphiphilic species formed by the interaction of nucleic acids, including calf thymus DNA (ctDNA), fish sperm DNA (fsDNA), and yeast RNA (yRNA), with Eu(III) in the presence of oil-soluble trioctylphosphine oxide (TOPO), are adsorbed to the water/tetrachloromethane (H_2O/CCl_4) interface, giving rise to significantly enhanced TIR-RLS signals. It has been found that the enhanced TIR-RLS intensity at 348.0 nm is proportional to the concentration of thermally denatured ctDNA, fsDNA and yRNA in the range 0.002～2.5 $\mu g \cdot mL^{-1}$, 0.002～2.5 $\mu g \cdot mL^{-1}$ and 0.003～2.0 $\mu g \cdot mL^{-1}$, respectively and their limits of determination (3σ) are 0.16 $ng \cdot mL^{-1}$, 0.19 $ng \cdot mL^{-1}$ and 0.28 $ng \cdot mL^{-1}$, correspondingly. Complicated artificial samples with highly interfering backgrounds were determined satisfactorily.

2.5.1 Introduction

Light scattering techniques such as Raman and Mie scatterings have frequently been applied in analytical and physical chemistries.[1,2] In recent years, a new resonance light scattering (RLS) technique, established simply on detecting enhanced light scattering signals with a common spectrofluorometer,[3,4] has proved to be an important and powerful tool not only for the quantification of nucleic acids,[5～10] proteins,[11～13] metallic ions[14～16] and drugs[17] in artificial and real samples, but also for the characterization of the aggregation and assembly of biological and chemical species.[18～22] It is a pity, however, that it suffers from at least three disadvantages at least, including: (1) the tolerance levels of coexisting foreign substances are not satisfactory. The RLS signal of a scattered particle depends on its absorption features, size, shape, concentration and refractive index relative to the surrounding medium,[3～6] and is influenced significantly by those of coexisting foreign substances as a result; (2) the RLS technique is employed in aqueous media, which accordingly confines the use of oil-soluble reagents and its application in the recognition and interaction between hosts and guests with immiscible properties in the same way, occurring possibly in complex biologic systems such as in cell matrix. Although sometimes surfactants are introduced as emulgents to solve this problem successfully, corresponding interaction mechanisms are made much more complicated;[23] (3) investigations of orientation of molecules are developed with difficulty using polarized excitation light due to multiple light scattering components in solutions. Therefore, further studies are compulsory.

To overcome the disadvantages stated above, we coupled the RLS technique with total internal reflected light at an oil/water interface based on the following considerations: (1) the RLS technique is established on the basis of the fluctuation of the refractive indexes in an aqueous solution where a steep change occurs between the refractive index of the inner scattered particles and that of their outer atmosphere,[3,4] which gives rise to mini-interfaces between the inner scattered particles and their outer atmosphere. The occurrence of the adsorption will easily bring about a sharp fluctuation of refractive indexes at the interfacial region; (2) the liquid/liquid interface is somewhat similar to an enlarged surface of a scattered particle and the refractive indexes play the same role as they do in a bulk phase; (3) hosts and guests with immiscible properties can encounter and interact at the liquid/liquid interface and the corresponding amphiphilic species can be adsorbed and enriched by the interface.[24] Thus recognition and interaction of hosts and guests with immiscible properties can be solved, and assays with high selectivity and sensitivity can be also expected; (4) an evanescent field is developed on the side of the optically rarer phase at the interface when a beam of light is incident from a medium of high refractive index to one of low refractive index and is totally reflected.[25] Since the intensity of the evanescent wave decays exponentially with increasing distance from the interface,[25] falling to undetectable levels within less than one wavelength,[26] the chemical species in the interfacial region can be highly selectively excited;[27] (5) oil-soluble reagents can be employed expediently. Furthermore, the interfacial region presents a good chance to study the orientation of molecules by means of polarized excitation light due to the relatively simple components in it. Therefore, total internal reflection of light at the interface can be coupled with RLS signals, *i.e.* total internal reflected resonance light scattering (TIR-RLS) signals, which can effectively disclose the information of the interface.

Quantitative analyses of nucleic acids are critical to both clinical tests and genetic diagnosis. Methods have been described mainly involving spectrophotometry,[28~30] spectrofluorimetry[31~34] and RLS techniques.[5~10] These methods, however, are generally established in aqueous bulks, and their selectivity and sensitivity are not satisfactory. Herein, we employ a TIR-RLS technique to determine nucleic acids at the H_2O/CCl_4 interface with high selectivity and sensitivity.

2.5.2 Experimental

2.5.2.1 Apparatus

TIR-RLS spectra and intensities were measured with a Hitachi F-2500 spectrofluorometer (Tokyo, Japan). In order to prepare a flat oil/water interface, an optical quartz cell (10 mm) was employed after a fresh coating treatment with a toluene solution containing 2% dichlorodimethylsilane on its lower inside wall so as to render it hydrophobic. The optical arrangement in the sample compartment was constructed as follows: two rightangled quartz prisms (10 mm × 10 mm × 10 mm, Huaguang Optics Co., Chongqing, China) were attached to the two sides of the optical cell facing the excitation light source and the fluorescence detector, respectively. The excitation beam passing through the prism and the cell wall was impinged upon the H_2O/CCl_4 interface with an incident angle of 72.6° (see the Electronic Supplementary Information (ESI)), sufficiently greater than its critical angle, 65.6°.

2.5.2.2 Reagents

The stock solutions of DNAs and RNA were prepared by dissolving commercially purchased calf thymus DNA (ctDNA, Beitai Biochemical Co., Chinese Academy of Sciences, Beijing, China), fish sperm DNA and yeast RNA (fsDNA and yRNA, Shanghai Institute of Biochemistry, Chinese Academy of Sciences, Shanghai, China) in water and stored below 4 °C. Their concentrations were determined according to the ab- sorbances at 260 nm. In this experiment, all the working solutions of nucleic acids were 25.0 $\mu g \cdot mL^{-1}$ (7.5×10^{-5} $mol \cdot L^{-1}$).

A 1.0×10^{-3} $mol \cdot L^{-1}$ Eu(III) stock solution was prepared by dissolving Eu_2O_3 (99.85%, Chemical Plant of

Peking University, Beijing, China) in diluted HCl. The concentration of the Eu(III) working solution was 1.0×10^{-4} mol·L^{-1}. A 1.0×10^{-2} mol·L^{-1} triocyctyl phosphine oxide (TOPO, E. Merck, Darmstadt) solution was prepared in tetrachloromethane. A 1.6×10^{-4} mol·L^{-1} working solution was prepared by diluting the stock solution with tetrachloromethane.

Britton–Robinson buffer solutions (pH 6.37～11.2) were used to control the acidity, while 0.1 mol·L^{-1} NaCl solutions were used to adjust the ionic strength. Nucleic acids were of biochemical-0 reagent grade, and all other reagents were of analytical-reagent grade without further purification. Doubly distilled water was used throughout.

2.5.2.3 Preparation of thermally denatured nucleic acid

Any thermally denatured nucleic acid solutions used in the study were obtained by submerging the calibrated flask, in which nucleic acid solutions had been added, in boiling water for 15 min, and then chilling the flask in ice water for 10 min to prevent the renaturation of the nucleic acids.

2.5.2.4 General procedures

An appropriate volume of sample or working solution of nucleic acids, 1.0 mL of buffer solution, and 3.5 ml of Eu(III) working solution were diluted to 10 ml with water and mixed thoroughly.

A 1.0 mL TOPO working solution and 1.0 ml of the Eu(III)– nucleic acid mixture were successively pipetted into a prepared optical quartz cell, blended thoroughly, and allowed to stand for 35 min before TIR-RLS measurements. The TIR-RLS spectra were obtained by simultaneously scanning the excitation and emission monochromators of the spectrofluorometer from 220 to 700 nm with $\lambda_{ex} = \lambda_{em}$ and the intensities were measured at 348 nm. The spectral bandwidth of the excitation and emission wavelengths was kept at 5.0 nm during the measurements.

2.5.3 Results and discussion

2.5.3.1 Spectral characteristics

As Fig. 1 shows, in the absence of thermally denatured ctDNA, the TIR-RLS intensities of the H_2O/CCl_4 interface are very weak in the region 280～630 nm even if the concentration of Eu(III) or TOPO increases. However, if a trace amount of thermally denatured ctDNA exists, a greatly enhanced TIR-RLS band in the range 330～380 nm characterized by the peak at 348.0 nm can be observed, indicating that a new chemical species has been formed and adsorbed to the interface.

At pH 8.69, Eu(III) can combine with ctDNA to create a binary complex, in which Eu(III) still possesses the ability to combine.[32] In such a case, TOPO, a hydrophobic and synergistic ligand in the CCl_4 phase, can interact with Eu(III). Then the binary hydrophilic complex changes into a ternary amphiphilic species, repelled from both the aqueous and the CCl_4 phases, which, however, can be adsorbed to the interface with the same amphiphilic property and consequently result in a greatly enhanced RLS signal.

2.5.3.2 Optimization of the general procedures

Fig. 2 demonstrates the dependences of TIR-RLS signals of the H_2O/CCl_4 interface on pH values. It is obvious that the two curves are very similar except for the intensities. The similarities can be found in: (1) the TIR-RLS intensities are stable and at a maximum in the optimum pH range located from 7.96 to 8.95, which is most likely ascribed to the deprotonation of the phosphate group that facilitates the interaction between ctDNA and Eu(III); (2) both of the TIR-RLS intensities decrease below pH 7.96 and above pH 8.95. The former may be the result of the protonation of the phosphate group of ctDNA and the latter is most probably due to the gradual formation of insoluble europium hydroxide. The distinction of the intensities can adequately elucidate the nature of the interaction based on Eu(III) and thermally denatured ctDNA. The disassembly of the double-stranded structure of natural ctDNA makes the phosphate group more exposed, causing the interaction of Eu(III) with the phosphate group much easier. This result is analogical to reactions of lanthanide ions (Tb^{3+} and Eu^{3+}) or their complexes with single-stranded DNA and RNA,[35] displaying specific fluorescence enhancement effect.

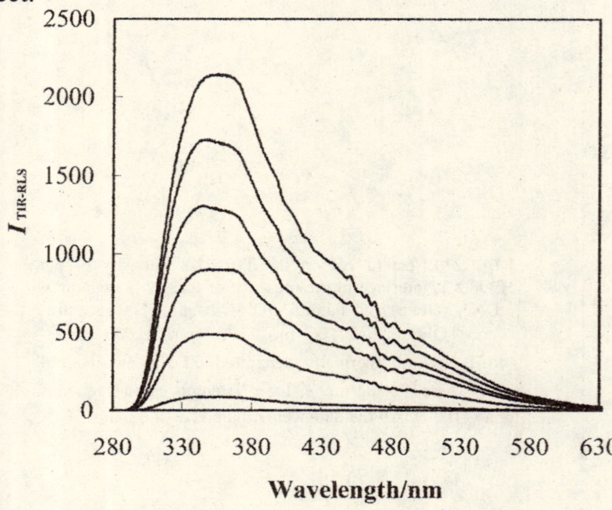

Fig. 1 TIR-RLS spectra of the amphiphilic species of Eu(III)–TOPO and thermally denatured ctDNA–Eu(III)–TOPO adsorbed at the H_2O/CCl_4 interface. Concentrations: TOPO, 1.6 × 10^{-4} mol·L^{-1}; Eu(II), 3.0 × 10^{-5} mol·L^{-1}; thermally denatured ctDNA (from top to bottom, μg·mL^{-1}), 2.5; 2.0; 1.5; 1.0; 0.5; 0.0. pH, 8.69. Ionic strength of the aqueous phase, 0.008.

At pH 8.69, the effect of ionic strength on the TIR-RLS intensity was tested. With ionic strength increasing, the TIRRLS intensity declines obviously. This is probably ascribed to the encumbrance of the combination of Eu(III) with thermally denatured nucleic acid resulting from the gradually increase of the shielding effect of charges on both Eu(III) and the phosphate group.

The relationships between the detection time and the TIR- RLS intensity have been studied. The TIR-RLS signals of both blank and sample are beyond the detection range of the spectrofluorometer about one minute after the interface becomes flat, and then rapidly declines to its detection range. Thirty minutes later, both of the TIR-RLS intensities of the sample and blank are almost stable. This perhaps results from the influence of the emulsification, which produces a lot of emulsion particles and greatly disturbs the TIR-RLS signal. However, the emulsion particles are so unstable that they will disappear in a short period of time. After about 90 min, the TIR- RLS intensities of the sample start to decline gradually, which is probably caused by the instability of the amphiphilic species at the H_2O/CCl_4 interface. In this research we let the interacting system stand motionless for 35 min in the quartz cell before measurements

2.5.3.3 Mole ratio of Eu(III)–thermally denatured ctDNA at the H_2O/CCl_4 interface

In the formation of amphiphilic species, Eu(III) functions as a bridge of the hydrophilic and hydrophobic parts. Consequently, its concentration should be considered. As our work shows, the TIR-RLS intensity strongly depends on Eu(III) concentration. When the Eu(III) concentration is below 8.5 × 10^{-6} mol·L^{-1}, the TIR- RLS intensity increases with increasing Eu(III) concentration. When the Eu(III) concentration is over 8.5 × 10^{-6} mol·L^{-1}, the TIR- RLS intensity is almost constant even if its concentration reaches 3.5 × 10^{-5} mol·L^{-1}. In this assay, 3.5 × 10^{-5} mol·L^{-1} Eu(III) was employed in order that as many amphiphilic species as possible could be produced at the H_2O/CCl_4 interface as many as possible. There is a turning point on the curve, where Eu(III) concentration is 8.5×10^{-6} mol·L^{-1}, indicating that the mole ratio of Eu(III) and thermally denatured ctDNA is 1.89: 1, which can also be obtained by keeping the total concentration of Eu(III) and thermally denatured ctDNA as 1.3×10^{-5} mol·L^{-1} while simultaneously changing the concentrations of the two interacting components. As our work shows, when the mole fraction of Eu(III) is 0.65, the TIR-RLS intensity reaches a maximum, revealing that their mole ratio is 1.86: 1, which is very similar to 1.89: 1. The mole ratios of Eu(III) with thermally denatured fsDNA and yRNA, which can be obtained in the same way, are 3.52: 1 and 3.45: 1, respectively, and are highly analogous to those of Tb(III) with thermally denatured ctDNA, fsDNA, and yRNA,[31] which are 1.67: 1, 3.33: 1, and 3.33: 1, respectively.

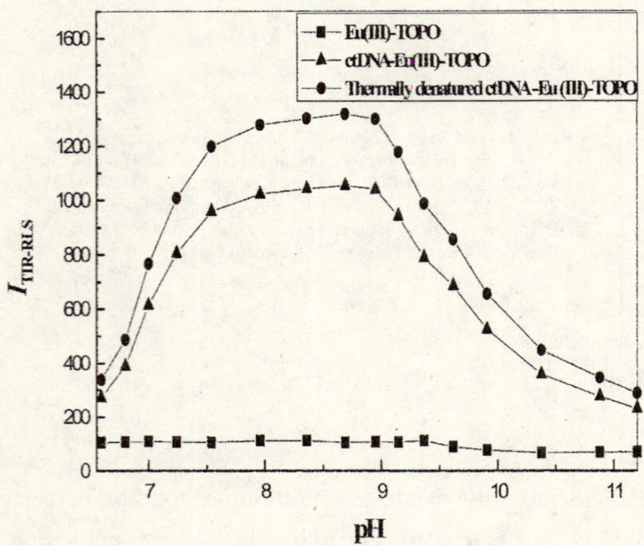

Fig. 2 Effect of pH on the TIR-RLS intensity of the H_2O/CCl_4 interface in the presence of thermally denatured ctDNA (circle) and natural ctDNA (triangle). Concentrations: TOPO, 1.6×10^{-4} mol·L^{-1}; Eu (III), 3.0×10^{-5} mol·L^{-1}; both thermally denatured ctDNA and natural ctDNA are 1.5 μg·mL^{-1}. Ionic strength of the aqueous phase, 0.009. All the data were obtained at 348.0 nm.

2.5.3.4 Selection of hydrophobic synergistic ligands

In order to form amphiphilic species, TOPO was employed to interact with Eu(III). However, other oil-soluble synergistic ligands, such as benzoylacetone, diphenyl guanidine, 1,10-phe- nanthroline and 4,7-diphenyl-1,10-phenanthroline, can also interact with Eu(III). So, selection of a proper ligand is necessary. It has been found that TOPO is the most suitable ligand. Besides, the dependence of the TIR-RLS intensity on the concentration of TOPO has also been tested when the concentrations of Eu(III) and thermally denatured ctDNA are both fixed. We have discovered that the TIR-RLS intensity is stable in the TOPO concentration range of 3.0×10^{-5}~6.0×10^{-5} mol·L^{-1}, and are still constant even though its concentration reaches 1.6×10^{-4} mol·L^{-1}. Therefore, in this work, 1.6×10^{-4} mol·L^{-1} TOPO was used so as to make as many amphiphilic species as possible form at the H_2O/CCl_4 interface as many as possible. It has been noticed that when the thermally denatured ctDNA concentration is fixed at 1.5 μg·mL^{-1}, the TIR-RLS intensity reaches the maximum when the concentrations of Eu(III) and TOPO are 8.5×10^{-6} mol·L^{-1} and 3.0×10^{-5} mol·L^{-1}, respectively. Accordingly, we consider that the mole ratio of TOPO and Eu(III) is 3.53 : 1.

2.4.3.4 Interference of coexisting foreign substances

With a tolerance level of 10%, the influences of coexisting foreign substances including common metal ions, sugars, amino acids, nucleotides, surfactants and proteins have been examined and listed in Table 1. The common metals ions can be allowed at very high concentrations. Especially, K^+, Na^+ and NH_4^+ can be allowed at more than 1.0×10^{-2} mol·L^{-1}. Sugars, β-CD, and amino acids can also be allowed over 11.5×10^{-4} mol·L^{-1}. In addition, proteins such as bovine serum albumin (BSA), human serum albumin (HSA) and γ-globulin (γ-IgG) can be allowed at 15 μg·mL^{-1} [21], 15 μg·mL^{-1} and 10 μg·mL^{-1}, respectively. Obviously, compared with other methods, the selectivity of TIR-RLS method is much better.[5~10,28~34] Therefore, we consider that this analytical approach can be applied to the direct determination of nucleic acids in samples with high interfering backgrounds.

However, Table 1 also shows that nucleotides and some anions such as PO_4^{3-} and $H_2PO_4^-$ can be allowed at very low concentration levels, which may be evidence that Eu(III) bonds with phosphate groups. Cation surfactants and anion surfactants were allowed at much lower concentration levels. The reason for the former may be that cation surfactants can also combine with nucleic acids to form another amphiphilic species, causing serious interferences as a result. The reason for the latter may be that anion surfactants can compete at the sites of the H_2O/CCl_4 interface region with amphiphilic species formed by thermally denatured nucleic acid, Eu(III) and TOPO.

2.5.3.6 Calibration curves and sample analyses

At pH 8.69 and ionic strength 0.008, the linear relationships of enhanced TIR-RLS intensity with the concentration of thermally denatured nucleic acids were obtained according to the standard procedure. All analytical parameters are presented in Table 2. It can be seen that the sensitivities of the TIR-RLS method for different nucleic acids have the following sequence: ctDNA > fsDNA > yRNA. Furthermore, the limits of detection (3s) are 0.16 ng·mL^{-1}, 0.19 ng·mL^{-1} and 0.28 ng·mL^{-1} for the three thermally denatured nucleic acids, correspondingly, showing the sensitivities of this method are much better than those of other methods.[5~10,28~34]

To test the present assay, six complicated artificial samples with high interfering materials were analysed. As Table 3 shows, the results are reproducible and reliable, which proves that the TIR-RLS method can be applied to the direct determination of nucleic acids in complicated samples with high interfering background.

2.5.4 Conclusion

In recent years, the specific phenomena of liquid/liquid interfaces have attracted the interest of many researchers in various fields such as structured array nanoparticle synthesis,[36,37] studies of kinetic mechanisms of synergistic extraction, chelate extraction and ion-pair extraction,[38~45] interface assembly,[46] material and electron transfer,[47~49] protein solvation and liquid films.[50~53] Therefore, it is very important to characterize liquid/liquid interfaces through constructing novel and simple spectroscopic techniques. Our work show that the present TIR-RLS technique is obviously superior to the RLS technique in terms of sensitivity, selectivity, the convenient use of oil-soluble reagents and the investigations of the recognition and interaction between hosts and guests with immiscible properties, and displays high promise in the analysis of samples with high background interferences. Therefore, the TIR-RLS tech- nique is a promising tool and has the prospect of developing into TIR-RLS microscopy in the future. We suppose that TIR-RLS analysis of interfaces may be used to analyze biochemical samples such as biomembranes[54] and nanoparticles synthesis.[36,37] In-depth study of nanoscale membranes will allow the recognition of unknown properties such as water at the edges.[53] In addition, similar to the RLS technique, the TIR-RLS technique can be applied to characterize assembly and aggregate with no color changes and no fluorescent reagents, obviously facilitating the investigations of liquid/liquid interfaces.

Table 1 Tolerance levels of coexisting foreign substances[a]

No.	Coexisting foreign substance	Concentration tolerated/10^{-4} mol·L^{-1}	Change in $I_{TIR\text{-}RLS}$ (%)	No.	Coexisting foreign substance	Concentration tolerated/10^{-4} mol·L^{-1}	Change in $I_{TIR\text{-}RLS}$ (%)
1	Ca(II), Cl^-	25	+7.7	21	Lactose	27	+8.2
2	Mn(I),Cl^-	30	+9.5	22	Maltose	11.5	+9.1
3	Cu(II), Cl^-	10.5	+8.8	23	Sucrose	15	+3.5
4	Ni(I), Cl^-	12	+7.2	24	β-CD	12	+4.8
5	Fe(III), Cl^-	20.5	−5.2	25	L-W	35	+4.5
6	Cr(III), Cl^-	16	+4.6	26	L-C	20	−8.2
7	Mg(I),Cl^-	60	+2.5	27	L-R	42	+6.1
8	Pb(I), Cl^-	55	−3.7	28	5'-AMP	0.003	+9.5
9	Zn(II), Cl^-	60	+5.9	29	5'-GMP	0.003	+8.6
10	Al(III), Cl^-	53	+3.8	30	5'-CMP	0.003	+8.7
11	Hg(I), Cl^-	64	−6.9	31	5'-UMP	0.003	+9.9
12	Co(II), Cl^-	54	−5.6	32	CTMAB	0.0015	+3.6
13	Cd(II), Cl^-	62	+7.6	33	CTMAC	0.0020	+6.1
14	$SO4^{2-}$, Na^+	3	−5.2	34	Zeph	0.0010	+7.7
15	$H_2PO_4^-$, K^+	0.001	+4.2	35	SDBS	0.03	−7.5
16	$PO4^{3-}$,Na^+	0.002	+2.3	36	SDS	0.05	−6.6
17[b]	K^+,Cl^-	120	−5.6	37	SLS	0.09	−4.6
18[b]	Na^+, Cl^-	200	−6.2	38[c]	BSA	15	+2.3
19[b]	NH_4^+, Cl^-	150	+7.7	39[c]	HSA	15	+5.6
20	Glucose	12	+6.4	40[c]	γ-IgG	10	+8.8

[a] Concentrations: TOPO, 1.6×10^{-4} mol·L^{-1}; Eu(III), 3.0×10^{-5} mol·L^{-1}; thermally denatured ctDNA, 1.5 μg·mL^{-1}. pH, 8.69. All the data were obtained at 348.0 nm. β-CD, β-cyclodextrins; L-W, L-tryptophan; L-C, L-cysteine; L-R, L-arginine; 5'-AMP, 5'-aderosine monophosphate; 5'-GMP, 5'-guanosine monophosphate; 5'-CMP, 5'-cytidine monophosphate; 5'-UMP, 5'-uridine monophosphate; CTMAB, cetyltrimethyl ammonium bromide; CTMAC, cetyltrimethyl ammonium chloride; Zeph, zephiramine; SDBS, sodium dodecyl benzene sulfonate; SDS, sodium dodecylsulfonate; SLS, sodium lauryl sulfate; BSA, bovine serum albumin; HSA, human serum albumin; γ-IgG, γ-globulin. [b] The ionic strength of the aqueous phase is 0.008 except for numbers 17, 18 and 19 where the ionic strength of the aqueous phase is 0.012, 0.020 and 0.015, respectively. [c] The concentration of proteins is represented by μg·mL^{-1}.

Table 2 Analytical parameters of the determination[a]

Nucleic acid	Linear range /μg·mL^{-1}	Linear regression equation /c, μg·mL^{-1}	LOD[b]/ 3σ, ng·mL^{-1}	Correlation coefficient
ctDNA	0.002–2.5	$\Delta I_{TIR\text{-}RLS}$ =6.5+ 868.2 c	0.16	0.9979 (n =7)
fsDNA	0.002–2.5	$\Delta I_{TIR\text{-}RLS}$ =3.7 + 749.0 c	0.19	0.9920 (n =7)
yRNA	0.003–2.0	$\Delta I_{TIR\text{-}RLS}$ = 4.6+ 425.6 c	0.28	0.9992 (n =5)

[a] Concentrations: TOPO, 1.6×10^{-4} mol·L^{-1}; Eu(III), 3.0×10^{-5} mol·L^{-1}. pH, 8.69. All the data were obtained at 348.0 nm. The ionic strength of the aqueous phase is 0.008. [b] Limit of detection.

Table 3 Determination results for complicated artificial samples with high interfering backgrounds[a]

Nucleic acids in samples/μg·mL^{-1}	Main additives[b]	Mean found value (n = 5)/μg·mL^{-1}	Recovery range (n = 5)	RSD
ctDNA (1.5)	Mg(II), Ca(I), Co(II), K(I), SLS, lactose, HSA	1.53	98.0～104.5	1.25
ctDNA (1.5)	β-CD, SDS, BSA. Hg(I), glucose, L-W, L-R	1.56	94.8～105.7	2.8
fsDNA (1.5)	Mg(II), Ca(I), Cr(II), β-CD, SDBS, CTMAB, maltose	1.48	96.5～101.2	1.97
fsDNA (1.5)	5'-AMP, 5'-GMP, 5'-CMP, Cd(I), SDS, lactose, L-C	1.54	97.3～105.6	2.53
yRNA (1.5)	Mal, SDS, Pb(I), HAS, Mn(I), Co(I), L-R	1.57	97.6～105.3	2.46
yRNA (1.5)	BSA, Sucrose, 5'-CMP, γ-IgG, glucose, Al(II), L-C	1.48	95.3～99.6	1.89

[a] Concentrations of TOPO and Eu(II) are 1.6×10^{-4} mol·L^{-1} and 3.0×10^{-5} mol·L^{-1}, respectively. pH, 8.69. All the data were obtained at 348.0 nm. The ionic strength of the aqueous phase is 0.008. [b] Concentrations of additives: Proteins, 1 μg·mL^{-1}; nucleotide, 5×10^{-8} mol·L^{-1}; b-CD, 1.0×10^{-4} mol·L^{-1}; metal ions: 5.0×10^{-4} mol·L^{-1}; surfactant, 3×10^{-8} mol·L^{-1}; carbohydrares including glucose, lactose, maltose and sucrose, 2×10^{-4} mol·L^{-1}; amino acids including L-W, L-C and L-R, 2×10^{-4} mol·L^{-1}.

In order to characterize the properties of liquid/liquid interfaces, we are now intending to consider new techniques such as polarized TIR-RLS technique, three-dimension TIR-RLS spectroscopy technique, TIR-RLS correction spectroscopy technique, TIR-RLS imaging technique and time-resolved TIR- RLS technique.

Acknowledgement

We greatly appreciate the financial support of the Excellent Young University Teachers Foundation directed under the Education Ministry of China (No. 2000-11-123) and the Municipal Science Foundation of Chongqing City.

References

[1] Z. H. Yu and L. Brus, J. Phys. Chem. B, 2001, 105, 1123.

[2] V. S. Marinov, Z. S. Nickolov and H. Matsuura, J. Phys. Chem. B, 2001, 105, 9953.

[3] R. F. Pasternack, C. Bustamante, P. J. Collings, A. Giannetto and E. J. Gibbs, J. Am. Chem. Soc., 1993, 115, 5393.

[4] R. F. Pasternack and P. J. Collings, Science (Washington, D.C.), 1995, 269, 935.

[5] C. Z. Huang, K. A. Li and S. Y. Tong, Anal. Chem., 1996, 68, 2259.

[6] C. Z. Huang, K. A. Li and S. Y. Tong, Anal. Chem., 1997, 69, 514.

[7] Z. X. Guo, L. Li, H. X. Shen and X. Cong, Anal. Chim. Acta, 1999, 379, 45.

[8] Y. T. Wang, F. L. Zhao, K. A. Li and S. Y. Tong, Anal. Chim. Acta, 1999, 396, 75.

[9] M. Wang, J. H. Yang, X. Wu and F. Huang, Anal. Chim. Acta, 2000, 422, 151.

[10] Y. F. Li, W. Q. Shu, P. Feng, C. Z. Huang and M. Li, Anal. Sci., 2001, 17, 693.

[11] C. Z. Huang, J. X. Zhu, K. A. Li and S. Y. Tong, Anal. Sci., 1997, 13, 263.

[12] C. Z. Huang, Y. F. Li, J. G. Mao and D. G. Tan, Analyst, 1998, 123, 1401.

[13] G. Yao, K. A. Li and S. Y. Tong, Anal. Chim. Acta, 1999, 398, 319.

[14] S. P. Liu, G. M. Zhou and Z. F. Liu, Chem. J. Chin. Univ., 1998, 19, 1040.

[15] S. P. Liu, Z. F. Liu and G. M. Zhou, Anal. Lett., 1998, 31, 1247.

[16] Y. K. Zhao, Q. E. Cao, Z. D. Hu and Q. H. Xu, Anal. Chim. Acta, 1999, 388, 45.

[17] S. P. Liu, H. Q. Luo, N. B. Li, Z. F. Liu and W. X. Zheng, Anal. Chem., 2001, 73, 3907.

[18] R. F. Pasternack, K. F. Schaefer and P. Hambright, Inorg. Chem., 1994, 33, 2062.

[19] E. Borissevitch, T. T. Tominaga, H. Imasato and M. Tabak, Anal. Chim. Acta, 1997, 343, 281.

[20] C. Z. Huang, K. A. Li and S. Y. Tong, Bull. Chem. Soc. Jpn., 1997, 70, 1843.

[21] J. Parkash, J. H. Robblee, J. Agnew, E. Gibbs, P. Collings, R. F.

[22] Pasternack and J. C. D. Paula, Biophys. J., 1998, 74, 2089.

[23] E. Borissevitch, T. T. Tominaga and C. C. Schmitt, J. Photochem. Photobio. A:Chem., 1998, 114, 201.

[24] J. H. Yang, C. L. Tong, N. Q. Jie, X. Wu, G. L. Zhang and H. Z. Ye, J. Pharm. Biomed. Anal., 1997, 15, 1833.

[25] H. Watarai and Y. Saitoh, Chem. Lett., 1995, 283.

[26] R. Clapp and R. B. Dickinson, Langmuir, 2001, 17, 2182.

[27] M. A. S. Vigeant, M. Wagner, L. K. Tamm and R. M. Ford, Langmuir, 2001, 17, 2235.

[28] R. Okumura, T. Hinoue and H. Watarai, Anal. Sci., 1996, 12, 393.

[29] Z. Huang, K. A. Li and S. Y. Tong, Anal. Chim. Acta, 1997, 345, 235.

[30] Z. Huang, K. A. Li and S. Y. Tong, Chin. J. Anal. Chem., 1997, 25, 1052.

[31] Z. Huang, Y. F. Li, H. Q. Luo, X. H. Huang and S. P. Liu, Anal. Lett., 1998, 31, 1149.

[32] Y. X. Ci, Y. Z. Li and W. B. Chang, Anal. Chim. Acta, 1991, 248, 589.

[33] Y. X. Ci, Y. Z. Li and X. J. Liu, Anal. Chem., 1995, 67, 1785.

[34] C. Z. Huang, Y. F. Li and S. Y. Tong, Anal. Lett., 1997, 30, 1305.

[35] C. G. Lin, J. H. Yang, G. L. Zhang, X. Wu, R. J. Han, X. H. Cao and

[36] Z. Q. Gao, Anal. Chim. Acta, 1999, 392, 291.

[37] S. Cross and H. Simpkins, J. Biol. Chem., 1981, 256, 9593.

[38] R. Aveyard and J. H. Clint, J. Chem. Soc., Faraday Trans., 1995, 91, 2681.

[39] Bresme and N. Quirke, Phys. Chem. Chem. Phys., 1999, 1, 2149.

[40] Watarai, K. Sasaki, K. Takahashi and J. Murakami, Talanta, 1995, 42, 1691.

[41] Watarai, K. Takahashi and J. Murakami, Solvent Extr. Res. Dev. Jpn., 1996, 3, 109.

[42] Y. Yulizar, A. Ohashi, H. Nagatani and H. Watarai, Anal. Chim. Acta, 2000, 419, 107.

[43] Y. Yulizar, A. Ohashi and H. Watarai, Anal. Chim. Acta, 2001, 447, 247.

[44] Y. Chida and H. Watarai, Bull. Chem. Soc. Jpn., 1996, 69, 341.

[45] Y. Saitoh and H. Watarai, Bull. Chem. Soc. Jpn., 1997, 70, 351.

[46] Watarai, Trends Anal. Chem., 1993, 12, 313.

[47] H. Freiser, Bull. Chem. Soc. Jpn., 1988, 61, 39.

[48] N. Fujiwara, S. Tsukahara and H. Watarai, Langmuir, 2001, 17, 5337.

[49] Shao, Y. H. ; M. V. Mirkin and J. F. Rusling, J. Phys. Chem. B, 1997, 101, 3202.

[50] H. Nagatani and H. Watarai, Anal. Chem., 1998, 70, 2860.

[51] B. Liu and M. V. Mirkin, J. Am. Chem. Soc., 1999, 121, 8352.

[52] S. K. Pal, J. Peon and A. H. Zewail, Proc. Natl. Acad. Sci. USA, 2002, 99, 1763.

[53] D. P. Tieleman, H. J. C. Berendsen and M. S. P. Sansom, Biophys. J., 2001, 80, 331.

[54] P. J. Rossky, Nature, 2001, 410, 645.

[55] L. F. Scatena, M. G. Brown and G. L. Richmond, Science (Washington, DC), 2001, 292, 908.

[56] L. E. Morrison and G. Weber, Biophys. J., 1987, 52, 367.

(Wei Lu, Cheng Zhi Huang and Yuan Fang Li, published in *The Analyst*, 2002, 127, 1392～1396)

2.6 Backscattering Light Detection of Nucleic Acids with Tetraphenylporphyrin–Al(III)–Nucleic Acids at Liquid/Liquid Interface

Abstract: A backscattering light (BSL) detection assembly is constructed and applied to the determination of nucleic acids with high sensitivity and selectivity based on the measurements of BSL signals at water/tetrachloromethane (H_2O/CCl_4) interface. In aqueous medium of pH 3, the binary complex of of Al(III)–DNAs could be formed by the interaction of Al(III) with the phosphate group of DNAs, which then could interact with tetraphenylporphyrin (TPP) in tetrachloromethane through liquid/liquid interaction, forming a ternary complex of TPP–Al(III)–DNAs at the interface. It was observed that greatly enhanced BSL signals occurred with maximum peak at 469 nm when the ternary complex of TPP–Al(III)–DNAs were absorbed to the liquid/liquid interface. The enhanced backscattering light intensity (I_{BSL}) is in proportion to the concentration of calfthymus DNA (ctDNA) and fish sperm DNA (fsDNA) in the range of 0.6～1200 ng·mL^{-1} and 1.1～1200 ng·mL^{-1}, respectively. The limits of determination (3σ) are 60 pg·mL^{-1} and 110 pg·mL^{-1}, correspondingly. Artificial samples with highly interference backgrounds were determined with the recovery ranging from 94.5% to 106.7%, and relative standard deviation (RSD) less than 2.4%.

Keywords: Backscattering light (BSL); Tetraphenylporphyrin (TPP); Nucleic acids; Al(III)

2.6.1 Introduction

Light scattering spectroscopy (LSS) is extensively used in physical sciences. It has been demonstrated that light scattering can provide structural and functional information about the tissue[1,2]. Backscattering signal is a wavelength-dependent oscillatory component, and its amplitude is related to cellularity or the population density of the epithelial nuclei. By analyzing the frequency and amplitude of this oscillatory component, the size distribution and density of epithelial nuclei can be extracted [2]. Polarized light scattering spectroscopy was reported that it could provide a direct experimental method for distinguish single-scattering component from the diffusive background[3]. Thus biomedical imaging with polarized light-scattering spectroscopy is developed to probe the structure of living epithelial cells in situ without needing tissue preparation or removal[4]. Mehrubeoglu et al. advanced a noninvasive in vivo optical technique, by diffusing reflectance spectroscopic imaging with oblique incidence, to successfully distinguish benign and cancer-prone skin lesions[5]. Therein oblique incidence has an advantage over normal incidence by gathering information from superficial layers without penetrating deep the tissue[6].

Resonance light scattering (RLS) technique, which was established by scanning the excitation and emission monochromator of a common spectrofluorometer to measure the enhanced scattering signals in the region of molecular absorption band, has been successfully exploited as a sensitive and selective tool to investigate the electronic and geometrical properties of aggregated chromophores, such as porphyrins[7～9], and chlorophyll[10]. It has proved to be an important and powerful tool either for the quantification of nucleic acids[11～14], proteins[15,16], metallic ions[17], and drugs[18] in artificial and practical samples, or for the characterization of the aggregation and assembly of biological and chemical species[19～21]. Since the spectral signals variations of single backscattering could afford the information about the size distribution, shape and refractive index of the scatterers[3], the fluctuation of the refractive index at the liquid/liquid interface indicates to us that the scattering of light at the liquid/liquid interface can be coupled with RLS measurements, and sensitively used to probe the interface properties. Absorption and reaction at the liquid/liquid interfaces have recently become attractive subjects in the fundamental studies of solvent extraction of metal ions, the detection of liquid-membrane separation, ion-selective electrodes, optical sensors, and counter current chromatography[22]. We formerly coupled the RLS technique with total internal reflected light (TIR) at the liquid/liquid interface, and successfully developed a highly selective and sensitive method of determination of chlortetracycline, human serum albumin, nucleic acids, and thiamine[23~26]. Liquid/liquid interfaces are also suitable for model systems to study processes that occur at biological and artificial membranes. Herein, we display our attempt to develop a backscattering light (BSL) technique, with the aid of the operation procedure of resonance light scattering technique to measure the scattering signals by simultaneously scanning the excitation and emission monochromator of the spectrofluorometer without wavelength difference of the two monochromator, to detect the nucleic acids at the H_2O/CCl_4 interface considering that tetraphenylporphyrin (TPP) is a highly hydrophobic chelate reagent with a very large molar absorptivity of 4.70×10^5 $dm^3{\cdot}mol^{-1}{\cdot}cm^{-1}$ at 418.0 nm in tetrachloromethane, and has high promise for use on the interface studies to investigate the protonation and the demetalaltion of metalloporphyrin at the interface[27,28], and the formation of the supramolecular sensitizer[29].

2.6.2 Experimental

2.6.2.1 Apparatus

BSL spectra and intensities measurements were con- ducted on a Hitachi F-2500 spectrofluorometer (Tokyo, Japan) by simultaneously scaning the excitation and emission monochromator of the spectrofluorometer with $\Delta\lambda$ = 0. The sample chamber of the spectrofluorometer was changed and mounted our designed optical assembly as shown in Fig. 1. The optical assembly consists of two parts. One is the oblique incidence section, in which a right-angle prism is attached to the cell facing the excitation monochromator in order to guide the excitation to illuminate the scatterers at the H_2O/CCl_4 interfaces in the cell. The other is the transmission signal section, which is composed of three total reflecting prisms attached together by optical glue. In order to lessen the energy losses of the light signals, the bevel of the prism is aluminum film plated. The BSL signals of the analyte concentrated at the interface passed through the total reflecting prism and are detected by the emission monochromator.

A Techcomp UV-8500 spectrophotometer (Hong Kong, PR China) was used for absorption measurements. A pH-3C digital pH meter (Xiaoshan Scientific Instrument Plant, Zhejiang, PR China) was used to measure the pH values of the aqueous solutions, and MVS-1 vortex mixter (Beide Scientific Instrument Ltd., Beijing, PR China) was used to blend the solutions in volumetric flasks.

In order to prepare a flat oil/water interface, an optical quartz cell was employed after a fresh coating treatment with a toluene solution containing 2% dichlorodimethylsilane on its lower (8.0 mm) inside wall so as to make it hydrophobic. It has proved that the flat interface of the lower inside wall after one hydrophobic pretreatment could undergo repetitive use more than 500 time.

2.6.2.2 Reagents

The stock solutions of DNAs were prepared by dissolving commercially purchased calf thymus DNA (ctDNA, Beitai Biochemical Co., Chinese Academy of Sciences, Beijing, PR China), fish sperm DNA (fsDNA, Shanghai

Institute of Biochemistry, Chinese Academy of Sciences, Shanghai, PR China) in water and stored at 0～4 °C, and 24 h or more was needed for the dissolution, accompanied by occasional gentle shaking. Their concentrations were determined according to the absorbances at 260 nm. All working solutions of DNAs were 10.0 μg·mL^{-1}.

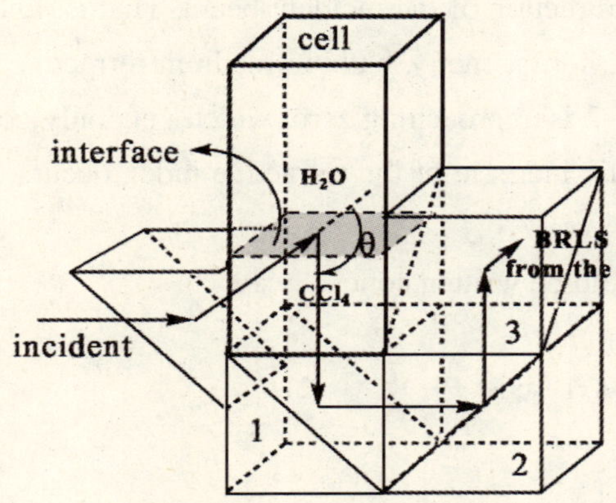

Fig. 1 Optical assembly for the backscattering light (BSL) measurements at the liquid/liquid interface. 1, 2, and 3: total reflecting prism.

Free base porphyrin, *α*, *β*, *γ*, *δ*-tetraphenylporphine (TPP) synthesized in our laboratory according to literature[30] and identified by ^{1}HNMR and IR, was dissolved in tetrachloromethane. The concentration of the solution was determined according to its absorbance at 419.0 nm (the Soret maxima) by using $\varepsilon = 4.7\times10^5$ M^{-1}·cm^{-1} in tetrachloromethane [30]. Its work solution is 2.0×10^{-6} mol·L^{-1}. The stock solution of Al(III) was prepared by dissolving 1.759 g $KAl(SO_4)_2\cdot12H_2O$ in 1000 mL doubly distilled water.

Britton–Robinson buffer solutions (pH 1.81～5.72) were used to control the acidity of the aqueous solutions, while 0.5 M KCl solutions were used to adjust the ionic strength. Nucleic acids were of biochemical reagent grade, and all other reagents were of analytical-reagent grade without further purification. Doubly distilled water was used throughout. All measurements were performed at room temperature (25±2 °C).

2.6.2.3 Standard procedure

Appropriate volume of sample or working solution of nucleic acids was placed in a 10 mL volumetric flask, and then 1.0 mL of buffer solution added. After vortexed, 1.0 mL of Al(III) working solution was added. The mixture was vortexed again and diluted to 10 mL with doubly distilled water and then mixed thoroughly. A 0.80 mL TPP working solution was pipetted into a dry optical quartz cell, along with 2.0 mL of the aqueous solution mixture. The mixture was vortexed thoroughly, and then allows standing for 20 min. The optical quartz cell was mounted on the assembly for BSL measurements. The BSL spectra were obtained by scanning simultaneously the excitation and emission monochromators of the spectrofluorometer from 300 to 600 nm with $\lambda_{ex} = \lambda_{em}$, and I_{BSL} was measured at 469.0 nm using a slit width of 5.0 nm for both excitation and emission with the luminescence mode.

2.6.3 Results and discussion

2.6.3.1 General considerations for BSL assembly design

The scattered light intensity by a spherical particle illuminated by monochromatic light can be expressed as Rayliegh scattering law[33,34]

$$I = \frac{8\pi^4 a^6 n_{med}^4 I_o}{d^2 \lambda_0^4}\left|\frac{m^2-1}{m^2+2}\right|^2 (1+\cos^2\theta) \qquad (1)$$

where I_0 is the intensity of incident monochromatic light, a is the particle radius, n_{med} is the refractive index of the medium surrounding the particle, d is the distance between the particle and the position where the scattered light is detected, m is the relative refractive index of the bulk particle material, and θ is scattering angle which is decided by the detection direction and the forward direction of the incident beam. That is, light-scattering properties of a particle depend on composition, size, shape, homogeneity, bathing medium refractive index, and the scattering angle. When the denominator of Eq. (1) $m^2 + 2$ is approaching zero, which generally occurs at the wavelength of the molecular absorption region where dramatic increase of the refractive index occurs, greatly enhanced light scattering then could be observed.

Considering the scattering angle, Eq. (1) could be written concisely as

$$I = K(1+\cos^2\theta) \qquad (2)$$

Where

$$K = \frac{8\pi^4 a^6 n_{med}^4 I_o}{d^2\lambda_0^4}\left|\frac{m^2-1}{m^2+2}\right|^2 \qquad (3)$$

which is a constant related to the intensity of the incident beam and the refractive index of medium. As Eq. (2) demon- strates, the scattered light intensity is greatly dependent on the scattering angle θ. For example, the scattered light in- tensity (I) is two times greater in the forward direction ($\theta = 0°$) or backward direction ($\theta = 180°$) than that at right angles to the incident beam ($\theta = 90°$).

Backward light-scattering spectroscopy has been demonstrated an effective means of detecting abnormalities in epithelial-cell nuclei associated with neoplasia, a precancerous state[31], and obtaining information about both the cell nuclei and smaller structures at various scattering angles[32]. Based on this consideration, we designed a new assembly as shown in Fig. 1 to detect backscattering light (BSL) signals at the liquid/liquid interface with θ larger than 90°. In this optical arrangement, the incident beam emitted from the Xe lamp of the spectrofluorometer passed through the prism and reached to the liquid/liquid interface. According to the Snell law, the incidence angle is ca. 72.6° and sufficiently greater than the critical angle of 65.6° for the occurrence of total internal reflection at the H_2O/CCl_4 interfaces as the variation of refractive index between the oil and water phases. Thus an evanescent field was developed on the side of water phase at the interface[23,35]. Therefore, the BSL signals with the scattering angle θ of 107.4° resulting from the scatterers at the interface illuminated by the incidence beam can be detected with the aid of three holophotes as shown in Fig. 1.

2.6.3.2 Spectral characteristics of the interaction

Fig. 2 displays the BSL spectral features from the interfaces of ctDNA, TPP–Al(III), TPP–ctDNA, and TPP–Al(III)–ctDNA. It can be seen that the BSL signals of ctDNA, TPP–ctDNA and TPP–Al(III) were very faint in the range of 300～600 nm. However, the greatly enhanced BSL signals of TP –Al(III)–ctDNA could be observed in the range of 440～470 nm characterized by the maximum scat- tering peak at 469 nm, and I_{BSL} increases with increasing nucleic acids concentration. Since the intense absorption of the TPP at 418 nm (the Soret band), the minimum BSL peak appears at 420 nm due to the strong absorption of the scattered light by TPP. Although the BSL signals of TPP–ctDNA are stronger than that of TPP–Al(III), they are still weaker than those of TPP–Al(III)–ctDNA in the range of 300～600 nm, indicating that interaction in the TPP–Al(III)–ctDNA system has occurred and the formed scatterers are adsorbed to the interface. Similar BSL could be obtained for

TPP–Al(III)–fsDNA.

In the aqueous solution, Al(III) can interact with ctDNA to form a binary complex of Al(III)–ctDNA[36]. The inner graph in Fig. 2 displays the Rayleigh scattering spectra features of the binary complex, which are mainly related to the non-corrected spectra sensitivity of the spectrofluorometer. Nevertheless, Al(III) still has the capability of combination in this complex with synergistic ligands. In the presence of TPP in CCl_4, the interaction of Al(III) with TPP results in the formation and adsorption of the ternary complex of TPP–Al(III)–ctDNA at the H_2O/CCl_4 interface. Since the ternary complex does not posses any absorption in the spectra region of 300～700 nm, the enhanced BSL signals should be ascribed to the common Rayleigh scattering non-corrected by the spectral sensitivity of the spectrofluorometer, not the enhaced resonace light scattering signals. As later will proved, linear relationships between I_{BSL} and the content of DNAs are obeyed in wide range, which further proves that the observed BSL signals should be ascribed to the common Rayleigh scattering. There is a possibility, however, the enhanced BSL signals results from the aggregation of DNA stimulated by the interaction with Al(III) and TPP from the insert on Fig. 2 since DNA has molecular absorption band in 240～290 nm region.

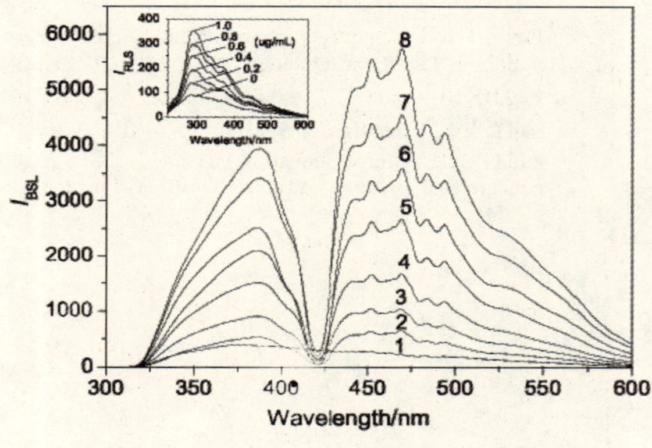

Fig. 2 BSL spectra of ctDNA (curve 1), TPP–Al (III) (curve 2), TPP–ctDNA (curve 3), TPP–Al (III)–ctDNA (curves 4–8) at the H_2O/CCl_4 interface. Inner graphic is the RLS spectra of the Al(III)– ctDNA in the aqueous phases. Concentrations: TPP, 1, 0; 2–8, 2.0 × 10^{-6} mol·L^{-1}; Al(III), 1 and 3, 0; 2, 4–8, 3.0 × 10^{-6} mol·L^{-1}; ctDNA (μg·mL^{-1}), 1, 0.5; 2, 0; 3, 0.5; 4, 0.2; 5, 0.4; 6, 0.6; 7, 0.8; 8, 1.0. pH 3, ionic strength, 0.003 mol·L^{-1}. Spectra are not corrected using the instrument sensitivity function.

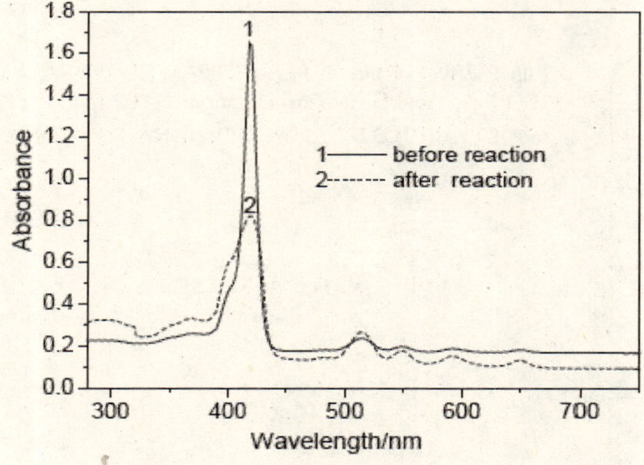

Fig. 3 The absorbance spectra variation of TPP in organic phases. Con- centration: TPP, 2.0 × 10^{-6} mol·L^{-1}, ctDNA, 0.5 μg·mL^{-1}, Al(III), 3.0 × 10^{-6} mol·L^{-1}. pH 3, ionic strength, 0.003 mol·L^{-1}.

We can infer this mechanism from the absorbency variation of TPP in CCl_4 solution as shown in Fig. 3. It shows the absorption spectra of TPP before and after the reaction. The absorbency of TPP at 418 nm (the Soret band) in organic phases evidently decline, indicating that the porphyrin molecule had reacted with the binary complex of Al(III)–ctDNA. The maximum absorption of TPP at 418 nm almost is consistent with the minimum scattering at 420 nm. We assume that the minimum in the intensity around 420 nm in the BSL spectra is surely due to absorption and scattering of incident light by porphyrin monomers in CCl_4 solution. Fig. 4 shows the BSL spectra variations of different concen- trations of TPP. Our results demonstrate that the BSL spectra vary with different TPP concentrations, and I_{BSL} withdraws when the concentration of TPP is in large excess of Al(III).

2.6.3.3 Optimization of the general procedures

The dependence of I_{BSL} on the pH of the aqueous medium was investigated. As Fig. 5 shows, the I_{BSL} of TPP–Al(III)–ctDNA varies with the pH of the aqueous medium and increases with the increase of pH values. The strongest signals can be found in the pH 3, and then I_{BSL} rapidly reduces instead with increasing values of pH. When pH is over 4.5, due to the hydrolysis of Al(III) into $Al(OH)^{2+}$, $Al_2(OH)_4^{2+}$, and $Al(OH)_3$, floccules could be observed and absorbed to interface, resulting in greatly enhanced $I_{BSL.}$ In this work, the aqueous solution acid was controlled with a Britton–Robinson buffer solution at pH 3.

At pH 3, the effect of ionic strength on the I_{BSL} was tested. As Fig. 6 shows, with ionic strength increasing, I_{BSL} declines evidently. We suppose that is due to the weakness of the combination of Al(III) with nucleic acid, resulting from the gradual increase of the shielding effect of charges on both Al(II) and the phosphate group. The whole determination was carried out with the ionic strength 0.0033 mol·L^{-1}.

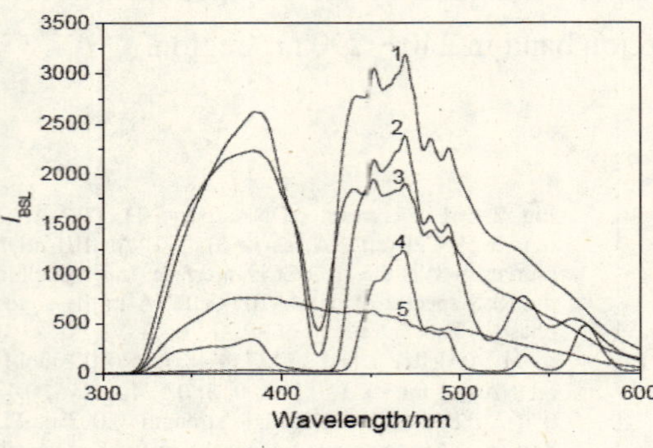

Fig. 4 The BSL spectra variation of the different concentrations of TPP. Concentration: TPP, 1, 2.0×10^{-6} mol·L^{-1}; 2, 2.0×10^{-7} mol·L^{-1}; 3, 2.0×10^{-5} mol·L^{-1}; 4, 2.0×10^{-4} mol·L^{-1}; 5, 0; ctDNA, 0.5 μg·mL^{-1}; Al(III), 3.0×10^{-6} mol·L^{-1}. pH 3, ionic strength 0.003 mol·L^{-1}. Spectra are not corrected using the instrument sensitivity function.

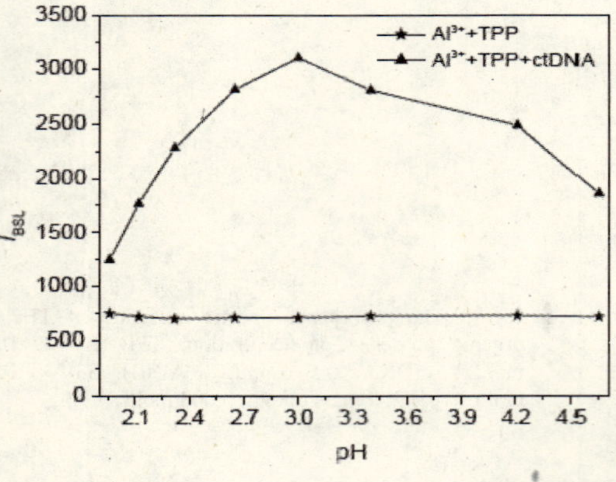

Fig. 5 Effect of pH on I_{BSL} of TPP–Al(III)–ctDNA at the H_2O/CCl_4 interface. Concentrations: TPP, 2.0×10^{-6} mol·L^{-1}; Al(III), 3.0×10^{-6}mol·L^{-1}; ctDNA, 0.5 μg·mL^{-1}.

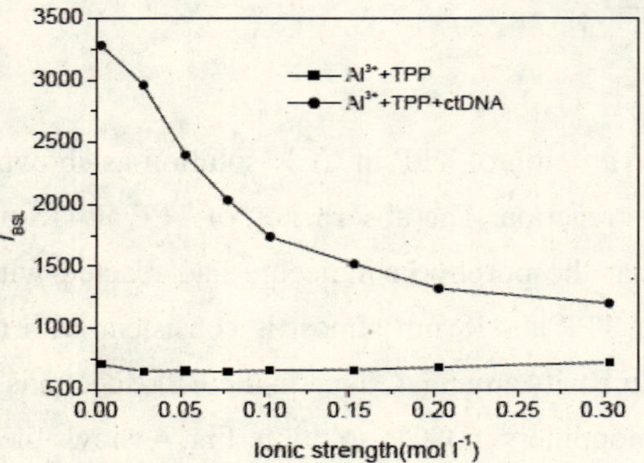

Fig. 6 Effect of ionic strength on $I_{BSL.}$ Concentrations: TPP, 2.0×10^{-6}mol·L^{-1}; Al(III), 3.0×10^{-6}mol·L^{-1}; ctDNA, 0.5 μg·mL^{-1}. pH 3 gradual increase of the shielding effect of charges on both Al(III) and the phosphate group. The whole determination was carried out with the ionic strength 0.0033 mol·L^{-1}.

The relationship of I_{BSL} with the interface height was studied. When the interface height was lower or higher, the incidence light would illuminate the portion of the interfacial scatters, resulting in the decrease of I_{BSL}. In this work, we employed the interface height of 0.80 cm.

2.6.3.4 Interference of coexisting foreign substance

With a tolerance level of 10%, the influences of coexisting foreign substances including common metal ions, sugars, amino acids, surfactants, and proteins have been examined and listed in Table 1. The common metals ions can be allowed at very high concentrations. Especially, K^+, Na^+ can be allowed at more than 2.5×10^{-2} mol·L^{-1}, and sugars can be allowed at 1.0×10^{-3} mol·L^{-1}. Proteins such as bovine serum albumin (BSA) and human serum albumin (HSA) can be allowed at 25.0 μg·mL^{-1}. These data show that, compared with other methods, the selectivity of this BSL method is much better[9~16,18]. Table 1 also shows that some cation surfactants and anion surfactants were allowed at much lower concentration levels. The reason may be that cation surfactants could also combine with nucleic acids to form another amphiphilic species, and anion surfactants can compete at the sites of the H_2O/CCl_4 interface region with amphiphilic species formed by TPP–Al(III)–ctDNA, causing serious interferences as a result. It was found that even if some macroscopic suspending substances existed in the aqueous phase, they couldn't disturb the determination. We suppose that it is because these particles cannot be adsorbed on the interface by the ternary complex, indicating that this technique can be used to study the interfacial reaction. Therefore, we consider that this analytical approach can be applied to direct determination of nucleic acids in samples with high interfering backgrounds[21,23~25].

Table 1 Tolerance levels of coexisting foreign substances

Foreign substances	Concentration (10^{-4} mol·L^{-1})	Change of I_{BSL} (%)	Foreign substances	Concentration (10^{-4} mol·L^{-1})	Change of I_{BSL} (%)
Co(III),Cl⁻	10	-7.8	Lactose	5.0	-4.69
Cd(II), Cl⁻	10	+5.6	Maltose	10	-3.25
Mg(II), Cl⁻	50	-5.8	Sucrose	15	+4.58
Ca(II), Cl⁻	20	-3.5	L-Phen	0.5	-1.0
Cr(III), Cl⁻	100	-5.6	L-Ser	0.1	+8.96
Ni(II), Cl⁻	25	-7.1	Glycin	0.5	-4.43
Pb(II), Cl⁻	50	-4.7	L-Lys	0.5	-3.44
Mn(II), Cl⁻	10	-6.98	SDBS	0.01	+2.8
Fe(III), Cl⁻	10	-9.6	CTMAB	0.01	+8.5
K(I), Cl⁻	250	-5.9	SDS	0.05	+2.6
Na(I), Cl⁻	500	+6.31	SLS	0.05	+3.9
Zn(I), Cl⁻	50	+3.9	BSA	25[a]	+3.4
Urea	50	-9.3	HSA	25[a]	+4.8

Notes: Values with superscript letter 'a' are in μg·mL^{-1}. Concentrations: TPP, 2.0×10^{-6}mol·L^{-1}; Al(III), 3.0×10^{-6}mol·L^{-1}; ctDNA, 0.5 μg·mL^{-1}; pH 3; ionic strength, 0.003 mol·L^{-1}

2.6.3.5 Calibration curves and sample analyses

According to the general procedures, the relationship of I_{BSL} at the interface and the concentration of ctDNA and fsDNA were constructed (Fig. 7). The enhanced I_{BSL} is in proportion to the concentration of ctDNA and fsDNA in the range of 0.6~1200 ng·mL^{-1} and 1.1~1200 ng·mL^{-1}, respectively, and the linear regression equations were $\Delta I = 693.8 + 4.96\times c$(ng·mL^{-1}; $r = 0.9998$; $n = 6$) and $\Delta I = 105.2 + 3.60\times c$(ng·mL^{-1}; $r = 0.9995$; $n = 6$), with their limits of determination (3σ) between 60 and 110 pg·mL^{-1}, correspondingly. These analytical parameters show that the sensitivities of this method are much high[11~13].

To test the present assay, four synthetic samples for ctDNA and fsDNA containing metal ions, sugars, amino acids, and surfactants were determined, and the results were given in Table 2. It can be seen that the recovery ranges from 94.5 to 106.7%, and R.S.D. is <2.4%. These values are very satisfactory for the determinations of synthetic samples, which proves that this method can be applied to the direct determination of nucleic acids in complicated samples with high interference background.

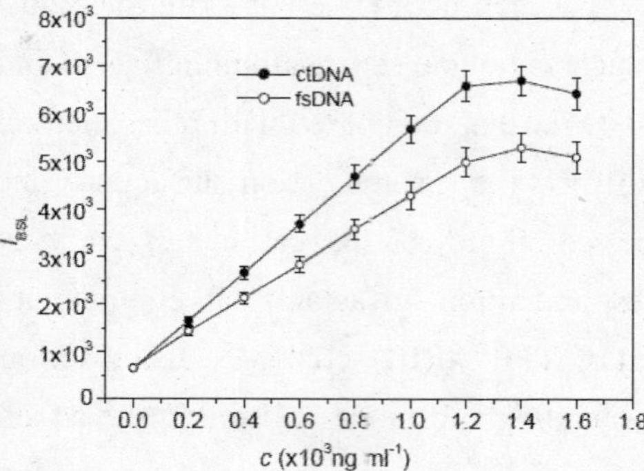

Fig. 7. Calibration graphs for the detection of ctDNA and fsDNA by BSL methods. Errors bars represent one standard deviation for four measurements. Concentrations: TPP, 2.0×10^{-6} mol·L^{-1}; Al(III), 3.0×10^{-6} mol·L^{-1}; pH 3, ionic strength, 0.003 mol·L^{-1}. The linear regression equations were $\Delta I = 693.8 + 4.96\ c(r = 0.9998;\ n = 6)$ and $\Delta I = 105.2 + 3.60\ c(r = 0.9995;\ n = 6)$, with their limits of determination (3σ) of 60 pg·mL^{-1} and 110 pg·mL^{-1}, correspondingly.

Table 2 Determination results for synthetic sample

Nucleic acids in samples (μg·mL^{-1})	Main interferences[a]	Found[b] (μg·mL^{-1})	Recovery range[b] (%)	R S D[b](%)
ctDNA (0.5)	Ni(II),Fe(III),Na(I), CTMAB, L-Lys	0.49	95.0–103.1	2.35
ctDNA (0.5)	Co(III),Cd(II),SDB, L-Ser, lactose	0.48	96.0–105.8	2.40
fsDNA (0.5)	Ca(II),Mg(II),maltose,L-Phen,SDBS	0.51	94.5–104.7	1.97
fsDNA (0.5)	urea,Mn(II),L-Lys,glycin, Zn(II)	0.49	97.3–106.7	2.28

[a] Concentrations: Ni(II), 1.0×10^{-4} mol·L^{-1}; Fe(III), 0.4×10^{-4} mol·L^{-1}; Na(I), 20×10^{-4} mol·L^{-1}; CTMAB, 0.04×10^{-6} mol·L^{-1}; L-Lys, 0.02×10^{-4} mol·L^{-1}; Co(III), 0.4×10^{-4} mol·L^{-1}; Cd(II), 0.4×10^{-4} mol·L^{-1}; SDB, 0.2×10^{-6} mol·L^{-1}; L-Ser, 1.0×10^{-4} mol·L^{-1}; lactose, 0.5×10^{-4} mol·L^{-1}; Ca(II), 0.8×10^{-4} mol·L^{-1}; Mg(II), 2.0×10^{-4} mol·L^{-1}; maltose, 0.4×10^{-4} mol·L^{-1}; L-Phen, 0.02×10^{-4} mol·L^{-1}; SDBS, 0.04×10^{-6} mol·L^{-1}; urea, 2.0×10^{-4} mol·L^{-1}; Mn (II), 0.4×10^{-4} mol·L^{-1}; L-Lys, 0.02×10^{-4} mol·L^{-1}; glycin, 0.02×10^{-4} mol·L^{-1}; Zn(II) 2.0×10^{-4} mol·L^{-1}.

[b] The results were obtained from five measurements. TPP, 2.0×10^{-6} mol·L^{-1}; Al(III), 3.0×10^{-6} mol·L^{-1}; ctDNA, 0.5 μg·mL^{-1}; pH 3; ionic strength, 0.003 mol·L^{-1}.

2.6.4 Conclusions

A remarkably sensitive and selective BSL technique at interface for nucleic acids assay has been developed. The TPP–Al(III)–ctDNA is a very simple supramolecular complex. Results of the greatly enhanced I_{BSL} at interface with the increasing concentration of nucleic acids reveal that this content of the supramolecular complex is proportional directly to trace amount of nucleic acids. The results obtained here indicated that BSL method is a very promising method and it provides a wider field of interface studies or the studies on turbid media. In addition, this technique is very appropriate to investigate recognition between hosts and guests with an immiscible property free from surfactants as emulsifiers because they can encounter and interact at liquid/liquid interfaces. And if coupled with the imaging BSL technique and polarization technique, it is possible to study the morphology of the complex at the liquid/liquid interfaces.

Acknowledgements

All authors herein are grateful to the supports of the National Natural Science Foundation of China (No.: 20275032), and the Municipal Science and Technology Committee of Chongqing, PR China.

References

[1] J.R. Mourant,I.J. Bigio, J. Boyer, R.L. Conn, T. Johnson, T. Shimada, Laser Surg. Med. 17 (1995) 350.

[2] L.T. Perelman, V. Backman, M. Wallace, G. Zonios, R. Manoharan, A. Nusrat, S. Shields, M. Seiler, C. Lima, T. Hamano, I. Itzkan, J. Van Dam, J.M. Crawford, M.S. Feld, Phys. Rev. Lett. 80 (1998) 627.

[3] V. Backman, R. Gurjar, K. Badizadegan, I. Itzkan, R.R. Dasari, L.T. Perelman, IEEE J. Sel. Top. Quantum Electron. 5(1999) 1019.

[4] R. Gurjar, V. Backman, L.T. Perelman, I. Georgakoudi, K. Badizadegan, I. Itzkan, R.R. Dasari, M.S. Feld, Nature 7(2001) 1245.

[5] M. Mehrubeoglu, N. Kehtarnavaz, G. Marquez, M. Duvic, L.V. Wang, Appl. Opt. 41 (2002) 182.G. Marquez, L.H. Wang, Opt.Express 1(1997) 454.

[6] R.F. Pasternack, C. Bustamante, P.J. Collings, A. Giannetto, E.J. Gibbs, J. Am. Chem. Soc. 115 (1993) 5393.

[7] P.J. Collings, E.J. Gibbs, T.E. Starr, O. Vafek, C. Yee, L.A. Pomerance, R.F. Pasternack, J. Phys. Chem. B 103 (1999) 8474.

[8] R.F. Pasternack, P.J. Collings, Science 269 (1995) 935.

[9] J.C. Paula, J.H. Robblee, R.F. Pasternack, Biophys. J. 68 (1995) 335.

[10] C.Z. Huang, K.A. Li, S.Y. Tong, Anal. Chem. 68 (1996) 2259.

[11] C.Z. Huang, K.A. Li, S.Y. Tong, Anal. Chem. 69 (1997) 514.

[12] Y.T. Wang, F.L. Zhao, K.A. Li, S.Y. Tong, Anal. Chim. Acta 396 (1999) 75.

[13] M. Wang, J.H. Yang, X. Wu, F. Huang, Anal. Chim. Acta 422 (2000) 151.

[14] C.Z. Huang, Y.F. Li, J.G. Mao, D.G. Tan, Analyst 123 (1998) 1401.

[15] C.Z. Huang, J.X. Zhu, K.A. Li, S.Y. Tong, Anal. Sci. 13 (1997) 263.

[16] Y.K. Zhao, Q.E. Cao, Z.D. Hu, Q.H. Xu, Anal. Chim. Acta 388 (1999) 45.

[17] S.P. Liu, H.Q. Luo, N.B. Li, Z.F. Liu, W.X. Zheng, Anal. Chem. 73 (2001) 3907.

[18] R.F. Pasternack, K.F. Schaefer, P. Hambright, Inorg. Chem. 33 (1994) 2062.

[19] C.Z. Huang, K.A. Li, S.Y. Tong, Bull. Chem. Soc. Jpn. 70 (1997) 1843.

[20] J.Parkash.J.H. Robble, J. Agnew, E. Gibbs, P. Collings, R.F. Pasternack, J.C.D. Paula, Biophys. J. 74 (1998) 2089.

[21] J. Gracia Fadrique, Langmuir 15 (1999) 3279.

[22] P. Feng, W.Q. Shu, C.Z. Huang, Y.F. Li, Anal. Chem. 73 (2001) 4307.

[23] P. Feng, C.Z. Huang, Y.F. Li, Anal. Biochem. 308 (2002) 83.

[24] W. Lu, C.Z. Huang, Y.F. Li, Analyst 27 (2002) 1392.

[25] W. Lu, C.Z. Huang, Y.F. Li, Anal. Chim. Acta 475 (2003) 151.

[26] H. Nagatani, H. Watarai, Anal. Chem. 68 (1996) 1250.

[27] H. Nagatani, H. Watarai, Anal. Chem. 70 (1998) 2860.

[28] R.H. Yang, K.A. Li, K.M. Wang, F.L. Zhao, N. Li, F. Liu, Anal. Chem. 75 (2003) 612.

[29] Y.E. Zeng, H.S. Zhang, Z.H. Chen, Handbook of Modern Chemical Reagents, Chemical Industry Press, Beijing, 4(1989).

[30] V. Backman, M.B. Wallace, L.T. Perelman, J.T. Arendt, R. Gurjar, M. Muller, G.Q. Zhang, G. Zonios, E. Kline, T. McGillican, S. Shapshay, T. Valdez, K. Badizadegan, J.M. Crawford, M. Fitzmaurice, S. Kabani, H.S. Levin, M. Seiler, R.R. Dasari, I. Itzkan, J. Van Dam, M.S. Feld, Nature 406 (2000) 35.

[31] V. Backman, V. Gopal, M. Kalashnikov, K. Badizadegan, R. Gurjar, A. Wax, I. Georgakoudi, M. Mueller, C.W. Boone, R.R. Dasari, M.S. Feld, IEEE J. Sel. Top. Quantum Electron. 7(2001) 887.

[32] J. Yguerabide, E.E. Yguerabide, Anal. Biochem. 262 (1998) 137～156.

[33] J. Yguerabide, E.E. Yguerabide, Anal. Biochem. 262 (1998) 157～176.

[34] L.E. Morrison, G. Weber, Biophys. J. 52 (1987) 367.

[35] C.X. Yang, Y.F. Li, P. Feng, C.Z. Huang, Chinese J. Anal. Chem. 30 (2002) 473.

(Yong Hong Wang, Hong Ping Guo, Ke Jun Tan, Cheng Zhi Huang,
published in *Analytica Chimica Acta*, 2004, 521, 109～115)

2.7 Directly Light Scattering Imaging of the Aggregations of Biopolymer Bound Chromium(III) Hydrolytic Oligomers in Aqueous Phase and Liquid/Liquid Interface

Abstract: Investigations of inorganic oligomers are important in both chemistry and physiology. In this contribution, we propose a laser induced light scattering imaging (LSI) and a total internal reflected light scattering imaging (TIR-LSI) technique, and apply them to characterize the interactions of inorganic oligomers with biopolymer in aqueous phase and at liquid/liquid interface, respectively. In aqueous medium, synthetic chromium(III) hydrolytic oligomers (CrHO) react with DNA, and the resultant binary could be extracted into the H_2O/CCl_4 interface in the presence of triocyctyl phosphine oxide (TOPO), forming a DNA–CrHO–TOPO ternary amphipathic complex at the interface with the associate constant of 1.32×10^3 $mol^{-1}\cdot dm^4$ for a given 1.0×10^{-4} $mol\cdot L^{-1}$ TOPO. Under the excitation of a 441-nm He–Cd laser light beam, the resultant light scattering and total internal reflected light scattering (TIR-LS) signals of the formed binary in aqueous phase and ternary at liquid/liquid interface could be easily captured using a common microscope coupled with a CCD camera. By digitally analyzing the CCD captures, we demonstrate that aggregations of the CrHO–DNA binary in aqueous phase and DNA–CrHO–TOPO ternary at liquid/liquid interface have occurred, respectively.

Keywords: Light scattering image (LSI) technique; Total internal reflection (TIR); Chromium(III) hydrolytic oligomers (CrHO); DNA

2.7.1 Introduction

It has reported that inorganic oligomers have shown physio- logical effects, and investigations on their species are important in the fields of chemistry, biochemistry, physiology and environics[1]. For example, the hydrolysis of environmental and biological concerned element of chromium has been of interest for many decades, and the trivalent chromium could form few members of the species of hydrolytic polymers containing monomer Cr^{3+}, dimer $Cr_2(OH)_2{}^{4+}$, trimer $Cr_3(OH)_4{}^{5+}$, and tetramer $Cr_4(OH)_6{}^{6+}$ in a hydrolysis process[2~7]. These trivalent chromium hydrolytic oligomers (CrHO) were reported to be relevant to protein binding such as collagen with the crosslinking efficiency of dimeric > trimeric > tetrameric [1]. In our previous work, we have demonstrated that the CrHO could induce the aggregation of DNA in bulk solution, turning out strong enhanced light scattering (LS) signals[8]. That indicates the CrHO species has strong physiological effect. Thus, we consider introduce liquid/liquid interface and investigate its actions in order to mimic this physiological and environmental element extracted into membrane.

In the past decade, resonance light scattering (RLS) technique, developed by using a common spectrofluorometer to measure the enhanced RLS signals occurred when a light beam with the wavelength close to the absorption region of species was applied to excite the species[9], has been found wide applications in the designation of bioassemblies and aggregation process[10~14], and can offer high sensitivity of analyte and simplicity of operation when the enhanced RLS signals employed for analytical purposes[15~19]. In order to improve the selectivity of RLS technique, we have introduced liquid/liquid interface [20] and proposed a total internal reflected resonance light scattering (TIR-RLS) technique to measure the molecular interactions of host-guest at liquid–liquid interface [21~24]. In principle, when a light beam passes through a liquid/liquid interface from optically denser to rarer phase, it may be total reflected from the interface when the incidence angle is larger than the critical angle, and develops an evanescent field on the side of the optically rarer phase at the interface. Thus, species extracted to the interface could be excited selectively and effectively in the amphipathic interfacial region of less than 200 nm thick, therefore, practical samples containing biopolymers[21～23], and drugs[18,24], could be detected with greatly improved sensitivity and selectivity. The problem is, however, the TIR-RLS technique still has limitations since it only discloses the average features of light scattering emission of all aggregation species, failing to display the nature of single scatterer in terms of the size and the distribution.

In order to investigate the scattered light of single light scatterer, we have developed a RLS imaging technique to characterize the light scattering emission in bulk solution, and found that the RLS imaging technique can yield a high sensitivity[25]. However, the RLS imaging technique is limited by instability since the scatterer in bulk solution is not static but in Brownian motion, making the light scattering signals related to the scatterers in the detection focus plane fluctuate[26]. That occurred to us to combine the total internal reflected light scattering (TIR-LS) at liquid/liquid interface with the light scattering imaging (LSI) technique to construct an immobile platform so that the scatterers could be stably immobilized or controlled for imaging. This combination is expected not only to display much higher sensitivity without the flaw of instability, but also provide more information of aggregations at the interface.

2.7.2 Experiential

2.7.2.1 Apparatus

The optical imaging system for total internal reflected light scattering imaging (TIR-LSI) is displayed in Fig. 1. The 441.6-nm light beam emitted from a He–Cd laser source (Shanghai Laser Technology Institute, China) was guided by coupling to one end of a total reflected quartz optical fiber (0.6 mm inner diameter, Laser Institute of Physics, Southwest University, Chongqing). The other end of the optical fiber was coupled to a quartz lens (f =12 mm) so that the light beam transmitted from the optical fibre could be focused. The output power of the laser source was calibrated and monitored in every measurement with a WL-4 Power Meter (Laser Institute of Physics, Southwest University, Chongqing) to ensure that the power supply is stable. The light beam was reflected to the water/tetrachloromethane interface with the incident angle of 70°, sufficiently greater than the 65.6° critical angle of the H_2O/CCl_4 interface, and the light spot of the laser beam at the interface was about 2 mm in diameter. An Olympus IX70 inverted microscope system (Olympus, Tokyo, Japan) coupled with a 10× objective (N.A. 0.10) was used to observe the light scattering imaging of species solution filled in a bottom-transparent square quartz sample cell (10 mm×10 mm×43 mm). To capture the observed LS images, a Cohu 4910 Series cooled CCD camera (Cohu, CA, USA), coupled with Scion Image software package for Windows 98, was employed.

TIR-LS spectra were measured with a Hitachi F-4500 spectrofluorometer (Tokyo, Japan). Considering the light scattering angle should be in accordance with that of the optical imaging system, the sample compartment of the spectrofluorometer has been modified as the displayed optical arrangement in Fig. 2, which is an improvement of our previous reports[21～24].

2.7.2.2 Reagents

Stock solutions of DNA were prepared by dissolving commercially purchased fish sperm DNA (fsDNA, Shanghai Institute of Biochemistry, Chinese Academy of Sciences, Shanghai) in deionized water (18.2Ω). The concentrations of DNA were determined according to the absorbance at 260 nm with ε_{DNA} = 6600 $M^{-1}\cdot cm^{-1}$ after establishing that the absorbance ratio of A_{260}/A_{280} was over the range of 1.80～1.90 for DNA[27]. In this experiment, all the working solutions of DNA were 10 μg·mL^{-1} (about 3.0×10^{-5} mol·L^{-1}). 1.0×10^{-3} mol·L^{-1} triocyctyl phosphine oxide (TOPO, E. Merck, Darmstadt) solution was prepared by dissolving 38.6 mg of the commercial product in 100 mL of tetrachloromethane, the working solution was prepared by diluting the stock solution to 1.0×10^{-4} mol·L^{-1} with tetrachloromethane. Stock solution of trivalent chromium was made by dissolving $CrCl_3·6H_2O$ in 18MΩ water, which is a deep blue solution. Fresh alkaline solutions should be prepared by dissolving the NaOH pellets in order to synthesize the chromium(III) hydrolytic oligomers (CrHO).

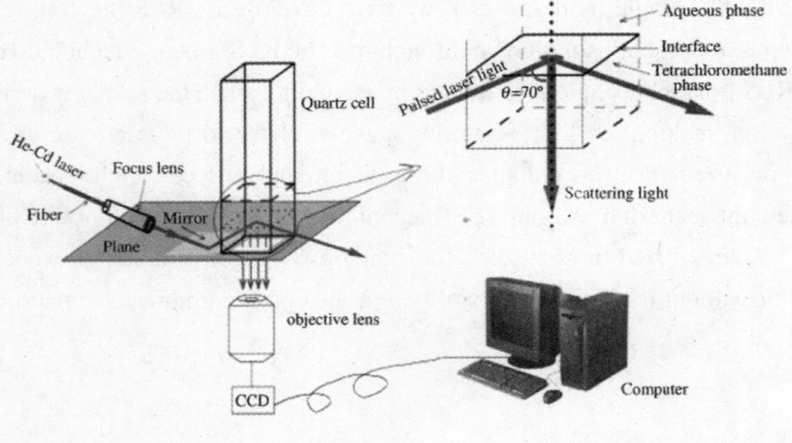

Fig. 1. Optical setup of the TIR-LSI (left), and the magnified schematic illustration of optical cell (upright) for the measurement of scattered light at the H_2O/CCl_4 interface under the total internal reflection configuration.

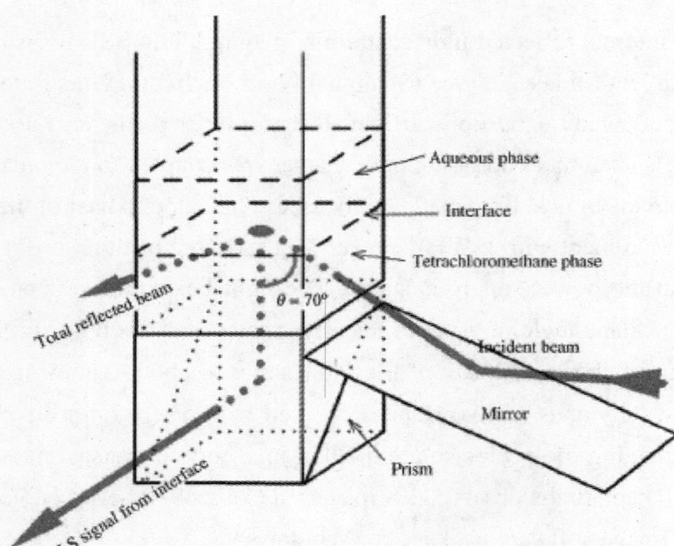

Fig. 2. The optical arrangement coupled in the sample compartment of spectrofluorometer for TIR-LS measurements at the H_2O/CCl_4 interface

2.7.2.3 Preparation of chromium(III) hydrolytic oligomers

The preparation of CrHO was similar to the report of Friese et al.[28]. It started by dropwise adding equal volumes of equimolar concentrations of NaOH to the blue chromium(III) solution of 0.2 mol·L^{-1} under rapid stirring. During the addition of alkaline solution, the blue chromium(III) solution changes to green, and becomes turbid with the formation of visible precipitate after 75% of the alkaline solution was added. Even though, the dropwise addition of alkaline was continued until the theoreticcally calculated amount was consumed. Then, the resultant green suspension was stirred rapidly for 4 h. During this period, the suspended green precipitates are gradually dissolved and give a green solution of pH 5.5. At last, the pH was adjusted to 3.5 with 1.0 mol·L^{-1} $HClO_4$ in order to get the maximum yields of CrHO[4,7], and the green color changes into blue green. The total concentration of chromium(III) species in the prepared CrHO solutionwas 0.1 mol·L^{-1}, andthen, dilutedto 1.0×10^{-3} mol·L^{-1} for use.

2.7.2.4 Procedures

One millilitre of Britton–Robinson buffer, 1.0 mL synthetic CrHO solution, and an appropriate volume of fsDNA solution were successively added into a 10 mL calibrated tube. The mixture in the calibrated tube was vortexed after each addition of the interacting additives, and then, diluted with water to 10.0 mL with thorough mixing at last. Then, 500 μL TOPO working solution and 500 μL of the CrHO–DNA aqueous mixture were transfered in sequence into a dry 10-mm optical quartz cell to form the liquid–liquid interface. The aqueous mixture and organic tetrachloromethane phase were stirred carefully and thoroughly, and left the mixture in the cell about 30 min prior to measurements in order to decrease the effect of bubbles during the stirring. Then, the cell was transferred for TIR-LS measurements in the same mode as measuring the RLS signals by scanning simultaneously the excitation and emission monochromators of the F-4500 spectrofluorometer from 200 to 700 nm with $\lambda_{ex} = \lambda_{em}$. The TIR-LS intensities were measured at 375 nm using a slit width of 5.0 nm for both excitation and emission. The interfacial image of DNA–CrHO–TOPO captured by CCD camera, was processed by Scion Image software package on Windows 98.

2.7.3 Results and discussions

2.7.3.1 TIR-LS spectral features

Fig. 3 displays that the TIR-LS signals of the CrHO–DNA binary complex at the H_2O/CCl_4 interfaces are very weak in the absence of TOPO in the organic phase. However, greatly enhanced TIR-LS signals could be observed if CrHO–DNA binary complex and TOPO are present in aqueous medium and tetrachloromethane phase, respectively. It was found that the enhanced TIR-LS signals get increased with increasing DNA content.

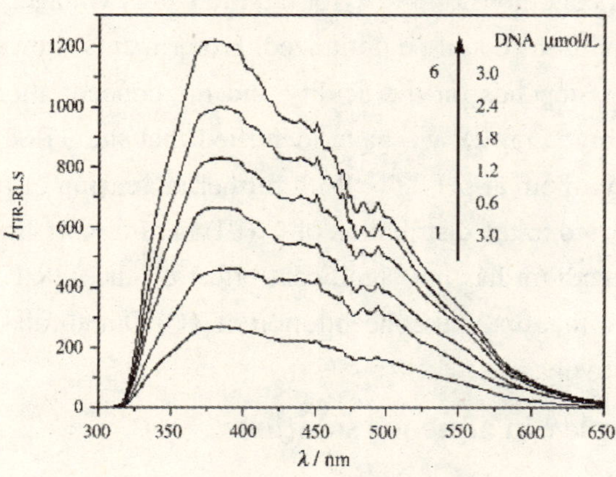

Fig. 3 TIR-LS spectra of CrHO–DNA (curve 1), and DNA–CrHO–TOPO (curve 2–6) at H2O/CCl4 interface. Concentration: TOPO: 1.0×10^{-4} mol·L^{-1}; Cr(III): 1×10^{-4} mol·L^{-1}; DNA (from curves 1 to 6): 3.0, 0.6, 1.2, 1.8, 2.4, 3.0 $\times10^{-6}$ mol·L^{-1}.

It is known that hydrolysis of Cr(III) could result in a distribution of oligomeric species formed via μ-hydroxo and μ-oxo bridges among the metal centers that lead to the formation of dimeric, trimeric, tetrameric, and higher order polymers from the Cr(III) monomer [28], making the various species of Cr(III) easily combine with DNA and form a binary complex of CrHO–DNA in the aqueous phase through electrostatic attraction, resulting in enhanced LS signals (Fig. 4). Even though, the coordination number of Cr(III) is unsaturated, the water molecules will occupy the coordination sites of Cr(III). If a synergistic ligand, such as TOPO, is added, the synergistic ligand will replace the coordinated water molecules to meet the requirements of the saturated coordination of the central Cr(III) ion, and then, Cr(III) ion acts as a bridge between the TOPO and DNA. Since the TOPO and

CrHO–DNA binary complexes are dissolved in CCl_4 and the aqueous phase respectively, the interfacial region of H_2O/CCl_4 system is amphipathic, thus DNA–CrHO–TOPO ternary complex is subsequently formed and exists at the interface, generating greatly enhanced TIR-LS signals. Fig. 4 shows that the LS spectra of aqueous phase containing CrHO–DNA complex before and after the addition of TOPO in tetrachloromethane phase. The greatly decreased light scattering signals of CrHO–DNA complex in the aqueous phase demonstrate that the transfer of CrHO–DNA binary complex from aqueous medium to amphipathic interface has occurred in the presence of TOPO in tetrachloromethane phase.

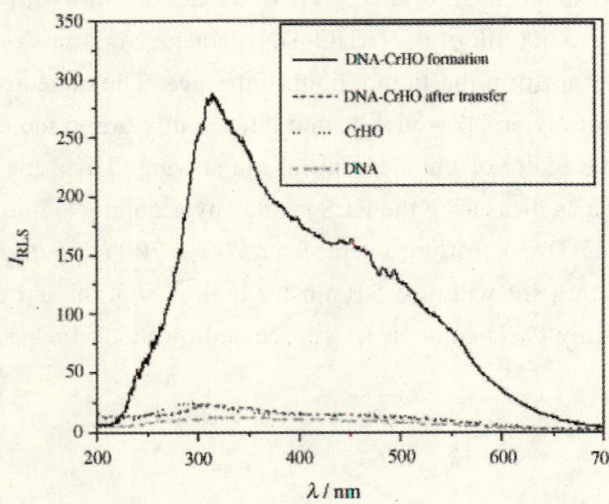

Fig. 4 LS spectra in aqueous phase containing CrHO–DNA complex before and after the binary transferred to the interface due to the addition of TOPO. Concentration: TOPO: 1.0×10^{-4} mol·L^{-1}; Cr(III): 1.0×10^{-4} mol·L^{-1}; DNA: 3.0×10^{-6} mol·L^{-1}.

The LS signals in aqueous medium (Fig. 4) and that from interface (Fig. 3) should not be ascribed to the resonance light scattering[9～11] since the characteristic light scattering wavelengths at 310 and 375 nm are far from the absorption region of both CrHO and CrHO–DNA which is characterized at 425 nm. These enhanced LS signals might be to be related to the instrumental conditions and the experimental conditions, which need further study in our following works. Under the optical instrumental conditions of 400 V for the PMT high voltage, and 5.0 nm slit width for excitation and emission, experimental conditions could be optimized. Experiments showed that the formation of the DNA–CrHO–TOPO ternary complex depends on the acidity and the concentration of Cr(III) in aqueous medium. With the homemade TIR assembly (Fig. 2), we have identified that the TIR-LS intensity of DNA–CrHO–TOPO ternary complex reaches its maximum at pH 2.56. With further increasing of pH, the TIR-LS intensity declines dramatically, which might be attributed to the distribution of Cr(III) in different oligomers with pH. On the other hand, ionic strength of the aqueous medium has not significant effect on the TIR-LS signal of the H_2O/CCl_4 interface. In addition, experiments showed that optimal concentration of TOPO and total Cr(III) should be 1.0×10^{-4} mol·L^{-1} and 1.0×10^{-4} mol·L^{-1}, respectively.

2.7.3.2 Features of CrHO–DNA complex in aqueous solution

To show the LS features of CrHO–DNA complex in bulk solution first, we applied the LS imaging system[25] to observe the image of CrHO–DNA complexes in bulk solution. The three-dimensional (3D) images (Fig. 5) were obtained by analyzing the surface plot of original LS image using Scion Image software. These images clearly showed the distribution of the number and light scattering intensity. The counts of these scatterers in each image were statistically estimated with a five-difference variation of LS intensity using Scion Image software, and then the distribution of light scattering intensity of the single scatterer over the range of 25～85 could be obtained (Fig. 6). The *N*-value (counts/piece) is the total numbers of the scatterers for every five-difference variation of LS intensity in each piece of image, and the I_{LS} is the intensity of the each scatterer calculated by Scion Image software.

Directly observations (Fig. 5) and analyses on the statistic data (Fig. 6) show that the numbers of scatterers with light inten- sity ranging from 25 to 30 get increased from C to F in Fig. 6 with increasing DNA concentration, and the scatterers with the LS intensity higher than 60 could only be seen clearly in E and F in Fig. 6, indicating the enlargement of the CrHO–DNA binary complex in higher DNA concentration. The augment tendency of the amount of the species and the LS intensity of single scatterer with increasing DNA display that CrHO–DNA binary complex has aggregation tendency since the increasing LS intensity of the single scatterer discloses the enlargement of the aggregation species [9]. This information of the aggregation process of single bioassemblies in bulk solution, however, is generally impossible to be detected just by measuring the LS intensity of the total light scatterers in bulk solution with the common RLS technique since it only reflects the average light scattering features of all scatterers.

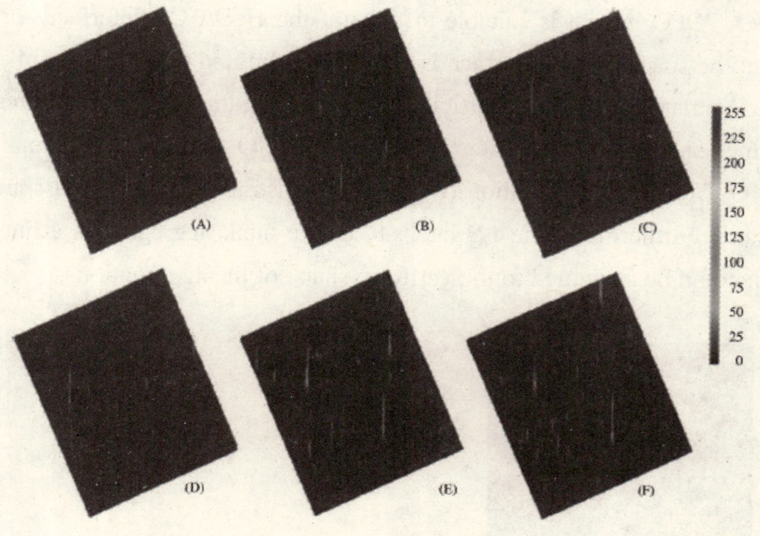

Fig. 5 The 3D LS image of CrHO–DNA aggregations in aqueous solution. Concentrations: Cr(III): 1.0×10^{-4} mol·L^{-1} except B where no CrHO added; DNA (from A to F): 0, 3.0, 0.6, 1.2, 2.4, 3.0×10^{-6} mol·L^{-1}.

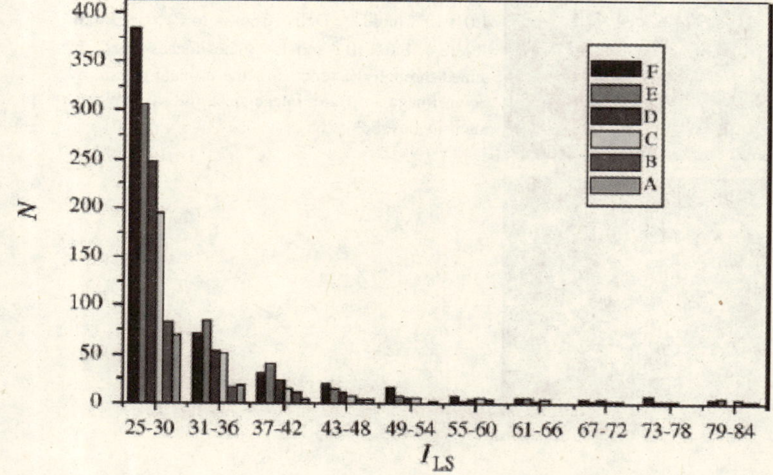

Fig. 6 The light scattering intensity distribution of the image in Fig. 5. Con- centrations: Cr(III): 1.0×10^{-4} mol·L^{-1} except B where no CrHO added; DNA (from A to F): 0, 3.0, 0.6, 1.2, 2.4, 3.0×10^{-6} mol·L^{-1}.

2.7.3.3 Interfacial aggregation of DNA–CrHO–TOPO ternary complex

To characterize the feature of the DNA–CrHO–TOPO complex, a microscopic imaging system based on TIR-LSI was established (Fig. 1). By introducing a 441.6 nm He–Cd laser to excite the DNA–CrHO–TOPO species, we could observe the LS signals at interface in situ. Fig. 7 shows the imaging of DNA–CrHO–TOPO complex with increasing DNA, indicating that DNA–CrHO–TOPO forms a hunk and variform shape, and this tendency gets stronger with increasing DNA, indicating that the aggregation of DNA–CrHO–TOPO has occurred. These features of the aggregations are not similar to the common aggregations species of organic chromophores[25], gold and silver nanoparticles[29,30].

As Fig. 8 shows, the CrHO–DNA aggregations in bulk solution have a symmetrical distribution and homogeneous shape, while the DNA–CrHO–TOPO aggregations at interface do not. These phenomena disclose the different shape and distribution of the same aggregation in different medium or phase. In aqueous phase, the aggregations could be well dispersed by water medium, presenting small and homogeneous scattering particles. In the presence of TOPO, however, the CrHO–DNA binary complex is extracted into the liquid/liquid interface in the form of a ternary complex of DNA–CrHO–TOPO, which is suitable to exist at the H_2O/CCl_4 interface for their amphipathic property. The occasion is that the space of the interface is much more limited than that of bulk solution, and then, the ternary complexes agglomerate from single particle to large aggregations, displaying the variform shape as Fig. 7 shows. Under the same conditions, the LS intensity of DNA–CrHO–TOPO aggregations at the interface is much higher than that of CrHO–DNA in bulk solution (Fig. 8), demonstrating the original source of strong LS signals from H_2O/CCl_4 interface. Furthermore, the LS intensity of the hunk aggregations at interface does not show uniform distribution, which could be attributed to the variform shape of the aggregations.

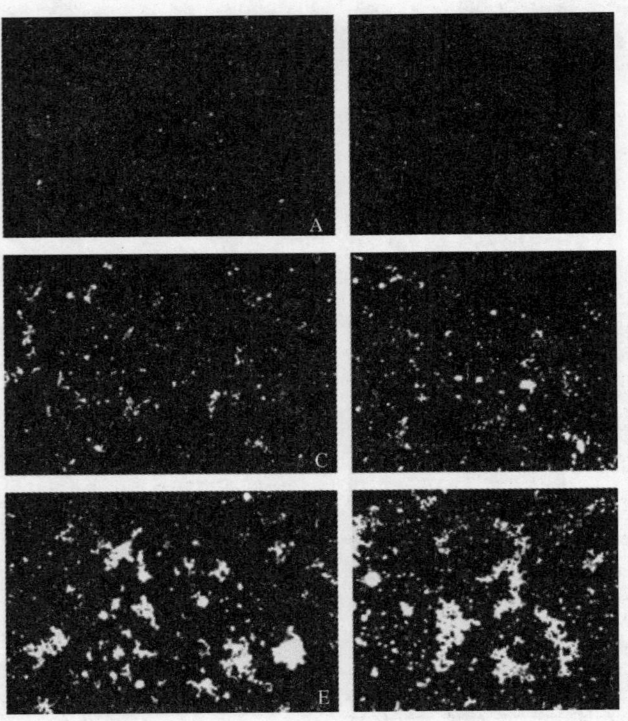

Fig. 7 TIR-LSI picture of DNA–CrHO–TOPO. Concentration: TOPO: 1.0×10^{-4} mol·L^{-1}, Cr(III): 1.0×10^{-4} mol·L^{-1}, DNA (from A to F): 0, 0.3, 0.6, 1.2, 2.4, 3.6×10^{-6} mol·L^{-1}. The images were obtained through the process of the original picture by Scion Image software. Image size: 768×512 pixels; intensity threshold: 26.

To intensively study the aggregating process, we monitored the time curve of the interfacial feature of DNA–CrHO–TOPO ternary complexes. It has demonstrated that the process of aggregation at the interface is time-dependent, that is why we should stand about 30 min, waiting for the stability of the aggregation process in our previous detection of ligands[21~23].

2.7.3.4 Equilibrium of DNA–CrHO–TOPO ternary complex at interface

According to the optimized experimental procedures, the linear relationship between the TIR-LS intensity at the interface and the total concentration of DNA can be established over the range of $0.5\sim3.6\times10^{-6}$ mol·L^{-1} for fsDNA with the equation $\Delta I = 8.31 + 309.15[\mathrm{D}]_{tot}$, where the correlation coefficient *(r)* is 0.998 for five measurements *(n* = 5), and $[\mathrm{D}]_{tot}$ is expressed as 10^{-6} mol·L^{-1}.

According to the 1:1 binding ratio of CrHO and DNA (Fig. 9), we can establish a stoichiometric model for the interaction of CrHO and DNA in aqueous phase,

$$[\mathrm{D}]_a + [\mathrm{C}]_a \longleftrightarrow [\mathrm{DC}]_a \quad (1)$$

where $[\mathrm{D}]_a$, $[\mathrm{C}]_a$, $[\mathrm{DC}]_a$ are free concentration of DNA, CrHO and CrHO–DNA in aqueous medium, respectively. Similar to the aqueous phase,

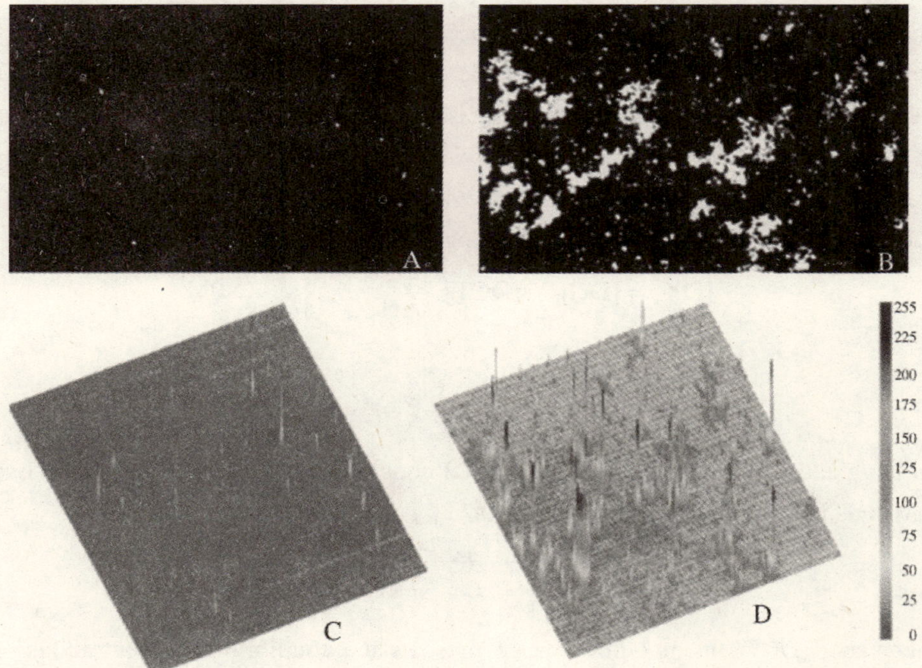

Fig. 8 The LS image (A and B) and 3D LS display (C and D) of CrHO–DNA aggregations in bulk solution (A and C), and the TIR-LS image of DNA–CrHO–TOPO aggregations at H2O/CCl4 interface (B and D). Concentration: TOPO: 1.0×10^{-4} mol·L^{-1}; Cr(III): 1.0×10^{-4} mol·L^{-1}; DNA: 3.0×10^{-6} mol·L^{-1}. Image size: 768×512 pixels; intensity threshold: 26.

when the DNA–CrHO interacts with TOPO at interface, a stoichiometric model could also be establish:

$$[\mathrm{DC}]_a + [\mathrm{T}]_{org} \xleftrightarrow{K_i} [\mathrm{DCT}]_i \quad (2)$$

$$K_i = \frac{[\mathrm{DCT}]_i}{[\mathrm{DC}]_a[\mathrm{T}]_{org}} \quad (3)$$

where $[\mathrm{DC}]_a$, $[\mathrm{T}]_{org}$, and K_i are free concentration of DNA–CrHO in the aqueous solution, TOPO in organic medium and the associate constant of interface interaction. $[\mathrm{DCT}]_i$ (mol·dm^{-2}) refers to the equilibrium concentrations of DNA–CrHO–TOPO at interface.

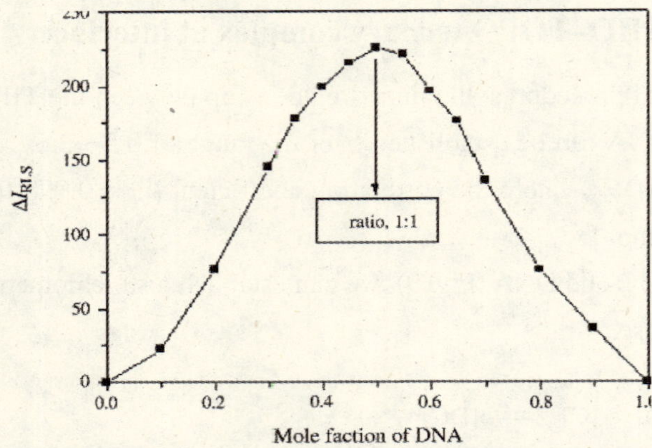

Fig. 9 Molar ratio of CrHO–DNA binding in aqueous solution. The concen-trations of DNA and CrHO were both changed simultaneously by kept the total concentration of 1.0×10^{-5} mol·L^{-1}; pH 2.56.

In the case of interfacial interaction, the total quantity of DNA and TOPO could be expressed as:

$$[\mathrm{D}]_{\mathrm{tot}}V_{\mathrm{a}}=[\mathrm{D}]_{\mathrm{a}}V_{\mathrm{a}}+[\mathrm{DC}]_{\mathrm{a}}V_{\mathrm{a}}+[\mathrm{DCT}]_{\mathrm{i}}S_{\mathrm{i}}+[\mathrm{D}]_{\mathrm{org}}V_{\mathrm{org}}+[\mathrm{DC}]_{\mathrm{org}}V_{\mathrm{org}} \quad (4\mathrm{a})$$

$$[\mathrm{T}]_{\mathrm{org}}V_{\mathrm{org}}=[\mathrm{T}]_{\mathrm{a}}V_{\mathrm{a}}+[\mathrm{DCT}]_{\mathrm{i}}S_{\mathrm{i}}+[\mathrm{T}]_{\mathrm{org}}V_{\mathrm{org}} \quad (4\mathrm{b})$$

where V_a, S_i, and V_{org} are the volume of aqueous phase (5.0×10^{-4} L), the interfacial area (1.0×10^{-2} dm^2) and the volume of organic phase (5.0×10^{-4} L), respectively. Since the solubility of DNA, CrHO–DNA in CCl_4 and TOPO in H_2O is very small, it is not necessary to consider the contributions from the DNA and CrHO–DNA in tetra-chloromethane phase, so dose the TOPO in aqueous phase. Furthermore, the CrHO is large excess in the present experimental conditions, and the free DNA can interact with CrHO to form DNA–CrHO completely. Thus, the free concentration of DNA in H_2O could be neglected. By neglecting the partitions of DNA and CrHO–DNA in CCl_4 phase, and TOPO in H_2O phase, we have Eq. (5) according to Eq. (4),

$$[\mathrm{D}]_{\mathrm{tot}}=[\mathrm{DC}]_{\mathrm{a}}+[\mathrm{DCT}]_{\mathrm{i}}\frac{S_{\mathrm{i}}}{V_{\mathrm{a}}} \quad (5\mathrm{a})$$

and

$$[\mathrm{T}]_{\mathrm{tot}}=[\mathrm{T}]_{\mathrm{org}}+[\mathrm{DCT}]_{\mathrm{i}}\frac{S_{\mathrm{i}}}{V_{\mathrm{a}}} \quad (5\mathrm{b})$$

If TOPO is large excess in the present experimental condition, we could get following linear function according to Eqs. (3) and (5) by substituting the $[T]_{org}$ with $[T]_{tot}$.

$$\log[\mathrm{DCT}]_{\mathrm{i}}=\log\frac{[\mathrm{T}]_{\mathrm{tot}}}{(1+K_{\mathrm{i}}\cdot[\mathrm{T}]_{\mathrm{tot}}\frac{S_{\mathrm{i}}}{V_{\mathrm{a}}})}+\log[\mathrm{D}]_{\mathrm{tot}} \quad (6)$$

On the other hand, $[DCT]_i$ in mol·dm^{-2}, which presents the equilibrium concentrations of DNA–CrHO–TOPO at interface, could be calculated from the total adsorption quantity of DNA–CrHO–TOPO at interface by following equation[24]:

$$[\mathrm{DCT}]_{\mathrm{i}}=\Gamma_{\mathrm{i}}\cdot\frac{\Delta I}{\Delta I_{\mathrm{max}}} \quad (7)$$

where Γ_i (mol·dm^{-2}) is the maximum adsorption concentration of DNA–CrHO–TOPO at interface, which can be estimated from the decrements of DNA–CrHO concentrations by measuring the LS intensity of aqueous solution before and after the interfacial interaction until the ΔI reaches the maximum (ΔI_{max}). ΔI is the enhanced TIR-LS intensity of DNA–CrHO–TOPO at interface when the concentration of DNA–CrHO equilibrated, while ΔI_{max} represents the enhanced maximum TIR-LS intensity of DNA–CrHO–TOPO compared to that in the absence of DNA. Thus, the $\Gamma_i/\Delta I_{max}$ could be calculated with a value of 1.78×10^{-10}.

Experiments have shown that a linear relationship exits between $\log(\Delta I_{TIR\text{-}LS})$ and $\log[D]_{tot}$, $\log(\Delta I_{TIR\text{-}LS}) = 8.43 + 0.988\log([D]_{tot})$ with $r = 0.998$ and $n = 5$ when $[D]_{tot}$ is expressed as 10^{-6} mol·L^{-1} (Fig. 10). Thus, we could establish a linear relationship between $\log[DCT]_i$ and $\log[D]_{tot}$ from Eq. (7),

$$\log[\mathrm{DCT}]_i = -1.44 + 0.988\log([\mathrm{D}]_{tot}) \qquad (8)$$

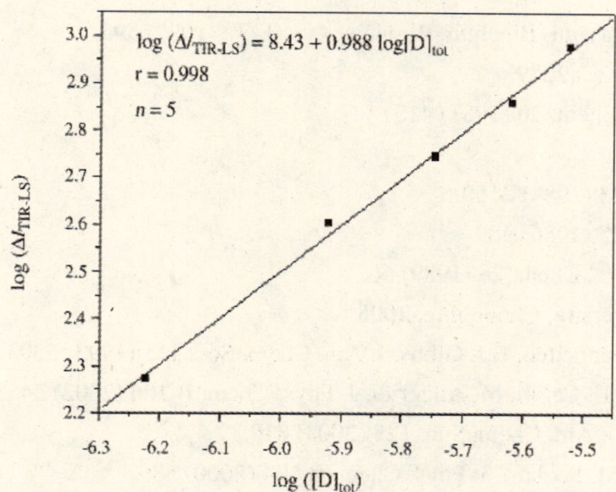

Fig. 10 Linear correlation between the $\Delta I_{TIR\text{-}LS}$ and the total concentration of DNA. $[\mathrm{D}]_{tot}$ should be expressed as 10^{-6} mol·L^{-1}. Concentration: TOPO: 1.0×10^{-4} mol·L^{-1}; Cr(III): 1.0×10^{-4} mol·L^{-1}; λ = 375 nm.

Making comparision could yield good identity between Eqs. (6) and Eqs (8) with the intercept of $b=-1.44$ for the following expression.

$$\log\frac{[\mathrm{T}]_{tot}}{(1+K_i\cdot[\mathrm{T}]_{tot}\dfrac{S_i}{V_a})}=b \qquad (9)$$

Thus, it is applicable to calculate K_i-value by substituting the values of $V=5.0\times10^{-4}$ L, $S_i=1.0\times10^{-2}$ dm^2.

$$K_i=\frac{1}{(10^{-b}-20)[\mathrm{T}]_{org}} \qquad (10)$$

K_i is dependent on the content of TOPO in organic phase. Therefore, it is very easy to deduce the K_i-value of the interfacial interaction of DNA–CrHO–TOPO for a given TOPO. Under the experimental conditions, the K_i-value is calculated to be 1.32×10^3 mol^{-1}·dm^4 for 1.0×10^{-4} mol·L^{-1} TOPO in the 500 μL tetrachloromethane, indicating that the extraction of the DNA bound CrHO from aquous medium to organic phase is effective.

2.7.4 Conclusions

By constructing a laser induced total internal reflecting light scattering imaging technique, we could observe the feature of DNA–CrHO–TOPO aggregations at H_2O/CCl_4 interface. With the imaging analysis of the imaging of DNA–CrHO–TOPO aggregations at interface, we demonstrate the self-assembled process of the aggregations from aqueous phase to interface. The CrHO–DNA aggregations have a symmetrical distribution and homogeneous shape in aqueous phase. When TOPO was added into oil phase, however, amphipathic ternary complex could form and exist stably at H_2O/CCl_4, resulting in the transfer of the chromium(III) hydrolytic oligomers bounded biopolymer from aqueous medium to interface, and aggregation species are presented. The large aggregations species at interface have a stronger scattering ability than in bulk solution, demonstrating the original source of strong light scattering signal from H_2O/CCl_4 interface.

Acknowledgments

Herein we are grateful to the supports from the National Natural Science Foundation of China (No. 20425517), and the Municipal Science and Technology Committee of Chongqing.

References

[1] J.R. Rao, R. Gayatri, R. Rajaram, B.U. Nair, T. Ramasami, Biochim. Biophys. Acta 1472 (1999) 595.

[2] M.E. Thompson, R.E. Connick, Inorg. Chem. 20 (1981) 2279.

[3] J.E. Finholt, M.E. Thompson, R.E. Connick, Inorg. Chem. 20 (1981) 4151.

[4] H. Stunzi, W. Marty, Inorg. Chem. 22 (1983) 2145.

[5] H. Stunzi, F.P. Rotzinger, W. Marty, Inorg. Chem. 23 (1984) 2160.

[6] F.P. Rotzinger, H. Stunzi, W. Marty, Inorg. Chem. 25 (1986) 489.

[7] H. Stunzi, L. Spiccia, F.P. Rotzinger, W. Marty, Inorg. Chem. 28 (1989) 66.

[8] H.P. Guo, A Thesis for MS Degree, Southwest University, Chongqing, 2005.

[9] R.F. Pasternack, C. Bustamante, P.J. Collings, A. Giannetteo, E.J. Gibbs, J. Am. Chem. Soc. 115 (1993) 5393.

[10] L.M. Scolaro, M. Castriciano, A. Romeo, S. Patane, E. Cefali, M. Allegrini, J. Phys. Chem. B 106 (2002) 2453.

[11] M.Y. Choi, J.A. Pollard, M.A. Webb, J.L. McHale, J. Am. Chem. Soc. 125 (2003) 810.

[12] N. Micali, F. Mallamace, A. Romeo, R. Purrello, L.M. Scolaro, J. Phys. Chem. B 104 (2000) 5897.

[13] R.F. Pasternack, E.J. Gibbs, D. Bruzewicz, D. Stewart, K.S. Engstrom, J. Am. Chem. Soc. 124 (2002) 3533.

[14] A.S.R. Koti, N. Periasamy, J. Mater. Chem. 12 (2002) 2312.

[15] C.Z. Huang, K.A. Li, S.Y. Tong, Anal. Chem. 68 (1996) 22593.

[16] Q.F. Li, X.G. Chen, H.Y. Zhang, C.X. Xue, Y.Q. Fan, Z.D. Hu, Fresenius J. Anal. Chem. 368 (2000) 715.

[17] L.J. Dong, R.P. Jia, Q.F. Li, X.G. Chen, Z.D. Hu, Anal. Chim. Acta 459 (2002) 313.

[18] W. Lu, C.Z. Huang, Y.F. Li, Anal. Chim. Acta 475 (2003) 151.

[19] S.P. Liu, P. Feng, Microchim. Acta 140 (2002) 189.

[20] J. Garcia-Fadrique, Langmuir 15 (1999) 3279.

[21] P. Feng, W.Q. Su, C.Z. Huang, Y.F. Li, Anal. Chem. 73 (2001) 4307.

[22] W. Lu, C.Z. Huang, Y.F. Li, Analyst 127 (2002) 1392.

[23] X.B. Pang, C.Z. Huang, Y.F. Li, W. Lu, Bull. Chem. Soc. Jpn. 76 (2003) 1941.

[24] C.Z. Huang, P. Feng, Y.F. Li, K.J. Tan, Anal. Chim. Acta 538 (2005) 337.

[25] C.Z. Huang, Y. Liu, Y.H. Wang, H.P. Guo, Anal. Biochem. 321 (2003) 236.

[26] X.H. Fang, W.H. Tan, Anal. Chem. 71 (1999) 3101.

[27] Z. Chen, J. Liu, D. Luo, Biochemistry Experiments, Chinese University of Sciences and Technology Press, Hefei, China, 1994.

[28] J.I. Friese, B. Ritherdon, S.B. Clark, Z. Zhang, L. Rao, D. Rai, Anal. Chem. 74 (2002) 2977.

[29] J. Yguerabide, E. Yguerabide, Anal. Biochem. 262 (1998) 137.

[30] J. Yguerabide, E. Yguerabide, Anal. Biochem. 262 (1998) 157.

(Jian Ling, Cheng Zhi Huang, Yuan Fang Lim, published in *Analytica Chimica Acta*, 2006, 567, 143～151)

Chapter 3

Analytical Applications in Protein Detection of Light Scattering Technique

3.1 Determination of Protein Concentration by Enhancement of the Pre-resonance Light-scattering of *α*, *β*, *γ*, *δ*-tetrakis(5-sulfothienyl)Porphine

A method of protein determination with the limit of determination at nanogram levels is proposed by using a common spectrofluorometer to detect the intensity of preresonance light-scattering (PRLS). In the pH range 1.81～4.10, the interactions of *α*, *β*, *γ*, *δ*-tetrakis(5-sulfothie-nyl)-porphine, T(5-ST)P with proteins were studied. It was found that the interactions result in a strongly enhanced preresonance light-scattering signal at 472.0 nm. Mechanism studies showed that the enhanced preresonance light-scattering stems from the *J*-aggregation of T(5-ST)P in the presence of proteins. It was found that the *J*-aggregation process is speedy and is scarcely affected by temperature, which supplies a precise method for the determination of proteins. Different proteins in the range 0～7 $\mu g \cdot mL^{-1}$ can be determined with the limits of determination below 100 $ng \cdot mL^{-1}$ depending on the concentration of T(5-ST)P. The results of determination for synthetic samples were in agreement with the desired values, and the ones for human serum samples were identical to those obtained according to the Bradford method using CBB G-250.

Keywords: Proteins; *α*, *β*, *γ*, *δ*-tetrakis(5-sulfothienyl)porphine; preresonance light-scattering; J-Aggregation

The determination of proteins is very important in clinical tests and laboratory practice. There have been many methods to determine the content of proteins in samples, but the commonly used methods are the Biuret,[1] Bradford,[2] Lowry,[3] and Bromcre- sol Green (BCG).[4] The former three methods are often applied to the determination of the total content of proteins in samples, and the latter to the content of albumin. The Biuret method, although simple, reproducible and capable of modifications, is not sensitive; the Bradford method, although sensitive, is too complicated to operate. As to the BCG method, because the BCG–albumin complex may partly precipitate, turbidity and the 'negative baseline effect'[5] are often found. Recently, Li and coworkers[6~9] reported several sensitive methods based on the interactions of porphyrin with proteins, that can be used for the determination of micro amounts of albumin and globulin by spectrophotometry[6~8] and spectrofluorometry.[9]

Analogous to stray light, scattered light is one of the major interferences in fluorescent determination, and attempts have been made to eliminate it. It has not been effectively used for analytical purposes until now, although it has been highly applicable to polymer sciences.[10] Our present study shows that scattered light near the absorption band in a medium of aggregates, which can be detected by using a common spectrofluorometer, can be extensively applied to analytical determination.

According to the macroscopic fluctuation theory, scattered light originates from the fluctuation of the refractive index of a solution.[11] When the incident beam of light is in the far red where the absorption is quite small in an absorbing medium, the Rayleigh scattering law is obeyed for the molecular particles of a size 20 times smaller than the wavelength of the incident beam. In such cases, the contribution of the scattered light from the imaginary part of the refractive index is very small, and the Rayleigh scattering depends on the real part of the refractive index. However, if the wavelength of the incident beam is close to the absorption band of molecular particles, the refractive index varies steeply and the contributions to the scattered light both from the real and imaginary parts should be considered. So, enhanced Rayleigh light-scattering can be expected.[11] It has been proved that the enhanced Rayleigh light-scattering in an absorbing medium is convenient for the study of the motions of molecules in a very dilute solution, avoiding the use of high concentrations of solute.[12] The enhanced Rayleigh light-scattering of aggregated molecules can be detected even by using a common spectrofluorometer.[13~19] When the instrumental conditions of the spectrofluorometer were adjusted without marked variations, the enhanced intensity of Rayleigh light-scattering was found to be proportional to the concentration of the aggregated molecules.[13,14] Since all of the absorption processes are inherently associated with light-scattering, it is possible that the weak Rayleigh light-scattering of organic dyes can be enhanced through their binding with macromolecules, such as nucleic acids and proteins. By using a common spectrofluorometer to measure the intensity and spectrum of resonance light-scattering (it was formerly called resonance light-scattering technique[13~17]), we have established methods for the determination of nucleic acids with sensitivity at nanogram levels,[13~15] studied the aggregation of porphyrins[16,17] and monitored the formation of the suprahelical helixes of nucleic acids.[18,19]

Since the dependence of the resonance light-scattering on the contributions of the real and imaginary parts of the refractive index is different, the maximum resonance light-scattering observed or calculated theoretically often was found to be at the red end of the absorption band.[11,20~24] It is for this reason that all the reported resonance light-scattering methods of nucleic acids were established with the maximum resonance light-scattering wavelengths being located slightly at the red end of the absorption bands by using organic dyes.[13~18] In this work, however, we report a method of protein determination, by using a water soluble porphyrin, α, β, γ, δ-tetrakis(5-sulfothienyl)porphine, T(5-ST)P, with the resonance light-scattering peak being located at the blue side of the absorption band. It was found that the *J*-aggregation occurs in the presence of proteins and gives the *J*-absorption band at 490.2 nm, whereas the maximum resonance light-scattering of the *J*-aggregation was found at 472.0 nm. This kind of resonance light-scattering signal should strictly be called preresonance light-scattering[12] because the maximum resonance light-scattering signals are located outside the absorption band.

3.1.1 Experimental

3.1.1.1 Apparatus

Absorption spectra were obtained by using a Hitachi U-3400 spectrophotometer (Tokyo, Japan), while the preresonance light-scattering spectra and the intensities were recorded and measured with a Shimadzu RF-540 spectrofluorometer (Kyoto, Japan). An SA 720 laboratory instrument (Orion, Cambridge, MA, USA) was used to measure the pH values of the solutions.

3.1.1.2 Reagents

Stock solutions of proteins were prepared by dissolving commercial bovine serum albumin (BSA; Beitai Biochemical Co., Chinese Academy of Sciences, Beijing, China), human serum albumin (HSA; Sigma, St Louis, MO, USA), γ-globulin (γ-IgG; Serva, Heidelberg, Germany), pepsin (Pep; Fangcao Medical Industrial Co., Shanghai, China), α-chymotrypsin (Chy; Shanghai Chemical Reagent Distribution Co., Shanghai, China), lysozyme (Lys) and cellulase (Cel, Shanghai Institute of Biochemistry, Shanghai, China) in doubly-distilled water except γ-IgG, which was dissolved with the aid of a small volume of 0.1 $mol \cdot L^{-1}$ NaCl solution. All the working concentrations of proteins were 25 $\mu g \cdot mL^{-1}$.

The water-soluble free base porphyrin, T(5-ST)P, purchased from Touji Institute of Chemistry (Tokyo, Japan), was dissolved in doubly-distilled water. The working concentration of T(5-ST)P was 2.0×10^{-5} $mol \cdot L^{-1}$.

The working solution of Coomassie Brilliant Blue (CBB G-250, Fluka, Buchs, Switzerland) was prepared by dissolving 0.1000 g of the crystal in 50 ml of 95% ethanol, and then mixing with 100 ml 85% phosphoric acid. The mixture was then diluted to 1000 ml with doubly-distilled water. The concentration of the working solution was 1.17×10^{-5} $mol \cdot L^{-1}$.

Britton–Robinson buffer solution (pH 1.81, composed of 0.04 $mol \cdot L^{-1}$ H_3PO_4, 0.04 $mol \cdot L^{-1}$ HAc and 0.04 $mol \cdot L^{-1}$ H_3BO_3) was used to control the acidity, while 0.5 $mol \cdot L^{-1}$ NaCl solution was used to adjust the ionic strength of the aqueous solutions. All reagents were of analytical grade and used without further purification. Water used throughout was doubly distilled.

3.1.1.3 General procedures

Into a 10 mL calibrated flask were added an appropriate working solution of proteins, 1.0 mL of Britton–Robinson buffer solution and appropriate T(5-ST)P solution. The mixture was then diluted with doubly-distilled water to 10 mL and mixed thoroughly. All the absorption and preresonance light scattering measurements were obtained against the blank treated in the same way without proteins.

The preresonance light-scattering spectra were obtained by scanning simultaneously the excitation and emission monochromators of the RF-540 spectrofluorometer from 400.0 to 750 nm with a $\Delta\lambda = 0$ nm and the slit width 5.0 nm for excitation and emission. The intensities of preresonance light-scattering were measured at 472.0 nm.

3.1.1.4 Sample preparation and determinations

To test the method, the content of proteins in synthetic samples containing metal ions, carbohydrates, amino acids, and surfacetants were determined. Three human serum samples, obtained from three different donors of the Capital of Southwest Normal University, were diluted 200-fold with doubly distilled water before the determination. Reference results for the determination of human serum samples were obtained by using CBB G-250 according to the literature.[2] The main procedure for the reference determination was in 10 mL dry calibrated flasks with additions of 0～0.10 mL standard BSA or sample solution and some water, and then 5.00 mL of the GBB G-250 working solution. The total volume of the mixture was kept to 5.10 mL. The content of proteins in the sample was determined by measuring the absorbance at 595 nm against the reagent blank.

3.1.2 Results and discussions

3.1.2.1 Features of preresonance light-scattering spectra

Figs. 1 and 2 display the preresonance light-scattering spectra of T(5-ST)P, BSA and the mixture of T(5-ST)P and BSA. T(5-ST)P has weak preresonance light-scattering over the wavelength range 400～750 nm; even so, the preresonance light-scattering in the wavelength range 440～460 nm is weaker than that in the range 400～440 and 460～550 nm because of the strong Soret absorption of T(5-ST)P. BSA has rather weak preresonance light-scattering even if its concentration is higher than 20 $\mu g \cdot mL^{-1}$. However, a strong preresonance light-scattering signal can be observed for the mixture of BSA and T(5-ST)P with the maximum preresonance light-scattering at 472.0 nm. Shoulder peaks in the range 480～550 nm can be observed also. These enhanced preresonance light-scattering signals increase with increasing concentration of proteins (Fig. 1), and decrease with increasing concentration of T(5-ST)P (Fig. 2). In addition, a small shoulder peak at 436.0 nm can be found both from Fig. 1 and Fig. 2. As Fig. 2 shows, a minimum valley at 446.0 nm occurs between the shoulder peak at 436.0 nm and the main preresonance light-scattering peak centered at 472.0 nm, especially so when the concentration of T(5-ST)P is large. The appearance of the minimum valley, located identically with the exciton splitting signal as defined in the molecule exciton theory, which is generally associated with aggregation,[25] is indicative of porphyrin–porphyrin interactions in the presence of proteins.[15,16,18] In other words, the aggregation of T(5-ST)P occurs in the presence of proteins.

3.1.2.2 J-Aggregation of T(5-ST)P in the presence of proteins

The aggregation of T(5-ST)P in the presence of proteins can also be elucidated by the absorption spectra shown in Fig. 3. Because of the protonation of the two pyrrolic nitrogen atoms in the porphyrin macrocycle, T(5-ST)P, depending on the acidity of the solution, can have three chemical species: the free base species, H_2P^{4-}, and the two protonated species, H_3P^{3-} and H_4P^{2-}, (pK_{a1} = 5.49, pK_{a2} = 6.95, I = 0.1, 25 °C).[26] At pH 1.81, T(5-ST)P exists in the form of H_4P^{2-}, and has D_{4h} spectroscopic features. The Soret band and Q band locate at 452.1 and 690.5 nm, respectively. These absorption bands, according to White,[27] originate from the second excited singlet state (the Soret maxima), and the vibronic state, Q(1,0).

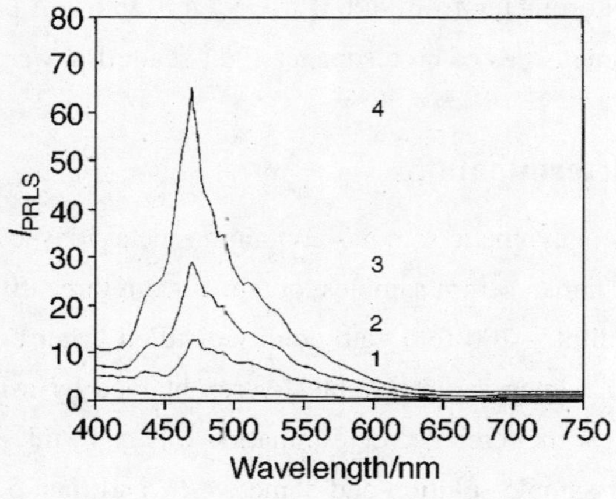

Fig. 1 Preresonance light-scattering spectra. Concentrations: BSA ($\mu g \cdot mL^{-1}$), 1, 0.0; 2, 1.0; 3, 2.0; 4, 5.0. T(5-ST)P, 1.2×10^{-6} $mol \cdot L^{-1}$; pH 1.81.

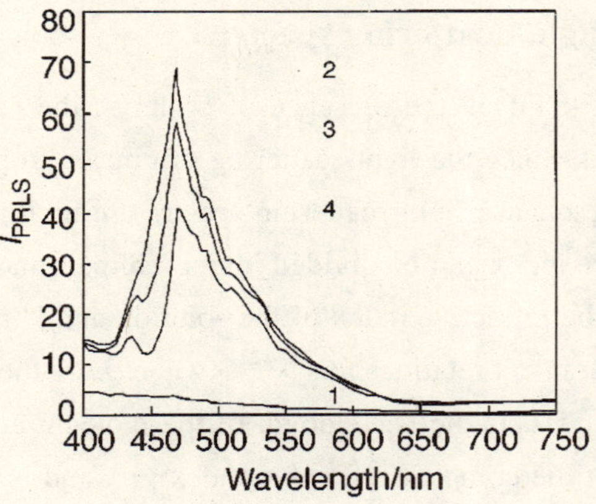

Fig. 2 The effect of the concentration of T(5-ST)P on the preresonance light-scattering spectra. Concentrations: T(5-ST)P ($\times 10^{-6}$ mol·L^{-1}): 1, 0.0; 2, 0.8; 3, 1.2; 4, 2.0. BSA: 2.0 μg·mL^{-1}; pH 1.81

As Fig. 3 shows, when proteins were added to T(5-ST)P solution, both the Soret and Q-bands decrease, giving a new weak absorption band at 490.2 nm. Three isosbestic points can be observed at 438.0, 472.1 and 645.0 nm (the inset spectra in Fig. 3 are more clear). Those isosbestic absorption points indicate species giving rise to the 490.2 nm absorption band originating from the species responsible for the 452.1 and 690.5 nm absorption bands. Since Beer's law is followed for the absorption of T(5-ST)P at 452.1 nm with its concentration, it is reasonable to assume that T(5-ST)P is monomeric under the same interacting acidity, ionic strength and concentration of T(5-ST)P and that the appearance of the 490.2 nm band is induced by proteins. So the species that is responsible for the 490.2 nm band in the presence of proteins must be the aggregates of T(5-ST)P. Therefore, it can be established that a similar monomer–aggregate equilibrium of T(5-ST)P to that of α, β, γ, δ-tetra (*p*-sulfophenyl) porphine (TPPS4) occurs in the presence of proteins.[15,16] The 490.2 nm band, located bathochromically compared with the absorption band of the parent species of organic dyes, is a *J*-aggregation band.[25,28,29] So the *J*-aggregation mechanism of T(5-ST)P in the presence of proteins can be established. As Fig. 3 shows, if the content of proteins is too large (over 10 μg·mL^{-1} for instance), the *J*-aggregates will dissolve in the microphase formed by the large amount of proteins, leading to the reappearance of the Soret band which is located hyperchromically compared with that in an aqueous medium.

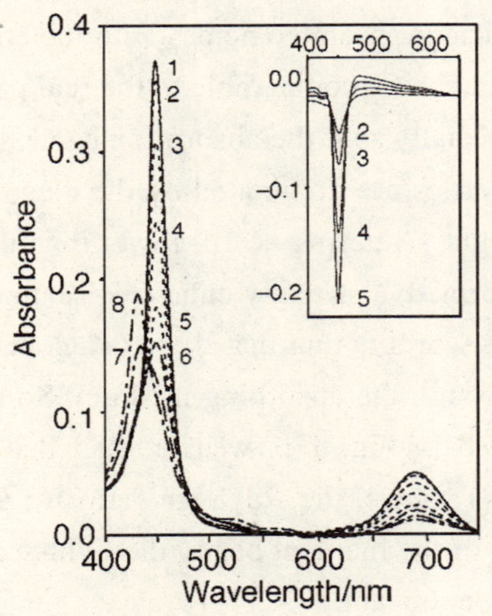

Fig. 3 The absorption spectra of the aggregation of T(5-ST)P in the presence of BSA. The spectra were obtained against the buffer blank except the inset spectra which were against the T(5-ST)P solution blank (curve 1). Concentration of BSA (μg·mL^{-1}): 1, 0.0; 2, 1.0; 3, 2.0; 4, 3.0; 5, 4.0; 6, 5.0; 7, 10.0; 8, 20.0. T(5-ST)P, 1.2 × 10^{-6} mol·L^{-1}; pH 1.81.

$$n = n_0 + \frac{2.303c\lambda_0^2}{2\pi^2}\int_0^{\infty}\frac{\varepsilon(\lambda)}{\lambda_0^2 - \lambda^2}\mathrm{d}\lambda \qquad (1)$$

3.1.2.3 Nature of the preresonance light-scattering spectra

With the ***J***-aggregation mechanism of T(5-ST)P in the presence of proteins, the features of preresonance light-scattering spectra can be easily understood. Since the light-scattering originates from the fluctuation of refractive index of a solution,[11] the present preresonance light-scattering spectra are no doubt associated with the fluctuation of refractive index *(m)*. The refractive index can be divided into a real part and an imaginary part and can be expressed as: [11] $m = n - ik$, where n is the refractive index of the solution and is related to the whole absorption spectrum of the molecule by Kronig–Kramers relationship,[20~21] where n_0 is the refractive index of the pure solvent, c is the molarity of the solution and λ_0 is the wavelength of the incident and scattering light; k is the factor that represents the imaginary part of the complex refractive index *(m)*, and is related to the quantum transition of the molecule which is responsible for the absorption band under consideration, and can be expressed as[21]

$$k = \frac{2.303\varepsilon c\lambda_0}{4\pi} \qquad (2)$$

Then we can get the Rayleigh ratio for 90° detection, $R(90°)$, which characterizes the intensity of the light-scattering of the system[22]

$$R(90^\circ) = \frac{4000\pi^2 n^2 c}{\lambda_0^4 N_A}[(\partial n/\partial c)^2 + (\partial k/\partial c)^2]C_V \qquad (3)$$

where N_A is the Avogadro constant, $\partial n/\partial c$ and $\partial k/\partial c$ are, respectively, the increments (per 1 M solute concentration) in the real part and the imaginary part of the refractive index. C_v is the Cabannes factor which accounts for the enhancement of the intensity of the light-scattering. By introducing n and k, we have

$$R(90^\circ) = \frac{(2.303)^2 \cdot 1000cn}{N_A}\left\{\left[\frac{1}{\pi}\int_0^\infty \frac{\varepsilon(\lambda)\mathrm{d}\lambda}{\lambda_0^2 - \lambda^2}\right]^2 + \frac{\varepsilon^2(\lambda_0)}{4\lambda_0^2}\right\}C_V \quad (4)$$

So, if the wavelength of an incident light beam is much removed from the absorption band, then $\partial k/\partial c \cong 0$, and the profile of light-scattering in the frequency region under consideration mainly depends on the real part of the refractive index; and if the wavelength of the incident beam coincides with the absorption band, the contribution to the light-scattering from the imaginary part can be comparable to the real part of the refractive index, and overlap the real part of the refractive index, especially so if the absorption band is an intense one. In such a case, the light-scattering is enhanced and its properties are dominated by the electronic transition of the absorption band; even though the total intensity of light-scattering is still lower than that of the solvent and it is difficult to detect.[11] However, if an aggregate is formed, a strongly enhanced scattering light can be detected even with a common spectrofluorometer.[13~17] It is worth noting that there is a concurrent loss of intensity in both incident and scattered beams as they pass through the absorbing medium. So the light-scattering in the Soret region of T(5-ST)P (440~460 nm) obtained in Fig. 1 is weaker than that outside the Soret bands (400~440, 460~550 nm). In addition, as eqn. (3) shows, the Rayleigh ratio for 90° detection is inversely proportional to the fourth power of the wavelength of the incident beam, the light-scattering in Fig. 1 and Fig. 2 decreases with increasing wavelength of the incident beam.

According to its relationship with ε, the imaginary part of the refractive index has a shape similar to the absorption spectrum; in contrast, the real part, as evaluated by the Kronig–Kramers integral, is very different.[20] Generally, the maximum enhanced resonance light-scattering often occurs at the red end of the absorption band which, according to Bauer *et al.*,[12] should strictly be called preresonance enhanced light-scattering. However, the 472.0 nm light-scattering peak in the present study, coinciding with the isosbestic point at 472.1 nm in the absorption spectrum, locates at the high energy side of the *J*-aggregation absorption band. It is possibly due to the strong absorption of the Soret band and the weak absorption of the *J*-aggregation band. The strong absorption of the Soret band can produce a large contribution to the scattering from the imaginary part and the weak *J*-aggregation band, however, can produce a small contribution. Since the Rayleigh ratio depends on the sum of the squares of the real and imaginary parts in the system, whether both parts are positive or not at the same time, the maximum of preresonance light-scattering should be located at the blue side of the *J*-aggregation. The shoulder peaks in the region 480～550 nm, can, to some extent, show the contribution from the *J*-aggregation band to the light-scattering.

3.1.2.4 Optimization of the general procedure

As stated above, the enhanced preresonance light-scattering signals result from the *J*-aggregation of T(5-ST)P induced by proteins. Generally, the aggregation of porphyrin is ascribed to the formation of the ion-pair of the cationic center on the porphyrin moiety, because of the protonation of the two pyrrolic nitrogen atoms in the porphyrin macrocycle, with one of the peripheral anionic groups of neighboring porphyrins, and the π–π interaction between porphryin systems.[28,29] So, changes of pH and ionic strength would affect the *J*-aggregation of T(5-ST)P in the presence of proteins. As Fig. 4 shows, the aggregation of T(5-ST)P decreases with increasing pH. This is possibly related to the isoelectric point of proteins. Proteins are positively charged when the pH is lower than their isoelectric points. By affecting the nature and quantity of the electric charges on proteins, pH has an effect on the *J*-aggregation of T(5-ST)P in the presence of proteins. So the lower the pH of the system, the more positive charges the proteins should have. Therefore the response of preresonance light-scattering is partly related to the isoelectric point of proteins and decreases with increasing pH. Fig. 5 shows that the intensities of the preresonance light-scattering for BSA, γ-Ig G and lysozyme, of the investigated six proteins, decrease initially with increasing the ionic strength, and then were found to remain constant when the ionic strength is higher than 0.18. The former part of the ionic strength curves can possibly be ascribed to the decrease of the statistical interaction between the porphyrin and the proteins because of the shielding effect of the charges both on the molecules of T(5-ST)P and proteins with increasing ionic strength. The flat part of the curves, however, possibly indicates the hydrophobic interaction between porphyrin macrocycles in the microphase formed by proteins.

It is worth noting that the aggregation of T(5-ST)P in the presence of proteins is very rapid and is not affected by temperature. All the data of preresonance light-scattering are stable at least in 2 h. This characteristic of the aggregation offers simplicity and reproducibility for the determination of proteins by using T(5-ST)P.

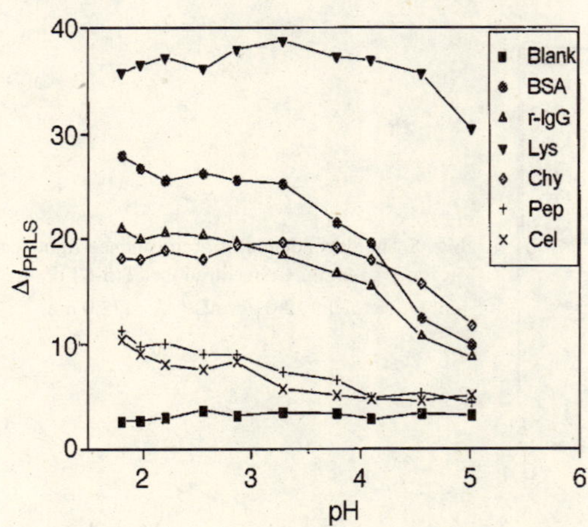

Fig. 4 The dependence of preresonance light-scattering on pH. Concentrations: T(5-ST)P, 1.2×10^{-6} mol·L^{-1}; proteins, 2.0 μg·mL^{-1}. $\lambda = 472.0$ nm.

3.1.2.5 Tolerance of nonprotein substances

The effects of substances including metal ions, amino acids, carbohydrates, and surfactants on the determination were tested by premixing BSA with the interfering substances. Table 1 shows that the common metal ions in fluids, such as Ca^{2+}, Mg^{2+}, Fe^{3+}, and NH_4^+ can be allowed with high concentrations (larger than 1.0×10^{-4} mol·L^{-1}); whereas those ions, such as Co^{2+}, Cr^{3+} and Cu^{2+} can be allowed only at very low concentration levels (lower than 1.0×10^{-7} mol·L^{-1}). However, all the interferences in the analysis of fluids, such as human serum samples, can be minimized by diluting with water. In addition, surfactant and amino acids, particularly L-Cys, L-Leu, L-Arg and L-His can be allowed at relatively high concentration levels.

3.1.2.6 Calibration curves

According to the general procedures, the relationship of the intensity of preresonance light-scattering with the concentration of proteins were obtained. It can be seen from Table 2 that when the concentration of T(5-ST)P is low, a linear relationship is followed. With increase in the concentration of T(5-ST)P the linear range is extended, and the sensitivity (slope of the linear regression equation) is reduced. The data obtained for some proteins such as lysozyme, α-chymotrypsin should be regressed in the form of two linear ranges in order to get good correlation coefficients. These data seem to follow a third order polynomial dependence. Fig. 6 shows the relationship of the intensity of preresonance light-scattering with the concentration of lysozyme. In fact, by using spectrophotometry, we found that the decrease of the absorbance at the Soret maxima with increasing concentration of proteins also follows a third order polynomial dependence (Fig. 7). It seems that the *J*-aggregation of T(5-ST)P in the presence of proteins, especially those proteins which have strongly enhanced preresonance light-scattering, follows a third order polynomial dependence.

In terms of the determination, although the *J*-aggregation follows a third order polynomial dependence, resulting correlation coefficients of the linear regression are acceptable and are larger than 0.9900 except for lysozyme, whose correlation coefficient is 0.9879 in the concentration range 0~5.0 μg·mL^{-1}. So proteins at nanogram levels can be determined (Tables 2 and 3). However, different proteins, as Table 3 shows, have different responses. Of those investigated, lysozyme has the strongest response and cellulase and pepsin have weak responses. It was reported earlier[13~17] that the enhancement effect of resonance light-scattering appears to depend on electrical properties of the individual chromophores, the strength of the electrical interaction between the chromophores and proteins, and the size of the thus-formed complex. Since the size and electrical charges of an individual protein molecule vary with the kind of protein, it can be concluded that the responses of preresonance light-scattering are protein-variability dependent.

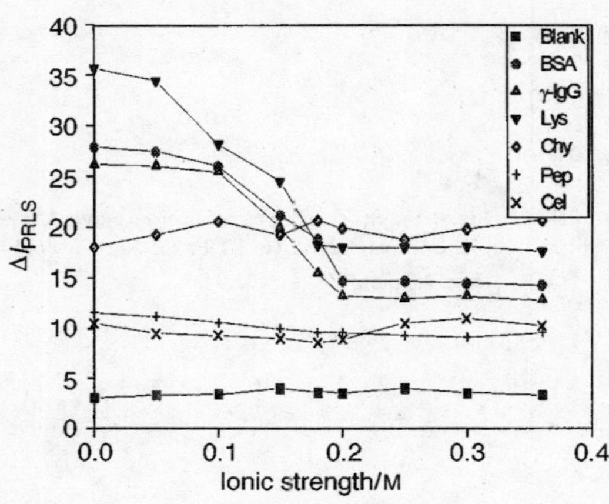

Fig. 5 The dependence of preresonance light-scattering on ionic strength. Concentrations: T(5-ST)P, 1.2×10^{-6} mol·L^{-1}; proteins, 2.0 μg·mL^{-1}. λ=472.0 nm.

Table 1 Tolerance of nonprotein substances in the determination of BSA

No.	Substance	Concentration*	Change in I_{PRLS} (%)
1	Al^{3+}, SO_4^{2-}	37.1	2.5
2	Ca^{2+}, Cl^-	99.8	-3.2
3	Cd^{2+}, Cl^-	0.44	-2.5
4	Co^{2+}, Cl^-	0.08	10.0
5	Cr^{3+}, Cl^-	0.04	3.5
6	Cu^{2+}, Cl^-	0.03	10.0
7	Fe^{3+}, Cl^-	179.1	-6.7
8	Hg^{2+}, Cl^-	0.1	-8.5
9	Mg^{2+}, Cl^-	100.0	-4.5
10	Mn^{2+}, Cl^-	72.8	3.2
11	NH_4^+, Cl^-	100.0	-6.9
12	Ni^{2+}, Cl^-	0.5	5.0
13	Pb^{2+}, $NO3^-$	2.4	-1.8
14	Zn^{2+}, Cl^-	30.6	1.8
15	NO_3^-, Na^+	161.3	6.9
16	NO_3^-, NH_4^+	64.5	-0.3
17	$H_2PO_3^-$	2.1	4.2
18	SCN^-, Na^+	34.4	-1.8
19	L-Try	8.0	6.2
20	L-Cys	80.0	-3.9
21	L-Asn	8.0	7.3
22	L-Leu	40.0	6.1
23	L-Glu	8.0	1.2
24	L-Gly	8.0	2.9
25	L-Arg	80.0	-6.3
26	L-His	80.0	8.9
27	L-Lys	8.0	3.4
28	L-Phe	8.0	6.6
29	L-Ser	8.0	6.9
30	L-Ala	8.0	2.4
31	L-Pro	32.6	4.1
32	Glucose	0.54	-2.9
33	Lactose	0.02	-9.1
34	Maltose	0.02	0.1
35	Sucrose	0.02	-7.7
36	β-Cyclodextrins	0.02	-2.7
37	SDS	0.25	-11.4
38	CTMAB	0.13	0.0
39	Zeph	11.5	-8.5
40	Gelatin	0.50	-0.6
41	Triton X-100	0.04	-5.4

* Concentration of nonprotein substances is expressed as $\times 10^{-6}$ mol·L^{-1} (No. 1~39), μg·mL^{-1} (No. 40) and % (v/v) (No. 41). Concentrations: T(5-ST)P, 1.2×10^{-6} mol·L^{-1}; BSA, 2.0 μg·mL^{-1}, pH 1.81. The relationship of the change in I_{PRLS} (%) and the % change in calculated concentration of BSA can be expressed as $\partial I_{PRLS}/I_0 = 14.2\ \partial c/c_0$, which was obtained according to the linear regression equation listed in Table 2, where the I_0 is the intensity of preresonance light-scattering when the concentration of BSA is c_0. $\partial I_{PRSLS} = I - I_0$.

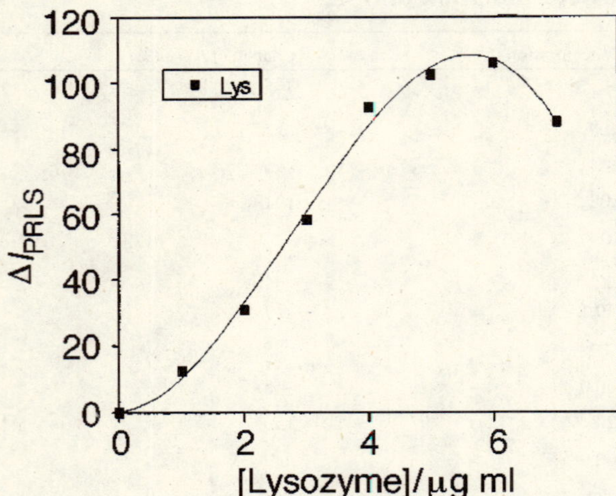

Fig. 6 The third order polynomial dependence of preresonance light-scattering on the concentration of lysozyme. The regression equation in the range 0–7.0 $\mu g{\cdot}mL^{-1}$ is ΔI_{PRLS} = $0.4 + 1.7c + 9.6c^2 - 1.1c^3$ (r = 0.9980). Concentration of T(5-ST)P, 1.2×10^{-6} $mol{\cdot}L^{-1}$; pH 1.81. λ = 472.0 nm.

3.1.2.7 Sample determination

Synthetic samples for various proteins containing metal ions, carbohydrates, amino acids and surfactants were determined, and the results are given in Table 4. It can be seen that proteins in synthetic samples can be determined with satisfactory results.

Since HSA and γ-IgG have different responses as shown in Table 3, errors will occur either by using HSA or γ-IgG as the standard for the determination of human serum samples. By using HSA as the standard to determine the mixture containing HSA and γ-IgG, we found that if the content of γ-IgG is lower than 50%, the error can be neglected assuming an acceptable determination error of 10% (Table 5). Table 6 displays the determination results for human serum samples with HSA as a standard, which was obtained from three different donors of the Capital of the Southwest Normal University and diluted 200-fold with doubly distilled water. By comparing the results of the present preresonance light-scattering method with the generally performed Bradford method using CBB G-250, it is clear that the determination for the total content of proteins is reliable, sensitive and practical.

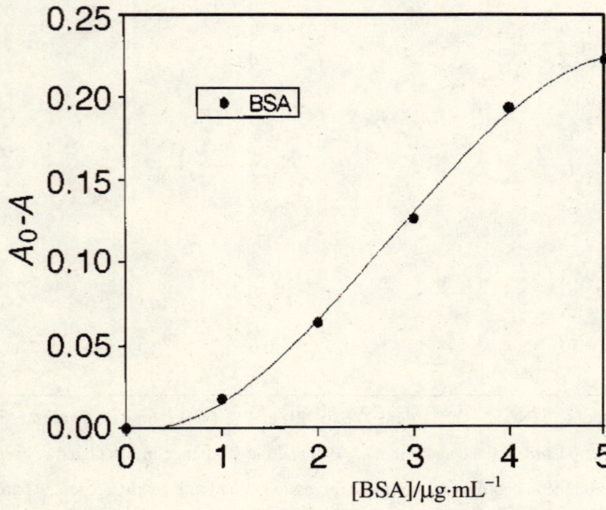

Fig. 7 The third order polynomial dependence of absorbance difference at the Soret maxima on the concentration of BSA. The regression equation in the range 0~5.0 $\mu g{\cdot}mL^{-1}$ is $A_0 - A = 0.001 - 0.110c + 0.028c^2 - 0.003c^3$ (r = 0.9995). Concentration of T(5-ST)P, 1.2×10^{-6} $mol{\cdot}L^{-1}$; pH 1.81. λ = 452.1 nm.

Table 2 Effect of the concentration of T(5-ST)P on the analytical parameters*

$C_{T(5\text{-}ST)P}$/μmol·L^{-1}	Linear range/μg·mL^{-1}	Linear regression equation/μg·mL^{-1}	Determination limit (3σ)/ng·mL^{-1}	Correlation coefficient (r)
0.4	0-1.5	$\Delta I = 0.4 + 16.0\ c$	10.1	0.9978
0.8	0-3.0	$\Delta I = 0.0 + 15.2\ c$	18.6	0.9985
1.2	0-5.0	$\Delta I = 2.0 + 14.2\ c$	26.4	0.9982
1.6	0-5.0	$\Delta I = 3.4 + 14.4\ c$	17.1	0.9918
2.0	0-6.0	$\Delta I = 3.2 + 13.0\ c$	18.9	0.9940
2.4	0-6.0	$\Delta I = 4.7 + 12.1\ c$	26.8	0.9960

* All the values were obtained by using BSA, pH 1.81.

Table 3 Analytical parameters for the determination of different proteins*

Proteins	Linear range/μg·mL^{-1}	Linear regression equation/μg·mL^{-1}	Determination limit (3σ)/ng·mL^{-1}	Correlation coefficient (r)
BSA	0-5.0	$\Delta I = 2.0 + 14.2\ c$	26.4	0.9982
HSA	0-5.0	$\Delta I = 1.8 + 14.0\ c$	26.8	0.9985
γ-IgG	0-5.0	$\Delta I = 1.2 + 11.8\ c$	31.8	0.9984
Lys	0-2.0	$\Delta I = 0.5 + 16.6\ c$	22.6	0.9985
	2.0-4.0	$\Delta I = -29.3 + 30.7\ c$		0.9980
Chy	0-2.0	$\Delta I = 0.4 + 5.2\ c$	72.1	0.9900
	2.0-7.0	$\Delta I = -29.9 + 17.9\ c$		0.9905
Prp	0.5-5.0	$\Delta I = 0.4 + 5.1\ c$	73.5	0.9970
Cel	0-7.0	$\Delta I = 0 + 4.8\ c$	78.1	0.9990

* Concentrations: T(5-ST)P, 1.2×10^{-6} mol·L^{-1}; pH 1.81

3.1.3 Conclusion

The presently reported method of protein determination by using T(5-ST)P, compared with the currently used four methods as stated in the introduction section, is very simple, sensitive, reproducible and does not involve complicated operations. Compared with the Biuret method, it can be used to determine the proteins at nanogram levels. It does not involve difficulties such as partial precipitation, which is usually found in the treatment of proteins by using phosphoric acid in the Bradford and BCG methods, that supplies a good reproducibility of the method. Although the T(5-ST)P method cannot supply a wide linear range because the intensity of preresonance lightscattering follows a third order dependence on the concentration of proteins, and involves extensive calibration, the use of this method can be performed in a short time even though it needs extensive calibration but has high efficiency, facility and sensitivity. However, this method cannot be used to determine the concentration of proteins in urine samples because the concentration of proteins is too low and the interferences of foreign substances cannot be eliminated by diluting the sample with doubly distilled water.

Table 4 Determination results for synthetic samples

Sample	Amount/μg·mL^{-1}	Nonprotein substances*	Found/μg·mL^{-1}, n= 5	Recovery (%, n= 5)	RSD† (%, n= 5)
BSA	24.9	Al^{3+}, Co^{2+}, Mn^{2+}, Pb^{2+}	24.5	99.5± 2.1	1.4
HSA	20.0	Carbohydrates	19.8	101.5± 3.0	1.3

Continued

Sample	Amount/μg·mL^{-1}	Nonprotein substances*	Found/μg·mL^{-1}, n= 5	Recovery (%, n= 5)	RSD† (%, n= 5)
γ-IgG	25.0	L-Pro, L-Leu, L-Cys	23.2	92.3± 3.7	2.1
Chy	25.0	β-CD, SDS, Triton X-100	24.1	100.0± 1.2	0.5
Lys	25.0	CTMAB, gelatin	24.8	105.0± 1.3	1.9

*1.9×10^{-4} mol·L^{-1} Al^{3+}, 4.0×10^{-7} mol·L^{-1} Co^{2+}, 5.0×10^{-4} mol·L^{-1} Ba^{2+}, 1.2×10^{-5} mol·L^{-1} Pb^{2+}; 1.0×10^{-8} mol·L^{-1} carbohydrates including glucose, lactose, maltose and sucrose; 4.0×10^{-6} mol·L^{-1} L-Pro, L-Leu and L-Cys; the concentration of Triton X-100, CTMAB and gelatin is 4.0×10^{-5} % (v/v). † Relative standard deviation for five measurements of samples. Concentrations: T(5-ST)P, 1.2×10^{-6} mol·L^{-1}, pH 1.81.

Table 5 Determination results for HSA and γ-IgG mixture

No.	Added/μg·mL^{-1}			Found/μg·mL^{-1}, n= 5	
	HSA	γ-IgG	R (%)*	HSA+γ-IgG	DR (%)†
1	22.5	2.5	10	25.1± 0.1	0.4
2	20.0	5.0	20	24.5± 0.1	-2.0
3	17.5	7.5	3.0	23.8±0.1	-4.8
4	15.0	10.0	40	23.1± 0.2	-7.6
5	12.5	12.5	50	22.8± 0.2	-8.8
6	10.0	15.0	60	21.6± 0.1	-13.6
7	7.5	17.5	70	19.8± 0.2	-20.8
8	5.0	20.0	80	18.2± 0.2	-27.2

Data were obtained by using BSA as the standard. * Ratio of γ-IgG to the mixture of BSA and γ-IgG. † Determination error, pH 1.81, T(5-ST)P, 1.2×10^{-6} M.

Table 6 Total content of proteins in human serum samples*

Sample	T(5-ST)P method		CBB G-250 method Found/mg·mL^{-1}
	Found/mg·mL^{-1} n= 5	Recovery (%, n = 5)	
1	74.7± 3.5	94.2 ± 2.2	73.6
2	71.8± 2.6	96.6 ± 3.1	73.4
3	69.3± 3.2	92.2 ± 1.8	71.4

* All the values of the T(5-ST)P method were obtained by using HSA as the standard at pH 1.81; T(5-ST)P, 1.2×10^{-6} mol·L^{-1}. Human serum samples were obtained from three different donors of the Capital of Southwest Normal University, and pretreated by diluting 200-fold with doubly-distilled water.

Acknowledgments

This project is supported by the Municipal Science Foundation of Chongqing for Young and Middle Scientists, and to which all the authors here are grateful.

References

[1] Zhang, L. X., and Wu, G. L., Advanced Biochemical Experiments, Advanced Education Press, Beijing, 1989, pp. 192.
[2] Wei, Y. J., Li, K. A.; and Tong, S. Y., Talanta, 1997, 44, 923.
[3] Zhang, J. X., and Halling, P. J., Anal. Biochem., 1990, 188, 9.
[4] Wei, Y. J., Li, K. A., and Tong, S. Y., Talanta, 1996, 43, 1.
[5] Zeng, W., Meng, X. J., Li, N., and Tong, S. Y., Anal. Chim. Acta, 1995, 316, 387.
[6] Tong, S. Y., and Li, N. Chin. Chem. Lett., 1993, 4, 1079.
[7] Li, N., and Tong, S. Y., Anal. Lett., 1995, 28, 1763.
[8] Li, N., and Tong, S. Y., Talanta, 1994, 41, 1657.
[9] Li, N., Li, K. A., and Tong, S. Y., Anal. Biochem., 1996, 233, 151.

[10] Zuo, J., The Principles and Applications of Laser Light Scattering in Polymer Science, Henan Science and Technology Press, Zhengzhou, 1994, p. 1.

[11] Miller, G. A., J. Phys. Chem., 1978, 82, 616.

[12] Bauer, D. R., Hudson, B., and Pecora, R., J. Chem. Phys., 1975, 63, 588.

[13] Huang, C. Z., Li, K. A., and Tong, S. Y., Anal. Chem., 1996, 68, 2059.

[14] Huang, C. Z., Li, K. A., and Tong, S. Y., Anal. Chem., 1997, 69, 514.

[15] Huang, C. Z., Zhu, J. X., Li, K. A., and Tong, S. Y., Anal. Sci., 1997, 13, 263.

[16] Huang, C. Z., and Li, Y. F., Bull. Chem. Soc. Jpn., 1998, 71, in the press.

[17] Pasternack, R. F., Bustamante, C., Collings, P. J., Giannetteo, A., and Gibbs, E. J., J. Am. Chem. Soc., 1993, 115, 5393.

[18] Huang, C. Z., Li, K. A., and Tong, S. Y., Bull. Chem. Soc. Jpn., 1997, 70, 1843.

[19] Huang, C. Z., Li, K. A., and Tong, S. Y., Chem. J. Chin. Univ., 1997, 18, 524.

[20] Anglister, J., and Steinberg, I. Z., Chem. Phys. Lett., 1979, 65, 50.

[21] Anglister, J., and Steinberg, I. Z., J. Chem. Phys., 1981, 74, 786.

[22] Anglister, J., and Steinberg, I. Z., J. Chem. Phys., 1983, 78, 5358.

[23] Stanton, S. G., Pecora, R., and Hudson, B., J. Chem. Phys., 1981, 75, 5615.

[24] Pecora, R., Dynamic Light Scattering, Plenum Press, New York, 1985, p. 80.

[25] Akins, D. L., Zhu, H. R., and Guo, C., J. Phys. Chem., 1994, 98, 3612.

[26] Zeng, Y. E., Zhang, H. S., and Chen, Z. H., Handbook of Modern Chemical Reagents, Vol. 4, Chemical Industry Press, Beijing, 1989, p. 793.

[27] White, W. I., in The Porphyrins, Vol. 5, ed. Dolphin, D., Academic Press, New York, 1978, p. 310.

[28] Ohno, O., Kaizu, Y., and Kobayashi, H., J. Chem. Phys., 1993, 99, 4128.

[29] Chandrashekar, T. K., van Willigen, H., and Ebersole, M. H., J. Phys. Chem., 1984, 88, 4326.

(Cheng Zhi Huang, Yuan Fang Li, Jian Guo Mao and Dai Gao Tan,
published in *The Analyst*, 1998, 123,1401～1406)

3.2 On the Factors Affecting the Enhanced Resonance Light Scattering Signals of the Interactions Between Proteins and Multiply Negatively Charged Chromophores Using Water Blue as an Example

Abstract: Electrostatic interactions of proteins, including bovine serum albumin (BSA), human serum albumin (HSA), γ-globulin (γ-IgG), α-chymotrypsin (Chy), lysozyme (Lys) and cellulase (Cel), with multiply negatively charged chromophores were investigated based on the measurements of the enhanced resonance light scattering (RLS) signals. Using triply negatively charged water blue (WB) as an example, the factors were discussed that affect the enhanced resonance light scattering signals of the interactions between proteins and the negatively charged chromophores. It was found that the enhanced RLS signals with the maximum light scattering peak at 346.0 nm in these interacting systems are strongly dependent on the isoelectric points of proteins and show adverse linear relationships with increasing ionic strength depending on the positive charges of the inorganic metal ions used to control the ionic strength of the medium, sufficiently disclosing that the electrostatic attraction performs an important role in the combination of proteins with WB. Linear responses were discovered between the enhanced RLS signals and the protein molecular weights (M_w), displaying the dimensions of scattered particles formed by proteins and WB make a key contribution to the RLS enhancements. An empirical equation is proposed which possibly displays the factors affecting the enhanced RLS signals of the interactions between proteins with negatively charged chromophores.

Keywords: Proteins; Water blue; Resonance light scattering (RLS) technique; Electrostatic interaction

3.2.1 Introduction

In recent years, resonance light scattering (RLS) technique has been more and more extensively applied for various analytical purposes in the quantification of proteins [1~7], nucleic acids [8~11], pharmaceutical drugs [12], sugars [13~15], surfactants [16] and metal ions [17] in artificial and real samples, and has become one of most important tools in characterizing the aggregation and assembly of biological and chemical species [18~21]. All these investigations have sufficiently shown that RLS technique is a favorite, powerful and promising tool due to its convenient manipulation, and high sensitivity.

In most investigations mentioned above, enhanced RLS signals are available when the interactions of analytes occur with corresponding organic probe reagents through electrostatic attraction. However, the interactions of the analytes with the biological targets depend on the nature of both components [22]. Thus, it is necessary to further understand the factors affecting the enhanced RLS signals of the interactions and characteristics of electrostatic force between analytes and the corresponding organic probe reagents, and also propitious to look for and synthesize novel and highly efficient probe reagents. Our previous studies [1,8,9,23] have indicated that enhanced RLS signals are relevant to the electrostatic attraction of the interacting components and the dimensions of the thus-formed scattered particles when the instrumental conditions maintain unchanged. In this contribution, we take the interactions of water blue (WB, Fig. 1 displays its molecular structure), a typical triply charged anionic triphenylmethane dye, with proteins as an example, and try to investigate the role of the electrostatic attraction played in the contributions to RLS enhancements.

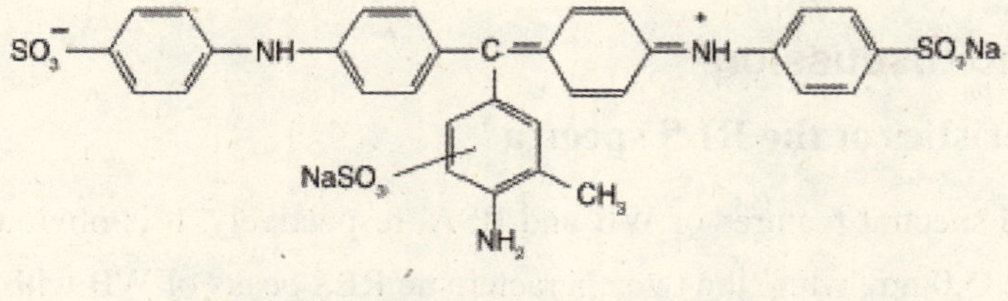

Fig. 1 Molecular structure of water blue (WB).

3.2.2 Experimental

3.2.2.1 Apparatus

RLS spectra and intensities were obtained with a Hitachi F-2500 fluorescence spectrophotometer (Tokyo, Japan), and the absorption spectra were measured by a Techcomp 8500 spectrophotometer (Hong Kong, China). A PHS-3C digital pH meter (Shanghai Dazhong Analytical Instruments Plant, Shanghai, China) and an MVS-1 vortex mixer (Beide Scientific Instrumental Ltd., Beijing, China) were used to detect pH values of aqueous solutions and blend the mixtures in volumetric flasks, respectively.

3.2.2.2 Reagents

Typical studies were carried out using commercial bovine serum albumin (BSA, Beitai Biochemical Co., Chinese Academy of Sciences, Beijing) and human serum albumin (HSA, Sigma, USA). For a comparison study, commercial γ-globulin (γ-IgG, Serva, Germany), lysozyme (Lys, Shanghai Institute of Biochemistry, Shanghai), α-chymotrypsin (Chy, Shanghai Chemical Reagent Distribution Co., Shanghai) and pepsin (Pep, Fangcao Medical Industrial Co., Shanghai) were also employed. 25.0 mg ml^{-1} protein solutions were all prepared by dissolving the commercial products in doubly distilled water, except for γ-IgG, with the aid of appropriate volumes of 0.1 $mol \cdot l^{-1}$ NaCl solution. Further dilution was made according to the necessity of the general procedure.

Water blue 1.0×10^{-4} $mol \cdot L^{-1}$ (WB, Shanghai Chemical Reagents Co., Shanghai) was prepared by directly dissolving the reagent in doubly distilled water. Britton-Robinson (BR) buffer solutions and NaCl solution were used to monitor the acidity and ionic strength of the interacting systems, correspondingly. Except that proteins were of biochemical-reagent grade, all other reagents were of analytical-reagent grade without further purification. Doubly distilled water was used throughout.

3.2.2.3 Sample

To test the proposed method, three fresh human urine samples, supplied by donors of our lab, were put into use. Mixtures of 10.0 mL of each fresh human urine sample with 0.0, 0.5, 1.5, 2.5, 3.5, 4.5, 5.5, 6.5 mL of 250.0 $\mu g \cdot mL^{-1}$ standard HSA working solution, were diluted to 25.0 mL with doubly distilled water. After that, 1.00 mL samples from these 25.0 mL diluted mixtures were also analyzed according to the general procedure.

3.2.2.4 General procedure

Into a 10 mL volumetric flask were added an appropriate volume of proteins working solution or sample solution, 1.0 mL of BR buffer solution and 1.0 mL WB solution. The mixture was vortex-mixed after each addition of the interacting additives, then diluted to the 10.0 mL scale mark with water and mixed thoroughly.

The RLS spectrum was obtained by scanning simultaneously ($\Delta\lambda$ = 0 nm) the excitation and emission monochromators of the spectrofluorometer from 220.0 to 520.0 nm, during which the spectral bandwidths of the excitation and emission monochromators were both kept at 5.0 nm. RLS intensity was measured at 346.0 nm.

3.2.3 Results and discussion

3.2.3.1 Characteristics of the RLS spectra

Fig. 2 shows the RLS spectral features of WB and BSA, respectively. It is obvious that the maximum RLS peak of BSA is located at 285.0 nm, while the two characteristic RLS peaks of WB with almost the same intensity are situated at 265.0 and 355.0 nm, correspondingly. Besides, the RLS signal of BSA is stronger than that of WB, but both are very faint over the scanning wavelength range of 220～520 nm. However, the RLS characteristics of the interacting systems of BSA and WB (from curve 3 to 6) are quite different from those of BSA and WB in the whole scanning region, obviously displaying that BSA has interacted with WB. Firstly, greatly enhanced RLS signals could be observed with the maximal RLS peak of the interacting system positioned at 346.0 nm.

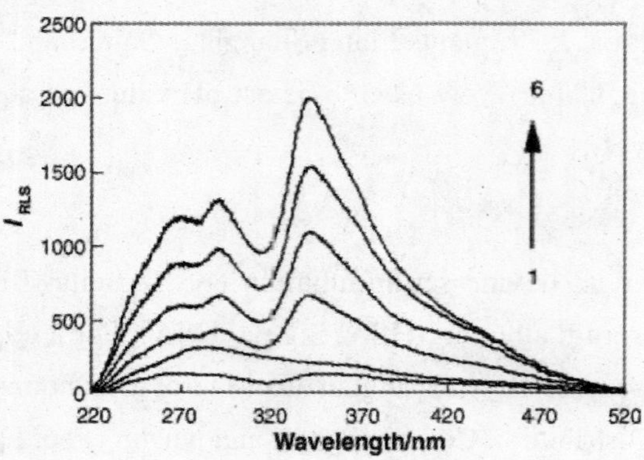

Fig. 2 RLS spectra of the interaction of WB and BSA. Line 1, WB; Line 2, BSA; Lines 3–6, BSA–WB. Concentrations: WB, 1.0×10^{-5} mol·L^{-1}, except for Line 2 without any WB; BSA (μg·mL^{-1}): 1, 0.0; 2, 10.0; 3, 2.0; 4, 4.0; 5, 6.0; 6, 8.0. pH, 2.09. Ionic strength, 0.001 mol·L^{-1}

Secondly, RLS shoulder peaks could also be found from 270 to 320 nm. In addition, it has been also found that the RLS signals of the interacting system increase proportionally with increasing BSA concentration, but change a little with the WB concentration in the range of 0.5×10^{-5} to 2.0×10^{-5} mol·L^{-1}, disclosing that the RLS signal of WB is enhanced by the presence of BSA. Compared with BSA, other proteins, including HSA, γ-IgG, Lys, Chy, show very similar RLS features when interacting with WB, with the exception of the RLS intensity varieties.

3.2.3.2 Effects of pH values in medium

In order to test the electrostatic attraction, we could adjust the pH of the medium so that the proteins are positively charged. Owing to the negatively charged –SO_3– group, it is not necessary to consider that adjusting pH-value of the medium should induce the change of charges on the molecular structure of WB in the pH range of 1.81～11.4. Thus, the properties of the biological target can define the required buffer conditions and ionic strength[22]. Therefore, the dependence of RLS signals of the interacting system of BSA and WB on the pH values mainly discloses the pH effect on the interactions related to proteins. As Fig. 3 shows, with the variation of pH-values, the RLS intensities of WB keep unchangeable, whereas those of the protein–WB mixtures present different traits. That is, the RLS intensities of the systems of WB with BSA, HSA, γ-IgG or Chy all lesson distinctly with the increasing pH value so that they nearly approach to the WB reagent blank level when the pH value reaches 4.78, 4.78, 5.33, 7.96, respectively, which are very close to their isoelectric points (pI_0), correspondingly (BSA, pI_0 = 4.9; HSA, pI_0 = 4.9; γ-IgG, pI_0 = 5.8; Chy, pI_0 = 8.1,[24]). For Lys–WB system, the RLS signals continue to be strong and do not change very much until the pH value gets 9.15. After that, RLS intensities also decline rapidly and come close to that of the reagent blank at pH 10.88, which is adjacent to the iso-electric point of Lys ($pI0$ =11.0, [24]) as well.

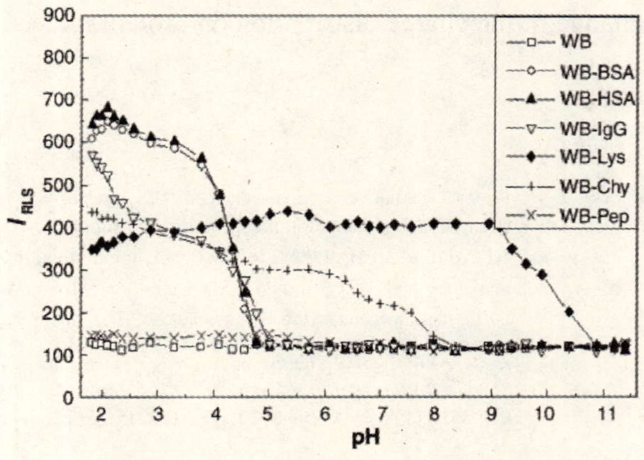

Fig. 3 Dependence of the RLS intensity on the pH values. Concentrations: proteins, 2 $\mu g \cdot mL^{-1}$; WB, 1.0×10^{-5} $mol \cdot L^{-1}$. λ = 346.0 nm. Ionic strength was kept at 0.009 by adding 0.1 $mol \cdot L^{-1}$ NaCl solution. The reagent blank solution is the mixture of WB and buffer.

Nevertheless, the RLS intensities of Pep–WB (Pep, pI_0 =1.0,[24]) system are just about the same as the reagent blank level in the whole pH range examined, disclosing that the interaction between Pep with WB does not occur.

Proteins permit to be positively charged and negatively charged when the pH of the medium is adjusted to be lower and higher than their pI_0 values, respectively. It is apparent that positively charged proteins can combine easily with the negatively charged WB, while negatively ones can not, so it is effortless to understand why the interactions of WB with BSA, HSA, γ-IgG, Chy or Lys have the similar RLS variation tendencies, and why in the whole pH range examined, the interactions of Pep with WB result in the approximately same signal levels as those of the WB blanks. Thus, above pH examinations disclose that the interactions of proteins with WB mainly proceed through charge-couple effect, not hydrophobic attraction. In other word, we can make a positively charged medium by adjusting the pH values of the medium in order to satisfy the electrostatic interaction between proteins and negatively charged chromophores.

In order to further investigate the role of electrostatic attraction, we tested different addition orders of reagents, including BSA–BR–WB, BSA–WB–BR and BR–WB–BSA. It was found that the sequence of BSA–BR–WB results in a higher enhanced RLS signal than other ways. We consider that it also results from the electrostatic attraction of these interacting components for mixing BSA, where the buffer first can provide the best pH medium for the change of the charged state of BSA, which is a key factor for the combination of BSA and WB, but other ways cannot do so or in the same way. For instance, when BSA and WB are mixed firstly, the pH of the solution is nearly neutral, which is not beneficial for the interaction of BSA with WB. The interactions of WB with HSA, γ-IgG, Lys, Chy have very analogical phenomena.

3.2.3.3 Effect of the ionic strength in the medium

The role of the charge-coupled effect played in the interactions of proteins with WB can be further confirmed by testing the effect of ionic strength [25]. As Fig. 4 shows, the enhanced RLS intensities of proteins–WB systems fall remarkably when the ionic strength (I_S) of the aqueous media, adjusted by 1.0 $mol \cdot L^{-1}$ NaCl solution, increases. Moreover, when the ionic strength is higher than 0.20 $mol \cdot L^{-1}$, the enhanced RLS signals of protein–WB are all scarcely detected, showing the combinations of proteins with WB have been held back. It is very interesting to notice that there are linear relationships between the RLS intensities and the ionic strength for different proteins, proving that electrostatic force plays an important part in the interactions of proteins with WB. The effect of the ionic strength can be evidently ascribed to the electrostatic attraction between proteins and WB because of the escalating shielding effect of the charges on both proteins and WB molecules, which blocks the formation of the combination products of protein–WB. In addition, the different slopes of the regression equations of different proteins with the increase of ionic strength show the change of the charge distribution on protein molecules.

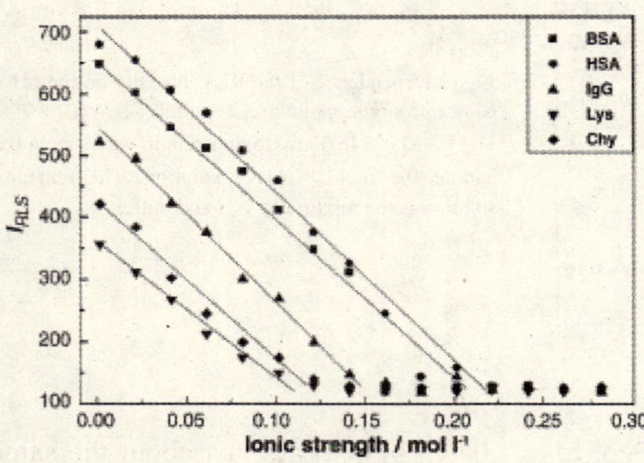

Fig. 4 Dependence of the enhanced RLS intensity on the ionic strength (I_S). Concentrations: proteins, 2.0 μg·mL^{-1}; WB, 1.0 × 10^{-5} mol·L^{-1}. pH, 2.09. λ = 346.0 nm. Ionic strength was adjusted by adding 1.0 mol·L^{-1} NaCl solution. Mixing WB with buffer solution made the blank solution. The linear regression equation for BSA, HSA, IgG, Lys and Chy are I_{RLS} = 655.3–2417I_S (r = 0.9970), I_{RLS} = 708.7–2599I_S (r = 0.9918), I_{RLS} = 539.6–2760I_S (r = 0.9971), I_{RLS} = 361.1– 2306I_S (r = 0.9988) and I_{RLS} = 432.6–2920I_S (r = 0.9935), respectively.

It was found that the decrease of the enhanced RLS intensity depends on the charge on the inorganic cations in the salts used for ionic strength control. As Fig. 5 shows, RLS intensities of proteins–WB systems drop much more rapidly when 1.0 mol l^{-1} multiply positively charged metal cation salts, such as $MgCl_2$ and $AlCl_3$, are put into use, further demonstrating the electrostatic attraction is a key factor in the combination of proteins with WB. The linear regression equations with the ionic strength controlled IA, IIA and IIIA metal ions including Na^+, K^+, Mg^{2+}, Ba^{2+} and Al^{3+} have similar intercept values (average value is 645.5, R.S.D. = 1.3%), while these controlled using IIB and VIB metal ions including Cd^{2+}, Zn^{2+} and Cr^{3+} have different intercepts, which are hardly interpreted and are possibly due to the electronic structure of the full filling and half filling orbits of these elements. On the other hand, the slopes of these regression equations are different depending on the charge'of the inorganic metal ions. From these slope data, we could get a regression of the slope data against the positive charges of the metal ions: S = 3191.8 – 777.2m (r = 0.9956, N = 8, P < 0.0001), where S is the slope values, m is the valence of the metal ions. That is an evidence to indicate that electrostatic interaction is an important factor in the interaction between WB and proteins.

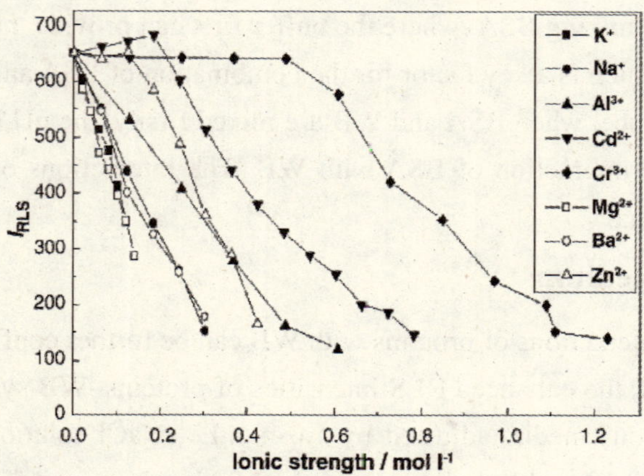

Fig. 5 Relationships between the RLS response levels and ionic strength of the aqueous media. Proteins, 2.0 μg·mL^{-1}; WB, 1.0 × 10^{-5} mol·L^{-1}. pH, 2.09. λ = 346.0 nm. Adding 1.0 mol·L^{-1} NaCl, KCl, $MgCl_2$, $CdCl_2$, $BaCl_2$, $ZnCl_2$, $AlCl_3$ and $CrCl_3$ solution to adjust the ionic strength of the media, respectively. The decay of each curve could be linearly regressed and the linear regression equations are I_{RLS} = 655.3 – 2417 I_{SNaCl} (r = – 0.9970, n = 7), I_{RLS} = 643.9 – 2490 I_{SKCl} (r = – 0.9959, n = 8), I_{RLS} = 652.8 – 1639 I_{SMgCl2} (r = – 0.9947, n = 6), I_{RLS} = 858.7 – 1571 I_{SCdCl2} (r = 0.9946, n = 6), I_{RLS} = 632.2 – 1553 I_{SBaCl2} (r = 0.9911, n = 6), I_{RLS} = 871.0 – 1630 I_{SZnCl2} (r = 0.9963, n = 6), I_{RLS} = 643.3 – 922 I_{SAlCl3} (r = – 0.9925, n = 6), I_{RLS} = 1017 – 876 I_{SCrCl3} (r = – 0.9820, n = 6), respectively. With these slope values together, we could have a regression equation of the slope data vis the positive changes of the metal ions: S =3191.8 – 777.2m (r = 0.9956, N = 8, P < 0.0001), where S is the slope values and m is the valence of the metal ions.

3.2.3.4 Dependence of RLS intensity on protein-variation

Under the optimum conditions described above, the relationships between the RLS intensity and the protein concentration have been investigated. From the results in Fig. 6, it can be seen that the slopes of these linear equations and linear ranges are dependent on protein-variability. In view of the fact that the dimension and electric charge state of an individual protein molecule vary with the kind of proteins, it is facile to understand that RLS responses are protein-variability dependent, shown in our work. As Fig. 7 shows, the slopes of the linear regression equations are proportional to the molecular weights of proteins (*M*w), indicating that the dimension of the combination products of proteins–WB is a dependent factor for the enhanced RLS intensity.

3.2.3.5 Theoretical discussion of the factors related to enhanced RLS signals

It was reported earlier[23] that the enhanced RLS signals appear to rely sensitively on electric properties of the individual chromophores, the strength of the electric interaction between the chromophores and biomolecules, and the dimension of the thus-formed complex. The effects of pH, ionic strength and the protein-variability, discussed above, further support that RLS technique can provide well valuable information as Ref. reported[23].

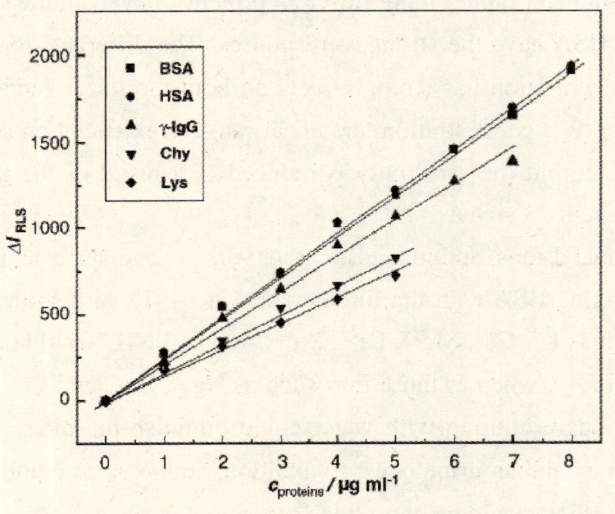

Fig. 6 Relationships between RLS intensities of protein–WB systems and the protein-variability. pH, 2.09. Ionic strength, 0.001 mol·L^{-1}. λ = 346.0 nm.

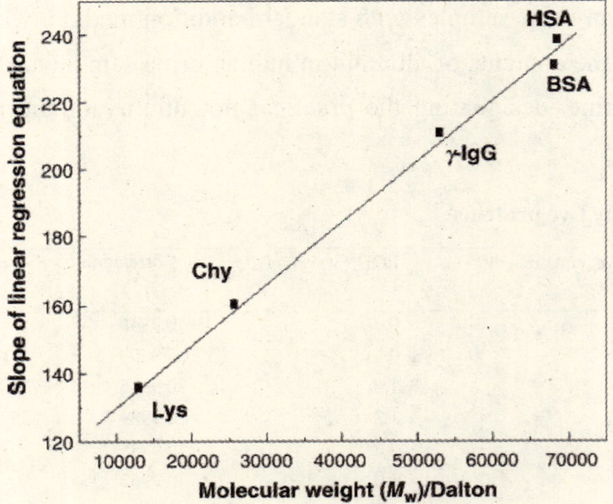

Fig. 7 Linear relationship between the RLS response levels and the molecular weight of proteins (*M*w). WB, 1.0 × 10^{-5} mol·L^{-1}. pH, 2.09. Ionic strength, 0.001 mol·L^{-1}. λ = 346.0 nm. The linear regression equation is S =113.9 + 1.78 × 10^{-3} *M*w (r = 0.9981), in which S is the slope of the linear regression equation in Table 2, and (*M*w) is the molecular weight of proteins.

According to Figs. 4 and 5, and the corresponding regression results, we could simply draw an empirical equation to show the effect of electrostatic interaction:

$$\Delta I = \alpha_{\mathrm{I}}(3191.8 - 777.2m)I_{\mathrm{s}} \qquad (1)$$

where α_I is a constant related to the intrinsic features of the metal ion used for ion strength control, *m*, the valence of metal ion, and I_S is the ionic strength quantitatively equal to the concentration of the singly charged metal ion. When $m = 1$, Eq. (1) is very simple; while *m* is larger than 1, the equation gets complicate.

In similar way, according to Figs. 6 and 7 and corresponding regression results, we could draw an empirical equation also and show the enhanced RLS signals have protein-variability:

$$\Delta I = \alpha_{\mathrm{P}} + (113.9 + 1.78 \times 10^{-3} M_{\mathrm{W}})c \qquad (2)$$

where α_P is a constant related to variety of proteins. For a given protein, a linear relationship could be constructed and thus protein assays could be made.

3.2.3.6 Analytical applications of the interaction between WB –proteins

As Fig. 6 and Eq. (2) show, the enhanced RLS intensity of WB by different proteins is in proportional to the concentration of proteins, and under the optimum conditions described above, the relationships between the RLS intensity and the protein concentration have been studied (Table 1). For different proteins, however, the sensitivity is different. Of these detected proteins, BSA and HSA have the strongest responses. The different slopes of the linear regression equations show that the WB concentration has strong effects on both the linear range and the sensitivity. For the same protein, with the escalating WB concentration, the linear range is extended on account of the strengthened ability to combine with the protein, but the sensitivity is reduced as a result of the increasing molecular absorption in the medium that weakens the RLS signals.

The effects of foreign substances, including metal ions, amino acids, carbohydrates, and surfactants, on this proteins assay method were investigated by premixing BSA with the foreign substances. Table 2 shows that the commonly observed metal ions in body fluids, such as K^+, Ca^+, Mg^{2+}, Fe^{3+}, Zn^{2+}, Al^{3+} and NH_4^+ could be allowed with high tolerant levels (more than 1.0×10^{-4} mol·L^{-1}), whereas those ions such as Hg^{2+}, Co^{2+} and Cr^{3+} could be allowed only at very low concentrations. Even though, diluting with water could diminish the interferences of these non-protein substances in real samples, such as human urine ones. In addition, amino acids could be tolerated at relatively high concentrations. Anionic surfactants could be permitted at very low levels.

Fig. 8 displays the determination results of human urine samples with standard addition method, where HSA was employed as the standard. The results show that the contents of albumin in human urine sample are in agreement with the standard values for normal human urine, designating the practical potentiality of the proposed method in clinical test.

Table 1 Analytical parameters for the determination of the five proteins

Proteins (μg·mL^{-1})	c_{WB} (10^{-5}mol·L^{-1})	Linear range (μg·mL^{-1})	Linearregression equation, ΔI (n = 5, μg·mL^{-1})	LOD[a](3σ/ng·mL^{-1})	Correlation coefficient (r)
BSA	0.5	0.01～6.5	25.2+208.2c	0.8	0.9946
	1.0	0.01～8.0	41.6+230.8c	0.8	0.9990
	1.5	0.01～9.0	60.8 + 165.3c	1.0	0.9975
	2.0	0.01～10.5	30.4+161.8c	1.2	0.9989
HSA	1.0	0.01～8.0	32.2+238.3c	0.6	0.9985
γ-IgG	1.0	0.01～7.0	18.6+210.2c	1.0	0.9962
Chy	1.0	0.01～5.0	25.7+ 160.4c	1.3	0.9975
Lys	1.0	0.02～6.5	44.6+ 135.9c	1.5	0.9990

[a]Limit of determination. pH, 2.09; ionic strength, 0.001 mol·L^{-1}; λ = 346.0 nm.

Table 2 Tolerance of foreign substances in the determination of BSA

No.	Non-protein substances	Concentration[a]	Change of I_{RLS} (%)	Non-protein substances	Concentration[a]	Change of I_{RLS} (%)
1	K^+, Cl^-	1500	-7.4	SO_4^{2-}, Na^+	720	-4.4
2	Ca^{2+}, Cl^-	350	-9.0	L-Cys	35	+2.9
3	Cd^{2+}, Cl^-	5.5	+5.2	L -Arg	72	+5.2
4	Co^{2+}, Cl^-	0.02	-9.9	L -Try	40	-4.0
5	Cr^{3+}, Cl	0.04	-6.4	L -Asn	50	-7.1
6	Cu^{2+}, Cl	0.08	+8.1	L -Glu	12	+6.3
7	Fe^{3+}, Cl^-	120	+5.4	Glucose	0.8	-7.3
8	Hg^{2+}, Cl^-	0.01	-7.1	Lactose	0.15	+6.2
9	Mg^{2+}, Cl^-	170	+2.9	Maltose	0.52	-3.5
10	Al^{3+}, Cl^-	15	+8.0	Sucrose	0.35	-4.9
11	NH_4^+, Cl^-	680	+4.8	SDBS	0.01	+10.2
12	Ni^{2+}, Cl^-	1.0	-7.3	SDS	0.02	+9.0
13	Pb^{2+}, Cl^-	0.45	+2.8	CTMAB	0.1	-5.5
14	Zn^{2+}, Cl^-	150	-9.5	β-CD	0.2	-7.9
15	NO_3^-, Na^+	100	-6.0	Zeph	8	-8.5
16	$H_2PO_4^-$, K^+	1200	-8.5	TritonX-100	0.07	+6.8

[a] The concentrations of non-protein substances are expressed by $\times 10^{-6}$ mol·L^{-1} (Nos. 1–30), and %(v/v) (No. 31). Concentrations: WB, 1.0×10^{-5} mol·L^{-1}; BSA, 2.0 μg·mL^{-1}; pH, 2.09; ionic strength, 0.001 mol·L^{-1}; λ=346.0 nm.

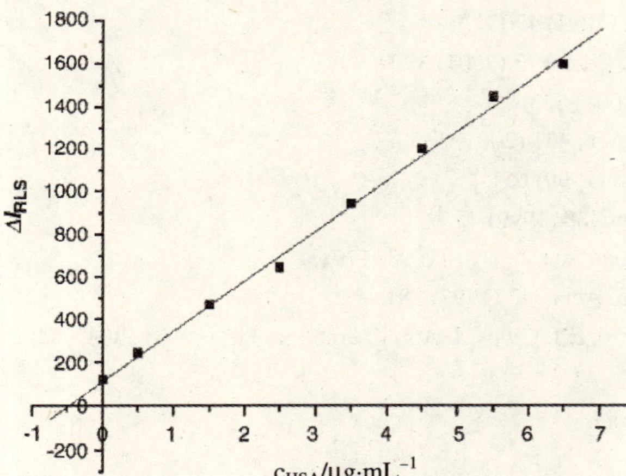

Fig. 8 Assay of human urine samples using standard addition method. Concentration: WB, 1.0×10^{-5} mol·L^{-1}. pH, 2.09. Ionic strength, 0.001. λ=346.0 nm. Three samples were analyzed. Their linear relationships can be regressed as ΔI=115.7+234.5c (r=0.9982, Sample 1, see the direct line in the figure), ΔI= 101.5+240.7c (r=0.9948, Sample 2, not shown in the figure), and ΔI=90.9+237.2c (r=0.9992, Sample 3, not show in the figure). Therefore, we could calculate that the content ofproteins in the three human urine samples are 12.3, 10.5 and 9.58 (mg·mL^{-1}), respectively. The data of ΔI_{RLS} were obtained against the WB reagent blank solution.

It is worth noting that white suspensions could be possibly observed if the dilution of the fresh human urine samples is not sufficient, and the assay will not offer correct results. In such a case, further dilutions of fresh human urine samples are necessary.

3.2.4 Conclusions

At pH 2.09, proteins, including BSA, HSA, γ-IgG, Lys and Chy, could combine through their protonated amine groups in amino acid residues with the anionic triphenylmethane dye, WB, resulting in WB molecules to aggregate on the proteins template and giving rise to considerably enhanced RLS signals characterized at 346.0 nm. This study indicates that the enhanced RLS signals are essentially associated with both the charge-couple effect between proteins and WB, demonstrating that highly negatively charged and molecular probe reagents should be considered in the study of proteins not only in search of but also in synthesizing novel RLS probes for proteins.

Acknowledgements

We are grateful to the support of the National Natural Science Foundation of China (NSFC, Nos.: 20425517, 20275032), and Chun Hui Program (No: [2004] 7–24) directed under the Ministry of Education of PRC, and the Municipal Science and Technology Committee of Chongqing.

References

[1] C.Z. Huang, Y.F. Li, J.G. Mao, D.G. Tan, Analyst 123 (1998) 1401.
[2] C.Q. Ma, K.A. Li, S.Y. Tong, Anal. Biochem. 239 (1996) 86.
[3] Q.E. Cao, Z.T. Ding, R.B. Fang, X. Zhao, Analyst 126 (2001) 1444.
[4] R.P. Jia, L.J. Dong, Q.F. Li, X.G. Chen, Z.D. Hu, Y. Nagaosa, Anal. Chim. Acta 442 (2001) 249.
[5] Y.T. Wang, F.L. Zhao, K.A. Li, Fresen. J. Anal. Chem. 364 (1999) 560.
[6] C.Q. Zhu, D.H. Li, Q.Z. Zhu, H. Zheng, Q.Y. Chen, H.H. Yang, J.G. Xu, Fresen. J. Anal. Chem. 366 (2000) 863.
[7] W. Lu, P. Feng, Y.F. Li, C.Z. Huang, Anal. Lett. 35 (2002) 227.
[8] C.Z. Huang, K.A. Li, S.Y. Tong, Anal. Chem. 68 (1996) 2259.
[9] C.Z. Huang, K.A. Li, S.Y. Tong, Anal. Chem. 69 (1997) 514.
[10] P. Bao, A.G. Frutos, C. Greef, J. Lahiri, U. Muller, T.C. Peterson, L.Warden, X.Y. Xie, Anal. Chem. 74 (2002) 1792.
[11] W. Lu, C.Z. Huang, Y.F. Li, Analyst 127 (2002) 1392.
[12] P. Feng, W.Q. Shu, C.Z. Huang, Y.F. Li, Anal. Chem. 73 (2001) 4307.
[13] S.P. Liu, H.Q. Luo, N.B. Li, Z.F. Liu, W.X. Zheng, Anal. Chem. 73 (2001) 3907.
[14] S.Z. Zhang, F.L. Zhao, K.A. Li, S.Y. Tong, Talanta 54 (2001) 333.
[15] S.Z. Zhang, F.L. Zhao, K.A. Li, S.Y. Tong, Anal. Chim. Acta 431 (2001) 133.
[16] S.P. Liu, G.M. Zhou, Z.F. Liu, Fresen. J. Anal. Chem. 363 (1999) 651.
[17] Y.K. Zhao, Q.E. Cao, Z.D. Hu, Q.h. Xu, Anal. Chim. Acta 388 (1999) 45.
[18] C.Z. Huang, Y.F. Li, N. Li, K.A. Li, S.Y. Tong, Bull. Chem. Soc. Jpn. 71 (1998) 1791.
[19] I.E. Borissevitch, T.T. Tominaga, H. Imasato, Anal. Chim. Acta 343 (1997) 281.
[20] R.F. Pasternack, C. Bustamante, P.J. Collings, A. Giannetto, E.J. Gibbs, J. Am. Chem. Soc. 115 (1993) 5393.
[21] R.F. Pasternack, P.J. Collings, Science 269 (1995) 935.
[22] D.W. Dixon, V. Steullet, J. Inorg. Biochem. 69 (1998) 25.
[23] Y.F. Li, C.Z. Huang, M. Li, Anal. Sci. 16 (2000) 1249.
[24] Z. Chen, J. Liu, D. Luo, Biochemistry Experiments, Chinese University of Sciences and Technology Press, Hefei, PRC, 1994, p. 345.
[25] Z.P. Li, K.A. Li, S.Y. Tong, Analyst 124 (1999) 907.

(Cheng Zhi Huang , Wei Lu, Yuan Fang Li, Yu Ming Huang,
published in *Analytica Chimica Acta* ,2006,556 , 469～475)

3.3 Determination of Proteins with α, β, γ, δ-tetrakis(4-sulfophenyl) Porphine by Measuring the Enhanced Resonance Light Scattering at the Air/Liquid Interface

Abstract: By attaching two right-angled prisms at a quartz cell of a common spectrofluorometer to change the propagation direction of the incident/emission light beams, a novel technique, reflected-light scattering (RFLS), was developed to detect the light scattering signals at the air/liquid interface. At pH 1.86 and ionic strength 0.04, the J- and H-aggregation of α, β, γ, δ-tetrakis(4-sulfophenyl)porphine that occurred at the interface in the presence of proteins, was assigned by measuring the enhanced resonance light scattering (RLS) signals characterized at 490.2 and 421.6 nm, respectively. With the enhanced RLS signals at 490.2 nm, a novel assay of proteins was established with the 3σ limit of detection being $18\sim70$ ng·mL^{-1}. The protein concentrations in synthetic samples and in human serum were determined with satisfactory results.

Keywords: α, β, γ, δ-Tetrakis(4-sulfophenyl)porphine; Proteins; Reflected-light scattering; Air/liquid interface

3.3.1 Introduction

Recently, the adsorption and molecular assembly structure at liquid interfaces has become attractive since the importance of their study in the fundamental fields of solvent extractions of metal ions, ion-selective electrodes, optical sensors, counter current chromatography[1,2] and the monolayer structure at the interfaces [3,4]. So, the development of surface-sensitive techniques and molecular probes, capable of yielding molecular assembly information about these interfaces, is of importance. Most existing surface techniques for measuring the interfacial properties, however, are constructed based on particle (electron, ion, or atom) scattering, which require samples in high vacuum and therefore are not suitable for use on vapor/liquid interfaces or buried liquid interfaces. Optical techniques, including infrared spectroscopy, Raman spectroscopy, ellipsometry, and Brewster angle microscopy are not intrinsically surface-specific[5,6]. Nonlinear optical spectroscopic techniques such as second harmonic generation (SHG)[7,8] and sum-frequency generation (SFG)[9] have appeared to be most successful and versatile. To measure the absorption and monolayer structure of the air/liquid interface in the presence of surfactants, a new neutron reflection technique has been developed and proved powerful if combined with surface tension measurements[3,4]. Such equipment, however, is expensive and complicated, limiting the spectral measurements of the characteristics of the interfaces to some degree[3,4]. So, new spectroscopic techniques need to be developed to selectively and sensitively probe the interactions that occur at the interfaces.

Scattered light originates from the fluctuations of the solution refractive index that consists of real and imaginary parts. If the wavelength of the incident beam is close to the absorption band of the molecular particles that exist as aggregates, enhanced resonance light scattering (RLS) can be expected [10,11] because of the fluctuation of the imaginary part of the refractive index. By using a common spectrfluorometer to measure the RLS signals in aqueous medium, Pasternack et al. [10,11] studied the aggregations of porphyrins in bulk aqueous solution and their assemblies on the template of biological molecules including nucleic acids and polypeptides[10~14].

Based on the enhanced RLS effects of proteins and nucleic acids on organic dyes[15,16], we have proposed assays of traces of these biological molecules in synthetic and practical samples. The fluctuation of the refractive index at the air/liquid interfaces indicates to us that the reflection of light at the air/liquid interface can be coupled with RLS measurements, and sensitively used to probe the interface properties. Herein, we display our attempt to use this refractive index-coupled technique, proposing a reflected-light scattering technique (RFLS) to measure the air/liquid interface where aggregation of *α, β, γ, δ*-tetrakis-(4-sulfophenyl)porphine ($TPPS_4$) occurred induced by proteins.

3.3.2 Experimental

3.3.2.1 Reagents

Seven commercial proteins were involved in the present experiments. Bovine serum albumin (BSA) and human serum albumin (HSA) were purchased form Sigma (St. Louis, MO), while *γ*-globulin (*γ*-IgG) was from Serva (Germany). Protamine sulfate (PTS) and lysozyme (Lys) were purchased from the Shanghai Institute of Biochemistry (Shanghai, China), while pepsin (Pep) was purchased from Fangcao Medical Industrial Co. (Shanghai, China). Stock solutions were prepared by dissolving directly the commercial proteins in doubly distilled water, except *γ*-IgG, which was dissolved with the aid of a few volumes of 0.1 $mol \cdot L^{-1}$ NaC1. All the working concentration of proteins were 10.0 $\mu g \cdot mL^{-1}$.

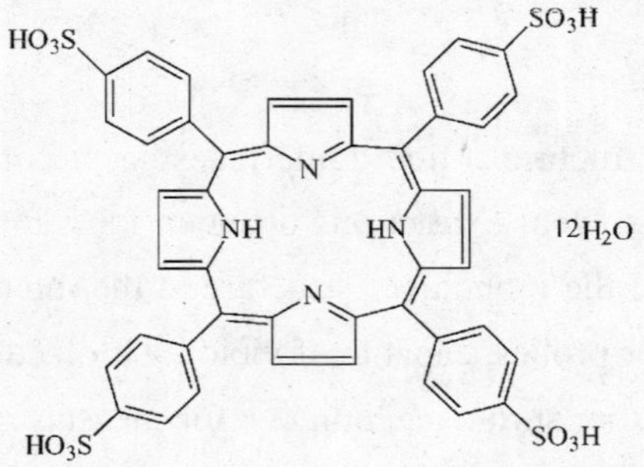

Fig. 1 Molecular structure of *α, β, γ, δ*-tetrakis (4-sulfophenyl) porphine ($TPPS_4$).

The water-soluble free base porphyrin, *α, β, γ, δ*-tetrakis-(4-sulfophenyl)porphine ($TPPS_4$, its molecular structure is displayed in Fig. 1), synthesized in our laboratory according to the literature [17] and identified by ^1H NMR and IR spectroscopy, was dissolved in doubly distilled water. The concentration was determined according to its absorbance at 413.0 nm (the Soret maximum) by using $\varepsilon = 5.1 \times 10^5\ M^{-1}\ cm^{-1}$ at pH 6.0[17]. The working concentrations were $2.0 \times 10^{-5}\ mol \cdot L^{-1}$. For comparison, Coomassie Brilliant Blue (CBB G-250, Fluka) was used for the detection of practical protein samples. Its working solution was prepared by dissolving 0.1000 g of the CBB G-250 crystals in 50 mL of 95% ethanol, and then mixing with 100 mL of 85% phosphoric acid. The mixture was diluted to 1000 mL with doubly distilled water. The concentration of the working solution was $1.17 \times 10^{-5}\ mol \cdot L^{-1}$.

A HCl–NaCl solution was used to adjust the pH values of the aqueous solution, while 1.0 M NaCl was used to control the ionic strength of the aqueous solution. All the reagents were of analytical grade and were used without further purification. Doubly distilled water was used throughout.

3.3.2.2 Apparatus and RFLS measurements

RFLS measurements were made with a F-4500 spectrofluorometer (Hitachi, Tokyo), whose optical arrangement in the sample compartment was constructed as the illustration in Fig. 2. Two right-angled NaCl. All the working concentration of proteins were 10.0 μg·mL^{-1}.

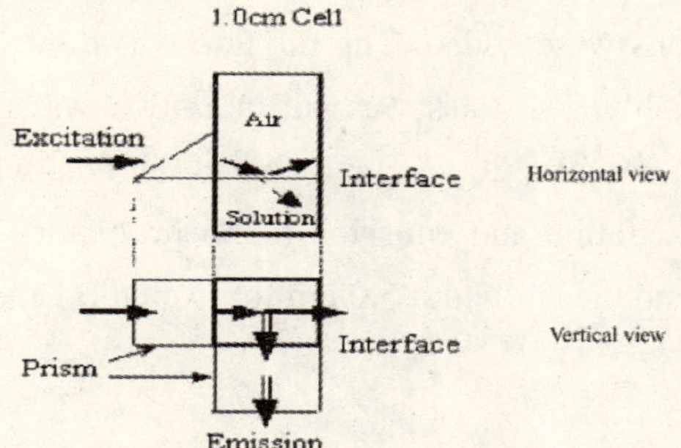

Fig. 2 Optical arrangements for the RFLS measurements at the air/liquid interface.

quartz prisms (10 mm × 10 mm × 10 mm, Huaguang Optics Co., Chongqing, China) were attached to the two sides of the cell holder facing the excitation light source and the fluorescence detector, respectively. So the incident excitation beam was introduced through the water phase and struck the interface with the incident angle θ_{in} = 46.4°, which was calculated according to the Snell equation

$$\frac{\sin\theta_{in}}{\sin\theta_{rr}} = \frac{n_2}{n_1}$$

where θ_{in} and θ_{rr} are the incident and refraction angles, n_2 and n_1 are the refractive indices of the optically rarer and denser phases (1.00 for air, 1.33 for water, and 1.50 for quartz). If the air/liquid interface is absolutely flat, the pressure of the liquid surface is zero because the surface tension points at the direction of the tangent line of the liquid surface. Since the refractive index of the liquid is larger than that of air, the incident beam from air to liquid is split into refracted and reflected beams at the interface. The refracted beam was transmitted in the liquid phase at θ_{rr} = 32.9°, while the reflected beam was emitted at the same angle as the incident beam: $\theta_{rl} = \theta_{in}$ = 46.4°.

To make a flat air/liquid interface in this experiment, the inside wall of the quartz cell was treated to produce a hydrophobic coating with a benzene solution of 2% dichlorodimethylsilane, so that the light beam can be reflected with the same reflecting angle as the incident angle.

An S-10A digital pH meter (Xiaoshan Scientific Instruments Plant, Zhejiang, China) was used to measure the pH values of the aqueous solutions, and an MVS-1 vortex mixer (Beide Scientific Instrumental Ltd., Beijing) was used to blend the solutions.

3.3.2.3 Preparation of samples

To test the method, the contents of BSA and γ-IgG in synthetic samples containing metal ions, amino acids, Triton X-100 and EDTA were determined. The total contents of HSA and γ-IgG in human serum samples, provided by four donors of the Capital of Southwest Normal University (Chongqing, China), which had been pretreated by diluting 2000-fold with doubly distilled water prior to the determination, were determined according to the general procedures. Reference values of the human serum samples were determined by using CBB G-250 according to the procedures in clinical tests[18]. The determination was made in 10 mL dry volumetric flasks in which 0～0.10 mL of standard BSA or sample solution was added, followed by some water, and then 5.00 mL of 1.2 × 10^{-5} mol·L^{-1} CBB G-250 working solution. The total volume of the mixture was kept to 5.10 mL. The contents of proteins in the samples were determined by measuring the absorbance at 595 nm against the reagent blank.

3.3.2.4 General procedures

Into a 10 mL volumetric flask were added $TPPS_4$ solution and some water to about 5 mL. The mixture was vortexed, and then protein and HCl–NaCl solutions were added. The mixture was diluted with doubly distilled water to the 10 mL scale mark and mixed thoroughly. The flask was put in a 50°C water bath, accompanied by occasionally manual shaking. The flask was taken out after 20 min, and cooled with tap water. The RFLS spectra were obtained by scanning simultaneously the excitation and emission monochromators of the F-4500 spectrofluorometer from 350 to 600 nm with $\Delta\lambda = 0$ nm and the slit width 5.0 nm for excitation and emission.

3.3.3 Results and discussion

3.3.3.1 Features of RFLS spectra

The aggregation properties of $TPPS_4$ in a variety of media has been well documented[12~14,19~27], giving J- and H-type aggregate species which are greatly different from their mother species depending on the environmental conditions. The conditions involve high $TPPS_4$ concentration, low pH values, high ionic strength and the presence of positive charged substances such as cation surfactants[22,23] or proteins[24,25]. As Li and Tong reported[24,25], J-and H-aggregation species of $TPPS_4$ can be found in the presence of proteins and the two aggregation species have characteristic absorption bands at 490.0 and 422.0 nm, respectively. Based on RLS measurement, we established the aggregation concept of $TPPS_4$ in the presence of proteins in aqueous medium: the characteristic RLS peak responsible for the J-aggregation is located at 490 nm, while the RLS peak for H-aggregation is at 422.0 nm[26,27].

Fig. 3 displays the RFLS features of $TPPS_4$ molecules at the air/liquid interface. It can be seen that the RFLS signal of $TPPS_4$ at air/liquid interfaces is very weak, and it becomes much weaker in the Soret region because of the strong absorption at its Soret band. If BSA is added to the $TPPS_4$ solution, however, enhanced RLS signals at the air/liquid interfaces are observed both at 490.2 and 421.6 nm. The two RLS peaks at the air/liquid interface are obviously identical to the findings of Pasternack et al. in bulk aqueous solution[10~14], and should be assigned to J- and H-aggregation, respectively[26,27]. The RFLS spectra of $TPPS_4$ in the presence of BSA have two RLS peaks at 490.2 and 421.6 nm, indicating that the J- and H-aggregation of $TPPS_4$ has occurred at the air/liquid interface. No significantly different RLS features can be found for the aggregation of $TPPS_4$ in the presence of BSA both at the air/liquid interface and in bulk aqueous solution except the RLS intensity. The two aggregations of $TPPS_4$, J- and H-, were also found to occur at the air/liquid interface in the presence of other proteins such as γ-IgG. With increasing protein concentration, both RLS peaks of all these protein-induced aggregation at 490.2 and 421.6 nm increase significantly, but no dependence of the wavelength location of the two characteristic RLS peaks on the protein variation and concentration could be found.

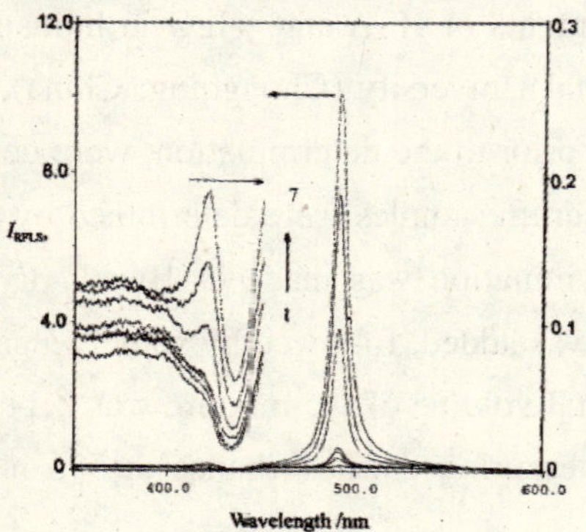

Fig. 3 RFLS spectra of the aggregation of $TPPS_4$ at the air/liquid interface in the presence of BSA. Concentrations: $TPPS_4$, 2.0×10^{-6} $mol\cdot L^{-1}$; BSA ($ng\cdot mL^{-1}$), 1, 0.0; 2, 150; 3, 300; 4, 450; 5, 600; 6, 800; 7, 1000. pH, 1.86; ionic strength, 0.04. The ordinate in the wavelength range from 350.0 to 450.0 nm are 40-fold enlarged.

3.3.3.2 Optimization of the general procedures

Fig. 4 displays the pH dependence of aggregation at the air/liquid interface induced by various proteins. Protamine sulfate displays the most strongly accelerative effect of the tested proteins, then lysozyme, but pepsin scarcely promotes the aggregation of $TPPS_4$ and fails to produce RFLS signals (not shown in Fig. 4). As Fig. 4 shows, proteins, including BSA, HSA, γ-IgG, PTS and Lys, have their own optimal pH to induce the aggregation of $TPPS_4$ at the air/liquid interface. The optimal pH value seems to relate to their isoelectric points, indicating that the aggregation of $TPPS_4$ can be encouraged by the protonation of proteins. That is in agreement with the findings of Pasternack et al. that the RLS intensity of the aggregate species depends on the aggregate size, strength of electronic coupling, and the aggregate geometry [14]. It is obviously that the protonation of proteins in a medium of pH lower than their isoelectric points will increase the strength of electronic coupling of the aggregation of $TPPS_4$.

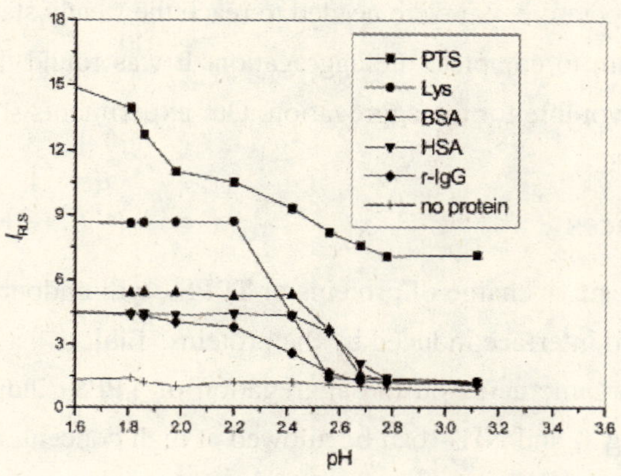

Fig. 4 Effect of pH on the aggregation of $TPPS_4$ in the presence of various proteins. Concentration: $TPPS_4$, 2.0×10^{-6} mol·L^{-1}; all the proteins were 700.0 ng·mL^{-1}; pH, 1.86; ionic strength 0.04.

We had reported that there are 2～3 protons participating in the aggregation of $TPPS_4$, independent of the kind of protein [27]. For a protein molecule unit, however, different numbers of aggregates are available since the aggregation number will increase with the molecule weight of the proteins. So, it can thus easily be understood that different proteins have different responses. Obviously, positive charge plays an important role in the aggregation process, so the effect of ionic strength of the medium should be considered. Fig. 5 shows that at ionic strength 0.04, the aggregation induced by both HSA and γ-IgG is nearly the same, but displays a great difference with increasing ionic strength.

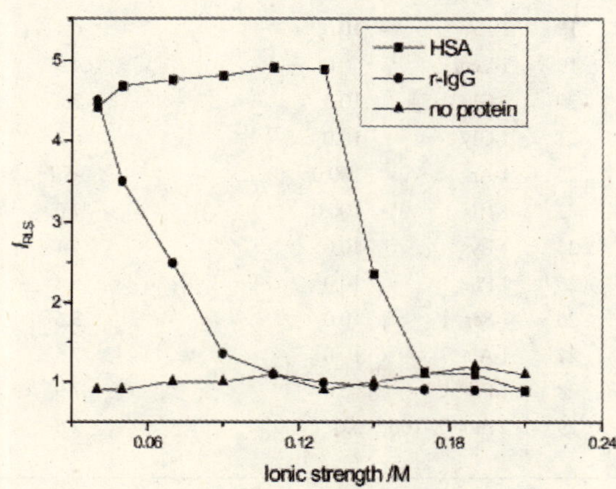

Fig. 5 Effect of ionic strength on the aggregation of $TPPS_4$ in the presence of HSA or γ-IgG. Concentrations and pH are the jsame as in Fig. 4.

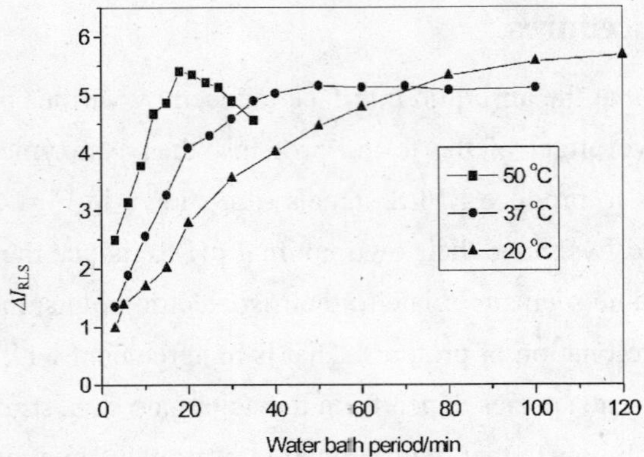

Fig. 6 Correlation between the aggregation rate and temperature. Concentration: $TPPS_4$, 2.0×10^{-6} mol·L^{-1}; BSA, 700 (ng·mL^{-1}); pH, 1.86; ionic strength, 0.04.

Fig. 6 shows the aggregation process at different temperatures. Increasing temperature is of benefit to the aggregation. If the aggregation proceeds at room temperature, 2 h were needed to reach the steady state. If aggregation proceeds at 50°C, however, it needs only 20 min to complete the aggregation. It was found that too high a temperature and too long a reaction period are not favorable for the aggregation. Our experiments showed that the optimal aggregation takes place in 20～25 min at 50°C.

3.3.3.3 Effects of non -protein substances

Non-protein substances, if they can affect the positive charge of proteins or $TPPS_4$, will undoubtedly exert an influence on the aggregation of $TPPS_4$ at the air/liquid interface induced by the proteins. Table 1 lists the effects of substances including amino acids, metal ions and organic acids on the aggregation of $TPPS_4$ induced by BSA. Common metal ions in body fluids, such as Ca^{2+}, Mg^{2+}, and NH_4^+ can be allowed at high concentrations ($>1.0 \times 10^{-4}$ mol·L^{-1}), whereas ions such as Co^{2+}, Cd^{2+}, Cr^{3+}, Cu^{2+}, and Pb^{2+} can be allowed only at very low concentrations ($<1.0 \times 10^{-7}$ mol·L^{-1}). However, dilution can minimize all the interferences in the determination of fluids, such as human serum samples. In addition, surfactants and amino acids, particularly l-Cys, l-Leu, l-Arg and l-His, can be allowed at relatively high concentration levels.

Table 1 Effects of non-protein substances on the determination of BSA

No.	Substance	Concentration $\times 10^{-6}$ (mol·L^{-1})	Change in I_{RLS} (%)	No.	Substance	Concentration (μg·mL^{-1})	Change in I_{RLS} (%)
1	Al^{3+}, SO_4^{2-}	15.0	7.1	16	l-Try	10.0	4.4
2	Ca^{2+}, Cl^-	20.0	5.3	17	l-Cys	100.0	-8.2
3	Cd^{2+}, Cl^-	2.0	-2.1	18	l-Asn	10.0	6.1
4	Cr^{3+}, Cl^-	1.5	2.1	19	l-Leu	50.0	4.9
5	Cu^{2+}, Cl^-	0.06	4.0	20	l-Glu	10.0	7.2
6	Co^{2+}, Cl^-	2.5	-4.2	21	l-Gly	10.0	5.2
7	Mg^{2+}, Cl^-	15.0	-3.5	22	l-Arg	100.0	-5.1
8	Mn^{2+}, Cl^-	10.0	-7.3	23	l-His	100.0	7.6
9	NH_4^+, Cl^-	2.0×10^4	-6.3	24	l-Lys	10.0	4.1
10	Ni^{2+}, Cl^-	1.0	6.4	25	l-Phe	10.0	5.8
11	Pb^{2+}, Cl^-	0.5	-4.4	26	l-Ser	10.0	3.6
12	Zn^{2+}, Cl^-	15.0	-1.7	27	l-Ala	10.0	7.5
13	EDTA	2.0	0.5	28	l-Pro	50.0	7.9
14	β-CD	50.0	-0.2	29[a]	Triton X-100	5.0	2.5
15	SDS	50.0	7.6				

[a]Concentration of Triton X-100 was expressed as %(v/v). Concentrations: $TPPS_4$, 2.0×10^{-6} mol·L^{-1}; BSA, 680 ng·mL^{-1}; pH 1.86; ionic strength 0.04.

3.3.3.4 Analytical parameters for the determination

Table 2 displays the analytical parameters for the determination of BSA by using different concentrations of $TPPS_4$. It is clear that there are two linear ranges (low and high linear ranges) for each concentration of $TPPS_4$. With increasing concentration of $TPPS_4$, the sensitivity (slope of the regression equation) of the low linear range decreases, while the sensitivity of the high linear range increases. However, if the concentration of $TPPS_4$ is too high, the sensitivity of the high linear range decreases again. We can therefore choose an appropriate concentration of $TPPS_4$ for analytical applications. All the results for the determination of samples in the present paper were obtained by using 2.0×10^{-6} mol·L^{-1} $TPPS_4$.

Table 2 Effects of $TPPS_4$ concentration on the analytical parameters[a]

Proteins	$c_{TPPS4} \times 10^{-6}$ (mol·L^{-1})	Linear range (ng·mL^{-1})	Regression equation (ng·mL^{-1})	Detection limit (3σ, ng·mL^{-1})	Correlation coefficient (r) (n = 6)
BSA	1.2	150～800	$\Delta I = 0.008c + 1.202$	18.0	0.9923
	1.6	30～300	$\Delta I = 0.0016c + 0.025$	22.0	0.9737
		300～800	$\Delta I = 0.016c + 6.072$		0.9898
	2.0	50–450	$\Delta I = 0.0015c + 0.171$	48.5	0.9857
		450～1000	$\Delta I = 0.017c + 6.546$		0.9950
	2.4	80～300	$\Delta I = 0.0011c + 0.250$	71.5	0.9660
		300～1000	$\Delta I = 0.018c + 5.078$		0.9904
HSA	2.0	50～450	$\Delta I = 0.0012c + 0.151$	53.5	0.9879
		450～1000	$\Delta I = 0.016c + 6.781$		0.9952
γ-IgG	2.0	70～450	$\Delta I = 0.0012c + 0.172$	66.5	0.9639
		450～1000	$\Delta I = 0.016c + 6.695$		0.9908
PTS	2.0	40～450	$\Delta I = 0.0015c + 0.150$	32.7	0.9889
		450～1000	$\Delta I = 0.036c + 10.280$		0.9947
Lys	2.0	40～450	$\Delta I = 0.0021c + 0.151$	40.3	0.9902
		450～1000	$\Delta I = 0.024c + 6.13$		0.9960

[a] All the values were obtained for pH, 1.86; ionic strength, 0.04.

Table 3 Determination results for synthetic samples containing non-protein substances

Protein samples	Non-proteins[a]	Found	Relative standard deviation (n = 5, %)	Recovery (n = 5, %)
8.46 μg·ml^{-1} BSA	Cu^{2+}, Pb^{2+}	7.92 ± 0.24	- 6.9	104.0
	Pro, Leu, Cys	8.62 ± 0.13	1.9	103.0
	Triton X-100, EDTA	8.31 ± 0.17	- 1.8	95.1
8.45 μg·ml^{-1} γ-IgG	Cu^{2+}, Pb^{2+}	8.54 ± 0.16	1.1	94.3
	Pro, Leu, Cys	8.04 ± 0.15	- 4.8	92.4
	Triton X-100, EDTA	9.01 ± 0.11	6.6	93.5

a Non-protein substances, 1.0×10^{-8} mol·L^{-1} Cu^{2+}; 1.0×10^{-7} mol·L^{-1} Pb^{2+}; 40 μg·mL^{-1} Pro, Leu, Cys; 4.0×10^{-5} % (v/v) Triton X-100; 8.4×10^{-5} mol·L^{-1} EDTA. Concentrations: $TPPS_4$, 2.0×10^{-6} mol·L^{-1}; pH 1.86; ionic strength 0.04.

Table 4 Determination results for a mixture of HSA and γ-IgG

No.	Added (μg·mL^{-1})				Found (μg·mL^{-1})	
	HAS	γ-IgG	HSA + γ-IgG	α (%)[a]	HSA + γ-IgG	DR (%)[b]
1	0.70	0.02	0.72	2.78	0.73± 0.01	1.39
2	0.55	0.15	0.70	21.43	0.71± 0.01	1.43
3	0.40	0.30	0.70	42.86	0.72± 0.01	2.86

[a]Ratio of γ-IgG to the sum of HSA and γ-IgG.

[b]Mean determination error (n = 5). All the results were obtained at pH 1.86 and ionic strength 0.04. $TPPS_4$, 2.0×10^{-6} mol·L^{-1}.

3.3.3.5 Sample determination

Synthetic samples for BSA or γ-IgG containing metal ions, amino acids, Triton X-100 and EDTA were analyzed. As can be seen in Table 3, the contents of BSA and γ-IgG in synthetic samples can be determined with good reproducibility.

Experiments showed that the RFLS responses for both HSA and γ-IgG are nearly equal (Table 4) at pH 1.86 and ionic strength 0.04. The determination results for the total content of HSA and γ-IgG inmixtures containing the two proteins at ionic strength 0.04 were satisfactory, using a standard solution of HSA. So, we herein propose an assay for the total content of proteins in human serum samples with HSA as the standard. Table 5 displays the determination results for human serum samples with HSA as the standard obtained from four different donors of the Capital of the Southwest Normal University. The samples were diluted 2000-fold with distilled water without other pretreatment. The results displayed in Table 5 are in good agreement with the reference values, that obtained with the common clinical method by using CBB G-250.

Table 5 Total content of proteins in human serum samples[a]

Sample	$TPPS_4$ method		CBB G-250 method ($mg \cdot mL^{-1}$)
	Found (n = 5, $mg \cdot mL^{-1}$)	Recovery (n = 5, %)	
1	75.8± 2.7	98.9	73.4
2	69.8± 2.5	95.7	71.1
3	67.4± 1.7	94.3	69.8
4	81.3± 3.2	93.2	82.1

[a] All the values for the $TPPS_4$ method were obtained at pH 1.86 and ionic strength 0.04 based on calibration with a HSA standard. $TPPS_4$, 2.0×10^{-6} $mol \cdot L^{-1}$.

It is clear that the determination of the total content of proteins is reliable, sensitive and practical.

3.3.4 Conclusions

The present assay of proteins based on the RFLS measurements is sensitive. As can be seen from Section 2, the RFLS technique provides a simple operation to measure the aggregation properties of TPPS4 at the air/liquid interface. Obviously, it is easy to characterize the interfacial features through the light scattering measurements. More importantly, the different features of the interfaces from the aqueous bulk medium supplies a simple way to establish highly selective methods. The present assay, for example, has better sensitivity and selectivity for protein assay than that of proteins in bulk aqueous solution with dyes such the biuret, Bradford, Lowry, and Bromcresol Green (BCG) methods[28]. The biuret method, although simple, reproducible and capable of modification, is not sensitive; the Bradford method, although sensitive, is too complicated to operate. As to the BCG method, because the BCG-albumin complex may partly precipitate, turbidity and the "negative baseline effect"[28] are often found. The present assay of proteins based on the measurements of RLS at the air/liquid interface can supply high efficiency, ease of use and sensitivity.

Acknowledgements

We greatly appreciate the financial support of the Excellent Young University Teachers Foundation directed under the Education Ministry of China (no. 2000-11), the National Natural Science Foundation of China (NSFC, no. 29875019), and the Municipal Science Foundation of Chongqing City.

References

[1] R. Osterbacka, C.P. An, X.M. Jiang, Z.V. Vardeny, Science 287 (2000) 839.
[2] P. Jungwirth, D.J. Tobias, J. Phys. Chem. B 102 (2000) 7702.
[3] S.R. Green, T.J. Su, J.R. Lu, J. Penfold, J. Phys. Chem. B 104 (2000) 1507.
[4] H. Yim, M. Kent, A. Matheson, R. Ivkov, S. Satija, J. Majewski, G.S. Smith, Macromolecules 33 (2000) 6126.
[5] J.R. Lu, Z.X. Li, R.K. Thomas, E.J. Staples, L. Thompson, I. Tucker, J.I. Penfold, J. Phys. Chem. 101 (1997) 10332.
[6] P.B. Miranda, Y.R. Shen, J. Phys. Chem. B 101 (1999) 3292.
[7] R. Seoane, J. Miñones, O. Conde, J. Miñones Jr., M. Casas, E. Iribarnegaray, J. Phys. Chem. B 102 (2000) 7713.
[8] V. Tsukanova, A. Harata, T. Ogaw, J. Phys. Chem. B 102 (2000) 7707.
[9] K.B. Eisenthal, J. Phys. Chem. 100 (1996) 12997.
[10] R.F. Pasternack, P.J. Collings, Science 269 (1995) 935.
[11] R.F. Pasternack, C. Bustamante, P.J. Colings, A. Giannetto, E.J. Gibbs, J. Am. Chem. Soc. 115 (1993) 5393.
[12] P.J. Collings, E.J. Gibbs, T.E. Starr, O. Vafeck, C. Yee, L.A. Pomerance, R.F. Pasternack, J. Phys. Chem. B 103 (1999) 8474.
[13] R.F. Pasternack, K.F. Shaefer, P. Hambright, Inorg. Chem. 33 (1994) 2062.
[14] J. Parkash, J.H. Robblee, J. Agnew, E. Gibbs, P. Collings, R.F. Pasternack, J.C. de Paula, Biophys. J. 74 (1998) 2089.
[15] C.Z. Huang, K.A. Li, S.Y. Tong, Anal. Chem. 68 (1996) 2259.
[16] C.Z. Huang, Y.F. Li, J.G. Mao, D.G. Tan, Analyst 123 (1998) 1401.
[17] Y.E. Zeng, H.S. Zhang, Z.H. Chen, Handbook of Modern Chemical Reagents, Vol. 4, Chemical Industry Press, Beijing, (1989) 786.
[18] D.A. Zhang, Experimental Handbook of Biological Molecules, Jilin University Press, Changchun, 1991, 327.
[19] R.F. Pasternack, P.R. Huber, P. Boyd, G. Engasser, L. Francessconi, E. Gibbs, P. Fasella, G. Gerioventura, L.C. De Hinds, J. Am. Chem. Soc. 94 (1972) 4511.
[20] O. Ohno, Y. Kaizu, H. Kobayashi, J. Phys. Chem. 99 (1993) 4128.
[21] D.L. Akins, H.R. Zhu, C. Guo, J. Phys. Chem. 98 (1994) 3612.
[22] Y. Moriya, N. Ogawa, T. Kumabe, H. Watarai, Chem. Lett. (1998) 221.
[23] C.Z. Huang, Y.F. Li, X.H. Huang, Acta Phys. Chim. Sinica 14 (1998) 731.
[24] S.Y. Tong, N. Li, Chin. Chem. Lett. 4(1993) 1079.
[25] N. Li, S.Y. Tong, Talanta 41 (1994) 1657.
[26] C.Z. Huang, J.X. Zhu, K.A. Li, S.Y. Tong, Anal. Sci. 13 (1997) 263.
[27] C.Z. Huang, Y.F. Li, N. Li, K.A. Li, S.Y. Tong, Bull. Chem. Soc. Jpn. 71 (1998) 1791.
[28] W. Zeng, X.J. Meng, N. Li, S.Y. Tong, Anal. Chim. Acta 316 (1995) 387.

(Cheng Zhi Huang, Yuan Fang Li, Ping Feng, published in *Analytica Chimica Acta*, 2001, 443, 73～80)

3.4 A Backscattering Light Detection Assembly for Sensitive Determination of Analyte Concentrated at the Liquid/Liquid Interface Using the Interaction of Quercetin with Proteins as the Model System

We report on the construction of a backscattering light (BSL) detection assembly based on detecting angle-dependent light scattering signals, by changing the sample chamber of a common spectrofluorometer. The BSL detection assembly was used to detect, with high sensitivity, the analyte concentrated at the liquid/liquid interface. We applied this assembly to study the interaction of proteins with quercetin in the presence of cationic surfactant. The species resulting from the interaction of quercetin with proteins, when concentrated at the H_2O/CCl_4 interface, generate enhanced BSL signals characterized at 376.0 nm which were found to be proportional to human serum albumin (HSA) and bovine serum albumin (BSA) in the range of 1～1250 ng·mL^{-1} and 2～1250 ng·mL^{-1}, respectively. Limits of determination (3σ) of 75 and 180 pg·mL^{-1} are reported for the two proteins.

3.4.1 Introduction

Resonance light scattering (RLS) enhancement is a very common phenomenon when the wavelength of a incident beam is close to the absorption band of aggregated chromophores.[1,2] The RLS technique, which was developed by scanning the excitation/emission monochromators of a common spectrofluorometer with $\Delta\lambda = 0$ nm, has found a variety of applications in the spectral assignments of molecular recognition and assembly.[1,2] For analytical purposes, this technique needs to be widely applied in the determination of nucleic acids,[3,4] proteins,[5,6] saccharides,[7,8] drugs,[9] surfactants,[10] and metallicions[11,12] in synthetic and practical samples. In order to improve the selectivity and sensitivity of RLS methods, we applied the RLS technique to detect totalinternal reflected light scattering signals at the liquid/liquid interface, and 1000-fold improved selectivity and sensitivity have been obtained.[5,9]

Recently, backward light-scattering spectroscopy (BLSS) has been demonstrated as an effective means of detecting abnormalities in epithelial-cell nuclei associated with neoplasia and a precancerous state based on detecting the size of cell nuclei to aid diagnosis of the disease.[13] A more recent implementation of BLSS has reported measurement of the spectrum of scattered light at various scattering angles to obtain information about both the cell nuclei and smaller structures.[14] These exciting reports prompted to us to further apply backward light-scattering (BLS) signals for quantification purposes, and thus herein we report on the design of a new assembly to detect backscattering light (BSL) signals of analyte concentrated at the liquid/liquid interface based on detecting angle-dependent light scattering signals.

Liquid/liquid interfacial binding has found applications in protein-based dispersions and emulsions encountered in food technology and two-phase enzymatic catalysis.[15,16] Interfacial binding or adsorption of proteins to surfaces and membranes is an important process in cell biology.[17～20] The detection of proteins at interfaces, however, is often accomplished by labeling the proteins with a fluorescent or radioactive tag. The surface plasmon resonance (SPR) technique offers a means of detecting unlabeled proteins on the basis of their mass altering the dielectric constant at the interface, but it requires a metal film in order to generate the plasmon wave,[21,22] and is greatly dependent on temperature.[23] In addition, the measurement is complicated if the protein is denatured at the metal surface. A metal surface such as gold may also be incompatible with supported lipid bilayers, which are useful as model membranes for studying protein–cell or protein–protein interactions.[24,25] Second harmonic generation (SHG), due to the effect of the adsorbed protein on the water molecules polarized near the charged interface,[26] has been applied at the solid/liquid interface. These methods, however, generally involve complicated equipment and need special pretreatment of samples. Herein we present a sensitive detection method of proteins based on detecting enhanced BSL signals of proteins adsorbed to the liquid/liquid interface, which is only accomplished using a common spectrofluorometer. We used the interaction of quercetin (QT) with proteins as a model system to exhibit the application of the newly designed assembly, considering that QT is one of the most abundant natural flavonoids found in a variety of common fruits and vegetables,[27] and it exhibits a broad range of biological activity connected to anticancer properties and antioxidative activity.[28] Thus, its interaction with proteins is important and worth studying.

3.4.2 Experimental

3.4.2.1 Apparatus

Backscattering light (BSL) spectra and intensities were measured with a Hitachi F-2500 spectrofluorometer (Tokyo, Japan). Fig. 1 illustrates the optical assembly we designed for this purpose, which was then mounted on the sample chamber of the spectrofluorometer. The assembly is composed of two parts. One is the oblique incidence part in which a mirror is used to reflect the incident beam emitted from the Xe lamp of the spectrofluorometer so as to illuminate the species acting as scatterers at the liquid/liquid interface. The other is the signal transmission part, which is composed of three holophotes attached together by optics glue, so that the BSL signals from the liquid/liquid interface in a 1 cm optical cell could be transferred to the emission monochromator of the spectrofluorometer. In order to make a flat interface, the 1 cm optical quartz cell (10.0 mm × 10.0 mm × 43.8 mm) in the assembly should be pretreated with a toluene solution containing 2% dichlorodimethylsilane on its lower inside wall so as to make it hydrophobic. A pH-3C digital pH meter (Xiaoshan Scientific Instrument Plant, Zhejiang, PRC) was used to measure the pH-values of the aqueous solutions.

3.4.2.2 Reagents

Stock solutions of proteins were prepared by dissolving human serum albumin (HSA, Shanghai Biochemical Institute, Shanghai, China) and bovine serum albumin (BSA, Baitai Biochemical Co, Chinese Academy of Sciences, Beijing, China). Working solutions of the two proteins were 5.0 μg·mL^{-1}.

Quercetin (QT, Shanghai Chemical Regent, PRC) solution was prepared with the aid of a small volume of 0.2 mol·L^{-1} NaOH solution, and the working solution is 8.0×10^{-5} mol·L^{-1}. Cetyltrimethylammonium bromide (CTMAB, Fluka AG, Switzerland) solution was prepared by dissolving CTMAB in doubly distilled water, and its working solution is 2.0×10^{-5} mol·L^{-1}. Britton-Robinson buffer solution (0.03 mol·L^{-1} H_3PO_4, 0.03 mol·L^{-1} HAc, 0.03 mol·L^{-1} H_3BO_3 and 0.04 mol·L^{-1} NaOH) was used to control the acidity, while 0.1 mol·L^{-1} NaCl solution was used to adjust the ionic strength of the aqueous phases. Proteins were of biochemical reagent grade, and all other reagents were of analytical grade used without further purification. Doubly distilled water was used throughout. All measurements were performed at room temperature (25 ± 2 °C).

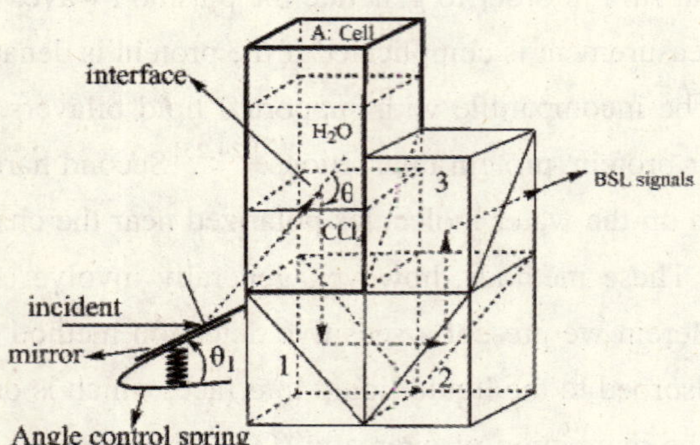

Fig. 1 Optical assembly mounted on the sample chamber of a common spectrofluorometer for BSL measurement at a liquid/liquid interface. A, optical cell; 1, 2, 3, homemade holophotes. The mirror was attached to the angle control spring. $\theta 1$ is the angle between mirror and the horizontal, and θ is the scattering angle decided by the direction of the incident beam and the BSL detection direction. By adjustment of the angle θ_1, different θ could be obtained.

3.4.2.2 Pretreatment of samples

Both artificial and practical samples were tested. As to the quantification of HSA in artificial samples, foreign substances such as metal ions, amino acids, and carbohydrates were added into HSA solutions and a series of artificial samples constructed. For practical samples, three human urine samples (freshly sampled from different healthy students of Southwest Normal University, PRC) were diluted 2-fold with doubly distilled water.

3.4.2.3 Standard procedure

1.0 mL CCl_4 solution was at first transferred to a dry optical quartz cell as the organic phase, then, 0.2 mL BR buffer solution, 0.4 mL QT solution, 0.6 mL CTMAB solution and protein working solution or protein sample solution were successively added to the cell. Appropriate water was then added so as to keep the aqueous phase volume at 2.0 mL. The two phases was thoroughly stirred and 20 min late, the optical quartz cell was mounted on the assembly for BSL measurements. The slit widths of both excitation and emission of the spectrofluorometer were kept as 5.0 nm, while the PMT voltage was kept as 400 V during the BSL measurements.

3.4.3 Results and discussion

3.4.3.1 General considerations for BSL assembly design

It is known that the electrons in a particle oscillate at the same frequency as the incident wave when the particle is exposed to an electromagnetic wave. The oscillating electron then radiates electromagnetic radiation with the same frequency as the oscillating electron. It is this secondary radiation that constitutes the scattered light, and the light intensity scattered by a spherical particle illuminated by a monochromatic light beam could be expressed as[29,30]

$$I = \frac{8\pi^4 a^6 n_{med}^4 I_0}{d^2 \lambda_0^4} \left| \frac{m^2 - 1}{m^2 + 2} \right|^2 (1 + \cos^2 \theta) \qquad (1)$$

where I_0 is the intensity of incident monochromatic light, a is the particle radius, n_{med} is the refractive index of the medium surrounding the particle, d is the distance between the particle and the position where the scattered light is detected, m is the relative refractive index of the bulk particle material, and θ is scattering angle which is decided by the detection direction and the forward direction of the incident beam. That is, lightscattering properties of a particle depend on its composition, size, shape, homogeneity, bathing medium refractive index, and the scattering angle.

As to the scattering angle, we can make a rearrangement of eqn. (1) and it could be written concisely as

$$I = K(1+\cos^2\theta) \quad (2)$$

Where $K = \dfrac{8\pi^4 a^6 n_{med}^4 I_0}{d^2\lambda_0^4}\left|\dfrac{m^2-1}{m^2+2}\right|^2$, which is a constant related to the intensity of the incident beam and the refractive index of medium. As for common RLS technique, the scattered light intensity is detected at 90°. However, as eqn. (2) demonstrates, the scattered light intensity is greatly dependent on the scattering angle θ, and the I-value is in fact in proportional to that of cos2θ. For example, scattered light signals in the forward direction (θ = 0°) or backward direction (θ = 180°) are two times greater than that at the right angle to the incident beam (θ = 90°). That is, the angle plays a very important role, and adjustment of the angle could result in different RLS signals. Thus we consider designing an assembly as shown in Fig. 1 so as to detect the BSL signals at these θ-values of larger than 90°.

We measured the relationship between the angular distributions and the BSL intensity using our assembly, and the results are shown in Fig. 2. It could be seen that the strongest BSL signals could be achieved when the light scattering angle is 154°. According to eqn. (2), the BSL intensity I_{BSL} linearly increases with increasing $\cos^2\theta$ in the range of 90° to 180°. According to the cosine function, $\cos^2\theta$ is directly proportional to θ and increases with increasing θ value. So the effect of θ on the I_{BSL} is similar to that of $\cos^2\theta$. We could see that the changes of I_{BSL} with θ in the range of 130°～154° displayed in Fig. 2 correspond to eqn. (2), and a linear relationship is available between the I_{BSL} and $\cos^2\theta$ with a regression coefficient (r) of 0.99. However, I_{BSL} decreases when θ is larger than 154°, which could be possibly ascribed to our assembly. With increasing θ angle, we should slowly heighten the quartz cell in order that the species at the interface could be excited with the incident beam. In such a case, the distance between the particle and the detection position d is slightly increased. According to eqn. (1), the intensity decreases with the second power of (d), and when angle θ is larger than 154°, the effect of distance between the scatterers and the detector possibly become more prominent and could not be negligible. Thus, weaker BSL signals could be detected at larger θ-values. In this experiment, we made the measurements at θ = 154°.

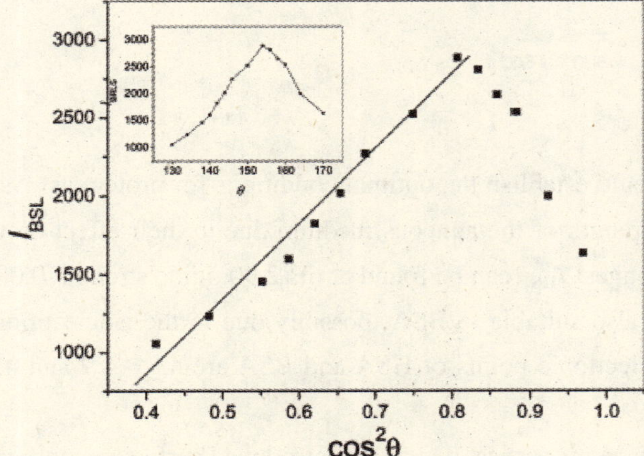

Fig. 2 Dependence of BSL signals on scattering angle θ and $\cos^2\theta$. Concentrations: QT, 1.6×10^{-5} mol·L^{-1}; CTMAB, 6.0×10^{-6} mol·L^{-1}; HSA added in aqueous medium, 500 ng·mL^{-1}. pH 2.90, ionic strength, 0.003 mol·L^{-1}. Linear regression equation: I = −1083 + 4792 $\cos^2\theta$ (r = 0.99, n = 9) in scattering angle range of 130～154°.

When the quartz cell is heightened, the species in a different field at the interface could be excited. Thus, in order to get identical BSL signals at the different θ-values, a flat oil/water interface should be required. For that purpose, we pretreated the 1 cm optical quartz cell with a toluene solution containing 2% dichlorodimethylsilane on its lower inside wall so as to make it hydrophobic.[16,20] It has proved that the flat interface of the lower inside wall after one hydrophobic pretreatment could undergo repetitive use more than 500 times.

Since the position of the incident beam through a spectrofluorometer is fixed, this decides the mirror height. Thus, in order to totally reflect the horizontal beam from the 150 W xenon lamp to the liquid/liquid interface, the height of the interface, which was decided by the volume of organic phase, should be constant. Our experiment shows that the optimal volume of organic phase is 1.0 mL.

In this assembly, the employment and adjustment of a mirror could result in a different incident angle so as to gain different θ-values. Thus, this assembly has the advantages of flexibility and minimizing the energy loss of incidence light by reflection, avoiding the light absorption and refractive artifacts compared with the optical prism. Simultaneously, the holophotes have been used to minimize the energy loss of incidence light and reduce the amount of background produced by light scattering from scratches, dirt, and aberrations.

3.4.3.2 Interaction of proteins with quercetin

Fig. 3 displays the BSL spectra of QT-CTMAB, CTMAB-HSA, QT-HSA, and QT-CTMAB-HSA at the H_2O/CCl_4 interface. It can be seen that the BSL signals of QT-CTMAB, QT-HSA, and CTMAB-HSA are very faint in the range of 300～650 nm. However, the BSL signals of QT-CTMAB-HSA are very strong in the range of 360～380 nm characterized by the peak at 376 nm, and the intensity of this characteristic signals (I_{BSL}) increases with increasing concentration of proteins. This indicates that new chemical species have formed and been adsorbed to the interface. QT-CTMAB-BSA shows similar BLS spectra.

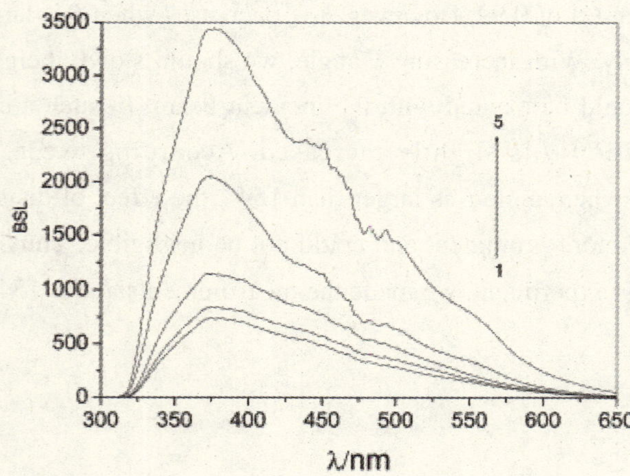

Fig. 3 BSL spectra of QT-CTMAB (curve 1), QT-HSA (curve 2), CTMAB-HSA (curve 3), and QT-CTMAB-HSA (curve 4, 5) at the H2O/CC14 interface. Concentrations: QT, 1.6×10^{-5} mol·L^{-1}; CTMAB, $6.0 \times 6\ 10^{-6}$ mol·L^{-1}; HSA added in aqueous medium (curves 1–5, ng·mL^{-1}), 0, 500, 500, 250, 500; pH 2.90, ionic strength, 0.003 mol·L^{-1}. Spectra are not corrected using the instrument sensitivity function.

By optimizing the general procedures, we could establish the optimal conditions for protein assays. The I_{BSL} of QTCTMAB-HSA varied with the pH, ionic strength of the aqueous medium due to their effect on the carried charges of the protein and quercetion, and the strongest I_{BSL} can be found at pH 2.90, ionic strength 0.003 mol·L^{-1}. Experiments show that this optimal condition is also suitable to BSA, possibly due to the isoelectionic point of BSA close to HAS, and it is known that the isoelectionic points of HSA and BSA are 4.7～4.9 and 4.9, respectively, and they carry the positive charges at pH 2.9.

Considering the effect of extraction of interface properties, herein we introduced surfactants into the interaction system, and tested the effect of anionic surfactant (SDBS, SLS), nonionic surfactant (Tween 20, Txiton X-100) and cationic surfactant (CTMAB, Zeph) on BSL intensity. It has proved that the highest backscattering intensity could be obtained in the presence of cationic surfactant. In this study, a common cationic surfactant CTMAB containing both a hydrophilic head and a hydrophobic tail was used for it is presumed to reside well at a liquid/liquid interface.[31, 32] Therefore, the synergistic adsorption of QT-HSA in the presence of CTMAB generates larger scattering species at the H_2O/CCl_4 interface, where CTMAB acts as a bridge of the organic phase and the aqueous phase.

It is important that the organic phase and the aqueous phase in the optical cell should be agitated thoroughly so that the interaction could complete sufficiently and expeditiously. Emulsification at the interface is thus unavoidable due to agitation. It is the emulsification in the aqueous after agitating that lead to the BSL signals becoming unstable and declined. The optimal standing time is established experimentally by monitoring the signals based on the time scan function of the spectrofluorometer. Experiments showed that allowing the mixture to stand 20 min could solve this problem. Steady BSL signals at the interface will then keep constant for 30 min, and decrease afterwards due to the desorption of the complex QT-CTMAB-proteins from the interface.

3.4.3.3 Calibration curves and sample detection

Eqn. (1) represents the light scattering of a single scatterer. For the species in the excited field of the incident beam, the total scattered light is the sum of the light scattering by the individual species.[33] Therefore, when experimental conditions have been set, eqn. (1) could be changed as,

$$I = K(1+\cos^2\theta)VN_A = K'c \quad (3)$$

where V is the volume of the sample consumed, and NA is Avogadro's constant. Thus, a simple function between the measured backscattering signals with the concentration of the analyte could be established. Experiments identify the linear relationships between the I_{BSL} of the system to the concentration of HSA, indicating that the detection of analyte using the BSL signal at the H_2O/CCl_4 interface is possible. As Fig. 4 shows, in the ranges 1～1250 ng·mL^{-1} for HSA and 2～1250 ng·mL^{-1} for BSA, the linear regression equations were ΔI_{BSL} = -288.2 + 6.0c (c, ng·mL^{-1}; r = 0.9997; n = 5) and ΔI_{BSL} = 974 + 4.9c (c, ng·mL^{-1}; r = 0.9983; n = 5), with the limits of detection (3σ) of 74.6 and 184 pg·mL^{-1}, respectively. The sensitivity is enhanced approximately 1000-fold than that of the RLS method of QT-HSA in the aqueous medium. With increasing QT concentration, the linear relationship range is extended (Table 1), while the sensitivity (slope of the linear regression equation) is reduced, indicating that the extraction of proteins from aqueous medium greatly improves the sensitivity.

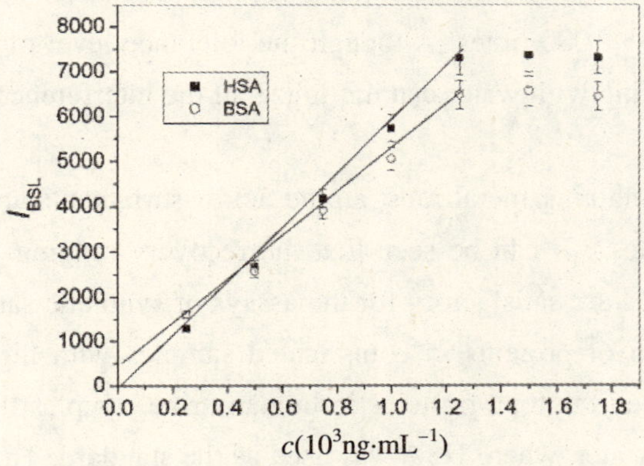

Fig. 4 Calibration graphs for the detection of HSA and BSA by BSL method. Error bars represent one standard derivation for four measurements. Concentrations: QT, 1.6 × 10^{-5} mol·L^{-1}; CTMAB, 6.0 × 10^{-6} mol·L^{-1}. pH 2.90, ionic strength, 0.003 mol·L^{-1}. The linear regression equations were ΔI = -288.2 + 6.0c (r = 0.9997; n = 5), ΔI = 974 + 4.9c (r = 0.9983; n = 5) in the ranges of 0.8–1250 ng·mL^{-1} for HSA and 1.8～1250 ng·mL^{-1} for BSA, respectively. The limits of detection (3σ) are 75 and 180 pg·mL^{-1}, respectively.

Table 1 Effect of the concentration of QT on the analytical parameters [a]

c_{QT} ($\times 10^{-5}$ mol·L^{-1})	Liner range (ng·mL^{-1})	Liner regression equation (ng·mL^{-1})	Limit of determinationCorrelation (3σ) (pg·mL^{-1})	Correlation coefficient (r)
2.0	1.6～1500	$\Delta I = -358.6 + 4.6c$	156.2	0.9986
1.6	0.8～1250	$\Delta I = -288.2 + 6.0c$	74.6	0.9997
1.2	1.7～800	$\Delta I = 156.6 + 5.3c$	169.5	0.9963
0.8	1.0～600	$\Delta I = 369.2 + 5.9c$	98.6	0.9985

[a] Concentrations: CTMAB, 6.0×10^{-6} mol·L^{-1}; pH 2.90, ionic strength, 0.003 mol·L^{-1}.

Table 2 Determination results for synthetic samples

Proteins in samples (μg·mL^{-1})	Main interferences[a]	Found (μg·mL^{-1}, n = 5)	Recovery range (%) (n = 5)	RSD (%) (n = 5)
HSA (0.5)	Fe^{3+}, Ni^{2+}, Na^+, Zeph, L-Lys	0.47	95.8～103.1	2.31
HSA (0.5)	Co^{3+}, Cd^{2+}, SDS, L-Ser, Lac	0.51	94.0～106.8	2.30
BSA (0.5)	Ca^{2+}, Mg^{2+}, Mal, L-Phen, SDBS	0.49	93.8～104.7	1.95
BSA (0.5)	Urea, Mn^{2+}, L-Lys, gly, Zn^{2+}	0.48	96.3～105.7	2.12

[a] Concentrations: Ni^{2+}, 1.0×10^{-4} mol·L^{-1}; Fe^{3+}, 0.4×10^{-4} mol·L^{-1}; Na^+, 10×10^{-4} mol·L^{-1}; Zeph, 0.04×10^{-4} mol·L^{-1}; L-Lys, 1.0×10^{-6} mol·L^{-1}; Co^{3+}, 0.4×10^{-4} mol·L^{-1}; Cd^{2+}, 0.4×10^{-4} mol·L^{-1}; SDS, 0.2×10^{-6} mol·L^{-1}; L-Ser, 0.4×10^{-6} mol·L^{-1}; lactose, 0.02×10^{-4} mol·L^{-1}; Ca^{2+}, 0.4×10^{-4} mol·L^{-1}; Mg^{2+}, 0.8×10^{-4} mol·L^{-1}; maltose, 0.2×10^{-4} mol·L^{-1}; L-Phen, 0.02×10^{-4} mol·L^{-1}; SDBS, 0.04×10^{-6} mol·L^{-1}; urea, 4.0×10^{-4} mol·L^{-1}; Mn^{2+}, 0.4×10^{-4} mol·L^{-1}; L-Lys, 0.01×10^{-5} mol·L^{-1}; glycin, 0.01×10^{-5} mol·L^{-1}; Zn^{2+}, 2.0×10^{-4} mol·L^{-1}. QT, 1.6×10^{-5} mol·L^{-1}; CTMAB, 6.0×10^{-6} mol·L^{-1}; HSA added in aqueous medium, 0.5 mg·mL^{-1}. pH 2.90, ionic strength, 0.003 mol·L^{-1}.

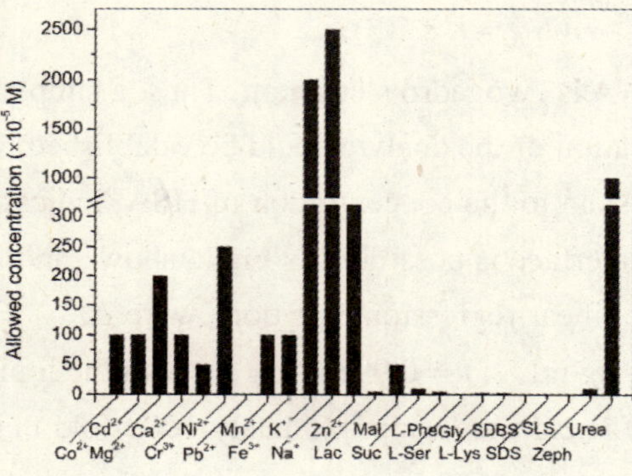

Fig.5 Tolerance levels of coexisting foreign substances with 5% determination error allowed. Coexisting foreign substances: All cations are prepared using chloride. Concentrations: QT, 1.6×10^{-5} mol·L^{-1}; CTMAB, 6.0×10^{-6} mol·L^{-1}. HSA added in aqueous medium, 500 ng·mL^{-1}. pH 2.90, ionic strength, 0.003 mol·L^{-1}.

The selectivity test of the present assay shows that the common metal ions are allowed at very high concentrations (Fig. 5). In particular, K^+ and Na^+ could be allowed at greater than 2.0×10^{-2} mol·L^{-1}. Compared with the RLS method of QT-HSA in bulk aqueous medium,[34] the ability to tolerate foreign substances such as glucose, lactose, sucrose, and maltose is enhanced about 10～1000 times. Although the tolerance level of Pb^{2+} and Cu^{2+} could be allowed only at lower concentrations, diluting with water can minimize all the interferences in the analysis of fluids, such as human urine samples.

Four synthetic samples for HSA and BSA containing metal ions, amino acids, surfactants and nucleic acid were determined, and the results are given in Table 2. It can be seen that the recovery ranging from 93.8%～106.8%, and RSD is lower than 2.31%. These values are satisfactory for the assays of synthetic samples, proving that this method can be applied to direct detection of proteins in complicated samples with high interference background. To test the present assay, we determined the total proteins in human urine samples that did not undergo any pretreatment except 2-fold dilution with water, where HSA was used as the standard. The detection results listed in Table 3 show that the contents of albumin in human urine samples are normal, indicating the practical potentiality of the present method in clinical tests.

Table 3 Total content in human urine samples

Sample	Found/μg·mL^{-1} (n = 5)	Added/μg ·mL^{-1}	Total content/μg·mL^{-1} (n = 5)	Recovery(%) (n = 5)	RSD (%) (n = 5)
1	12.6	5.0	17.8	96.3～102.6	3.5
2	5.8	5.0	10.5	97.8～103.2	2.8
3	8.6	5.0	13.8	98.1～102.3	2.6

[a] Concentrations: QT, 1.6 × 10^{-5} mol·L^{-1}; CTMAB, 6.0 × 10^{-6} mol·L^{-1}. pH 2.90, ionic strength, 0.003 mol·L^{-1}. Urine samples were freshly taken and diluted 2-fold.

3.4.4 Conclusions

Light scattering techniques are often used to determine the size of particles of known shape and composition,[34] but it has not been extensively applied to quantitative analysis. Herein we proposed a remarkably sensitive and selective backscattering light technique at the interface, and successfully applied it to proteins assay by collecting and analyzing the signals of species acting as scatterers at the interface with a common spectrofluorometer. It has showed that this technique has advantages of high sensitivity and selectivity due to the extraction and separation process through the liquid/liquid interface. As a result of greatly enhanced $_{IBSL}$ at the interface, this assembly shows high promise and could be applied to interface studies or solid scattering. It has the potential to investigate the recognition between hosts and guests with an immiscible property free from surfactants as emulsifiers at liquid/liquid interfaces. If coupled with the imaging technique and polarization technique, it could be used in the study of the morphology of the complex at liquid/liquid interfaces.

Acknowledgements

This research was supported by the National Science Foundation for Preeminence Youth in China (No: 20425517), the National Nature Science Foundation of China (NSFC, No: 20275032), Chun Hui Program (No: [2004]7～24) directed under the Ministry of Education of PRC, and the Municipal Science and Technology Committee of Chongqing.

References

[1] R. F. Pasternack, C. Bustamane, P. J. Collings, A. Giannetteo and E. J. Gibbs, *J. Am. Chem. Soc.*, 1993, 115, 5393.

[2] R. F. Pasternack and P. J. Collings, *Science*, 1995, 269, 935.

[3] C. Z. Huang, K. A. Li and S.Y. Tong, *Anal. Chem.*, 1996, 68, 2259.

[4] C. Z. Huang, K. A. Li and S.Y. Tong, *Anal. Chem.*, 1997, 69, 514.

[5] P. Feng, Y. F. Li and C. Z. Huang, *Anal. Biochem.*, 2002, 308, 83.

[6] B. S. Liu, H. Y. Zhang, H. L. Zhang and Y. Zhao, Spectrosc. *Spectral Anal.*, 2003, 23, 229.

[7] S. P. Liu, H. Q. Luo, N. B. Li, Z. F. Liu and W. X. Zheng, *Anal. Chem.*, 2001, 73, 3907.

[8] S. Z. Zhang, N. Li, F. L. Zhao, K. A. Li and S. Y. Tong, *Spectrochim. Acta, Part A*, 2002, 58, 273.

[9] P. Feng, W. Q. Shu, C. Z. Huang and Y. F. Li, *Anal. Chem.*, 2001, 73, 4307.

[10] C. X. Yang, Y. F. Li and C. Z. Huang, *Anal. Bioanal. Chem*, 2002, 374, 868.

[11] S. P. Liu, Z. F. Liu, M. Li, N. B. Li and H. Q. Luo, Fresenius' *J. Anal. Chem.*, 2000, 368, 848.

[12] X. Wu, L. Li, J. H. Yang, Y. B. Wang, S. N. Sun and N. X. Wang, *Microchim. Acta.*, 2003, 141, 165.

[13] V. Backman, M. B. Wallace, L. T. Perelman, J. T. Arendt, R. Gurjar, M. Muller, G. Q. Zhang, G. Zonios, E. Kline, T. McGillican, S. Shapshay, T. Valdez, K. Badizadegan, J. M. Crawford, M. Fitzmaurice, S. Kabani, H. S. Levin, M.

Seiler, R. R. Dasari, I. Itzkan, J. Van Dam and M. S. Feld, *Nature*, 2000, 406, 35.

[14] V. Backman, V. Gopal, M. Kalashnikov, K. Badizadegan, R. Gurjar, A. Wax, I. Georgakoudi, M. Mueller, C. W. Boone, R. R. Dasari and M. S. Feld, *IEEE J. Select. Topics Quantum Electron.*, 2000, 7, 887.

[15] J. L. Brash and P. W. Wojciechowski, *Interfacial Phenomena and Bioproducts*, Marcel Dekker, New York, 1996.

[16] M. Malmsten, *Biopolymers at Interfaces, Surfactant Science Series*, Marcel Dekker, New York, 1998, vol. 75.

[17] H. Lodish and J. E. Darnell, *Molecular Cell Biology*, W. W. Freeman and Co, New York, 1995.

[18] S. A. Tatulian, *Surface Chemistry and Electrochemistry of Membranes*, Marcel Dekker, New York, 1999.

[19] R. B. Gennis, *Biomembranes*, Springer-Verlag, New York, 1989.

[20] R. Freitag, *Biosensors in Analytical Biotechnology*, Academic Press, San Diego, 1996.

[21] R. L. Earp, R. E. Dessy and G. Ramsay, *Commercial Biosensors*, Wiley, New York, 1998, ch. 4.

[22] S. C. Schuster, R. V. Swanson, L. A. Alex, R. B. Bourret and M. I. Simon, *Nature*, 1993, 365, 343.

[23] C. E. Berger, T. A. M. Beumer, P. R. H. Kooyman and J. Greve, *Anal. Chem.*, 1998, 70, 703.

[24] A. A. Brian and H. M. McConnell, *Proc. Natl. Acad. Sci.*, 1984, 81, 6159.

[25] J. S. Salafsky, J. T. Groves and S. G. Boxer, *Biochemistry.*, 1996, 35, 14773.

[26] J. S. Salafsky and K. B. Eisenthal, *J. Phys. Chem. B*, 2000, 104, 7752.

[27] E. J. Middleton, C. Kandashwami and T. C. Theoharides, *Pharmacol. Rev.*, 2000, 52, 673.

[28] J. Peterson and M. Dwyer, *Nutr. Res.*, 1998, 18, 19958.

[29] J. Yguerabide and E. E. Yguerabide, *Anal. Biochem.*, 1998, 262, 137.

[30] J. Yguerabide and E. E. Yguerabide, *Anal. Biochem.*, 1998, 262, 157.

[31] R. R. Naujok, J. P. Hillary and R. M. Corn, *J. Phys. Chem.*, 1996, 100, 10497.

[32] M. C. Messmer, J. C. Conboy and G. L. Richmond, *J. Am. Chem. Soc.*, 1995, 117, 8039.

[33] C. F. Bohren and D. R. Hoffman, *Absorption and scattering of light by small particles*, John wiley & Sons, Inc, New York, 1998.

[34] P. Feng, X. L. Hu and C. Z. Huang, *Anal. Lett.*, 1999, 32, 1323.

(Cheng Zhi Huang, Yong Hong Wang, Hong Ping Guo and Yuan Fang Li,
published in *The Analyst*, 2005, 130, 200～205)

3.5 Flow-injection Resonance Light Scattering Detection of Proteins at the Nanogram Level

Abstract: A resonance light scattering (RLS) detection method for protein was developed, using a flow-injection system based on the enhancement of RLS signals from Biebrich scarlet (BS) by protein. The enhanced RLS intensities at 286.0 nm, in acidic aqueous medium, were proportional to the protein concentration over the range 0.005～18 μg·mL^{-1} and 0.008～16 μg·mL^{-1} for human serum albumin (HSA) and bovine serum albumin (BSA), respectively, with corresponding limits of detection (3σ) of 5.00 ng·mL^{-1} for HSA, and 7.80 ng·mL^{-1} for BSA. The method was successfully applied to the quantification of total proteins in human serum samples.

Keywords: flow injection resonance light scattering; Biebrich scarlet; proteins

3.5.1 Introduction

Quantitative analysis of proteins is important in clinical applications. The most commonly used method is staining–dye-based photometry, using dyes such as Coomassie brilliant blue (CBB)[1] and Folin phenol reagent[2]. Staining-dye-based photometric methods, however, generally suffer from limitations in terms of sensitivity, selectivity, stability and simplicity. Therefore, new assays, such as spectrophotometric[3,4], spectrofluorimetric[5,6], chemiluminescence [7,8], time-of-flight mass spectrometric [9] and electrochemical methods[10], have been developed.

Recently, Pasternack *et al.* used a spectrofluorometer to measure the light-scattering signals from aggregated species of π-staked molecules[11]. The RLS technique has now been applied to sensitive detection of proteins and nucleic acids[12,13], medicines[14], surfactants[15] and metal ions[16]. The reproducibility of a general RLS method, however, is not satisfactory for unstable dye-staining systems. Newly developed RLS techniques, including RLS imaging[17] and the total internally reflected RLS [14], although having much improved selectivity and sensitivity, still have not overcome the fluctuation of signals. Furthermore, it is not easy to perform automated analysis for these improved RLS techniques. Thus, it is necessary to develop new methods for coupled automated injection systems in order to overcome these shortcomings[18].

In this work, an automatic RLS method for proteins was developed using our flow-injection system, using Biebrich scarlet (BS) as the staining dye. Experiments show that strongly enhanced RLS signals resulting from the interaction of acidic Biebrich scarlet (BS) with protein, fluctuated and had poor reproducibility. After introducing the automatic flow injection system, however, stable RLS signals could be obtained. The method was used satisfactorily in protein determination in human serum samples.

3.5.2 Materials and Methods

3.5.2.1 Apparatus

RLS intensity and spectra were measured and recorded using a Hitachi F-2500 spectrofluorimeter (Tokyo, Japan), while the absorption spectra were obtained by using a Techcomp UV-8500 spectrophotometer (Hong

Kong, China). A flow cell with a 90 μL inner volume was used to measure the FI-RLS signals. pH values were measured with a PHS-3c pH meter (Chengdu, China), using a ND model peristaltic pump (Shanghai Instrumental Co, Shanghai, China) to drive the carrier liquid.

3.5.2.2 FI–RLS system

Fig. 1 shows the coupled detection assembly of our home-made flow-injection (FI) system. The FI unit was highly simplified, with only a solution delivery and a sample injection block. The injection block was made of an eight-way valve (Wenzhou, China), which was connected to a delivery vial (1) through a peristaltic pump (2) and to a piece of PTFE tube (5). The sample was introduced into an injection loop (7) through an injection port (4) using a peristaltic pump or a syringe (2). By turning the valve (8) clockwise, the injection sample was carried into the main stream and a second injection could be started again when the valve was reset.

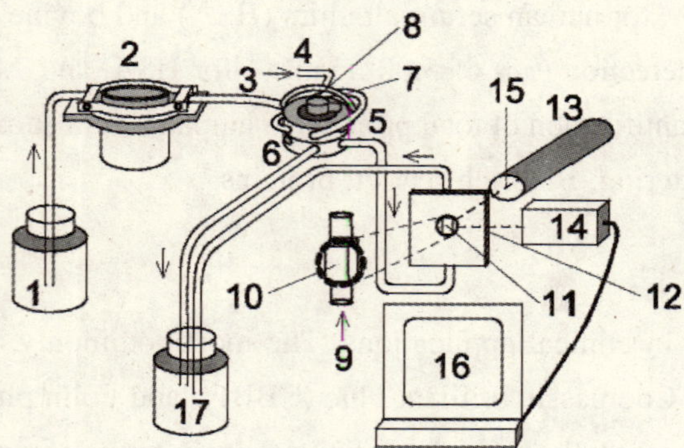

Fig. 1 Schematic diagram of FI-RLS assembly. 1, carrier solution vial; 2, peristaltic pump; 3, injection orifice of carrier solution; 4, inlet of sample; 5, injection outlet; 6, injection outlet of sample; 7, injection loop; 8, eight-way valve; 9, detection cell entrance; 10, amplified view of rectangular detection cell; 11, watching window; 12, slit; 13, Xe lamp; 14, PMT; 15, light beam; 16, computer; 17, waste vial.

A Hitachi F-2500 spectrofluorimeter was used for RLS signal detection, equipped with a 150 W Xe lamp light source (13), a 90 μL rectangular flow cell (10), a holder of the flow cell with a viewing window (11), a photomultiplier tube (PMT; 14), and a data acquisition and handling unit (16). All the reaction coils of the FI manifold were made of PTFE tube (i.d. 0.8 mm).

3.5.2.3 Reagents

Stock solutions were prepared by dissolving commercial bovine serum albumin (BSA; Beitai Biochemical Co., Beijing, China), human serum albumin (HSA; Sigma, USA), and γ-globulin (γ-IgG; Serva, Heidelberg, Germany) in doubly distilled water, except for γ-IgG, which was dissolved with the aid of a few mL of 0.1 mol·L^{-1} NaCl solution. Biebrich scarlet (BS, Shanghai Chemical Reagents Co., China) was dissolved in double-distilled water. BS working solution was 2.0×10^{-4} mol·L^{-1}. Britton–Robinson buffer was used to control the pH values of the carrier flow, while a 1.0 mol·L^{-1} NaCl solution was used to adjust the ionic strength. All reagents were of analytical grade and were used without further purification. The water used throughout was double-distilled.

3.5.2.4 Samples

Two human serum samples provided by the Hospital of Southwest Normal University (Chongqing, China) were diluted 50 000-fold with double-distilled water prior to injection, and without other pretreatment.

3.5.2.5 Procedure

The mixture of BS with Britton-Robinson buffer served as the carrier. Standard proteins or human serum samples were injected according to the flow path shown in Fig. 1.

All RLS measurements and absorption spectra were made against a reagent blank solution treated in the same way but without proteins. RLS spectra were made by simultaneously scanning excitation and emission ($\lambda_{ex}=\lambda_{em}$) monochromators of the spectrofluorometer from 220.0 to 600.0 nm. The RLS signals were detected at 286.0 nm with a 5.0 nm slit, and the working voltage of the PMT was 400 V.

3.5.3 Results and Discussion

3.5.3.1 Spectra features of BS–proteins interaction

Fig. 2 shows the RLS spectra of BS, BSA and BSBSA, which were obtained through the general RLS procedure. Both the RLS signals of BSA and BS were very weak over the wavelength range 220～600 nm. The RLS signals of their mixture, however, were very strong, and a characteristic RLS peak located at 286 nm could be observed, indicating an interaction between BS and protein. Experiments indicate that the RLS signals of the mixture increased with increasing protein concentration.

Fig. 3 shows the time-scanned FI-RLS spectra of BS-BSA with increasing BSA, and the baseline represents the carrier mixture of Britton–Robinson and BS. It could be seen that the addition of BSA induced very strong RLS signals, and the RLS signals could be reduced by injection of water instead of BSA, which is due to the effect of dilution on the interaction. Fig. 4 shows that BSA has a weak FI–RLS signal, corresponding to the results of Fig. 2. The RLS signals of BS-BSA increased with protein concentration and represent the interaction of BS and BSA, and it was found that the enhanced RLS intensities were proportional to the concentrations of proteins in a certain range. Experiments show that the RLS spectra of other proteins, such as HSA and γ-IgG, exhibit characteristics similar to those of BSA.

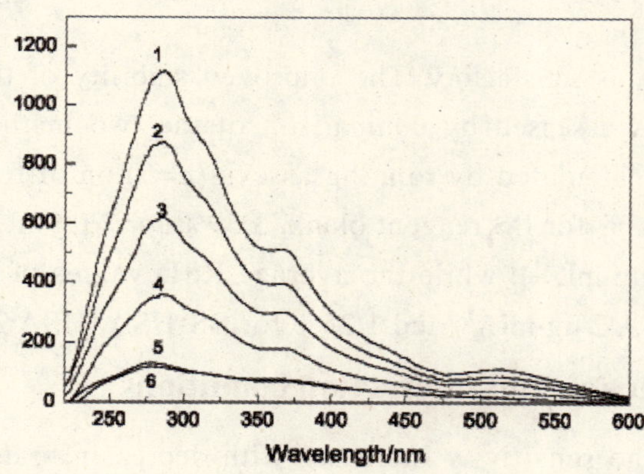

Fig. 2 RLS spectra 1–4, BS-BSA; 5, BSA; 6, BS. Concentrations: BS (except for 5, 0 mol·L^{-1}), 4.0 × 10^{-5} mol·L^{-1}; BSA (μg·mL^{-1}): 1, 4.0; 2, 3.0; 3, 2.0; 4, 1.0; 5, 5.0; 6, 0.0. pH 2.21, ionic strength, 0.12 mol·L^{-1}.

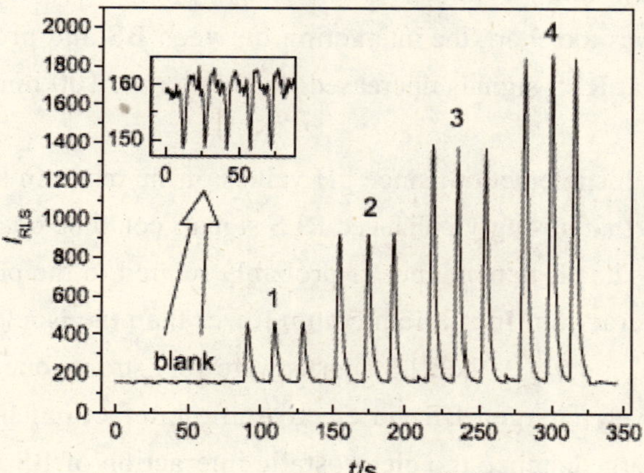

Fig. 3 Time-scanning of BS–BSA interaction. pH 2.21, ionic strength, 0.0018 mol·L^{-1}, carrier, BS + buffer. Concentrations: BS, 2.0 × 10^{-5} mol·L^{-1}; BSA (μg·mL^{-1}), blank, 0; 1, 4; 2, 8; 3, 12; 4, 16.

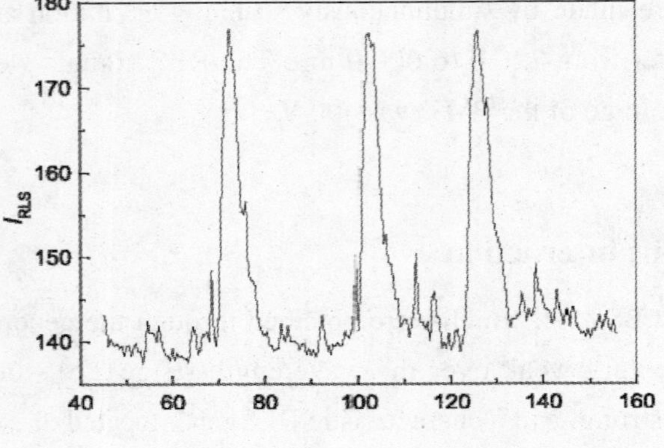

Fig. 4 Time-scanning of BSA. Carrier, BR buffer; concentration of BSA, 5.0 μg·mL^{-1}.

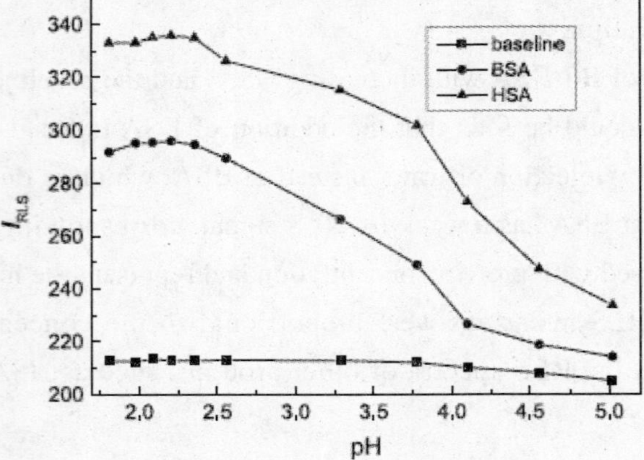

Fig. 5 Effect of pH on the interaction between BS and proteins. Concentration: BS, 2 × 10^{-5} mol·L^{-1}; all proteins are 2 μg·mL^{-1}; ionic strength, 0.0018 mol·L^{-1}.

Fig. 3 and Fig. 4 show that the stability is satisfactory. The improved stability of the FI-RLS method compared to the general RLS method was assessed by comparison of the two methods, using relative standard deviations (RSD). The RSD was calculated by running assays *(n*=5) on different days. The average RSD values of general RLS were 2.43% for BS reagent blank, 3.39% for 2 μg·mL^{-1} BS-BSA (BSA 2 μg·mL^{-1}) and 2.85% for BS-HSA (HSA 2 μg·mL^{-1}), while the average RSD values of FI-RLS were 0.79% for BS reagent blank, 1.16% for BS-BSA (BSA 2 μg·mL^{-1}) and 1.25% for BS-HSA (HSA 2 μg·mL^{-1}).

3.5.3.2 Optimization of flow injection and interaction conditions

The experimental results show that the sensitivity increases with decreasing rate of carrier stream flow (we used 3.5 mL·min^{-1} as the carrier flow rate), and that the sensitivity was independent of the length of the reaction coil. If the reaction coil length was too short, the interaction between BS and protein was incomplete. If too long, however, it was found that RLS signals decreased. In this work, 100 mm PTFE tube was used.

Acidity is an important factor affecting this interaction, since pH values of the medium strongly affect the electric charge of proteins. Figure 5 shows that strongly enhanced RLS signals could be obtained when values of the medium were in the range 1.81～2.36. The pH dependence is probably related to the positive charges of proteins and BS, due to an electrostatic interaction. In acidic medium lower than the isoelectric points (pI_0) of proteins (BSA, pI_0= 4.9[19], HSA, pI_0=4.7～4.9[19]), the RLS signals were very strong, due to the fact that the positively-charged protein reacts with negatively-charged BS via electrostatic interaction. In an aqueous medium at a pH near the pI_0, the protein is uncharged, hence the electrostatic interaction of BS and the protein is very weak and this results in very weakly enhanced RLS intensity.

Due to the electrostatic interaction between BS and proteins, the effect of ionic strength of the medium is strong, due to a shielding effect. Figure 6 shows the dependence of RLS signals of protein–BS interactions on the ionic strength. The RLS signals of BS-proteins are decreased with increasing ionic strength, which could be ascribed to the electrostatic interaction, since the shielding effect of the charges on the molecules of BS and proteins with increasing ionic strength is increased. The increase of baseline with ionic strength is due to the self-aggregation of BS. As Fig. 6 shows, the RLS signals of BS-HSA and BS-BSA reach maximum when the ionic strength is 0.0018 mol·L^{-1}.

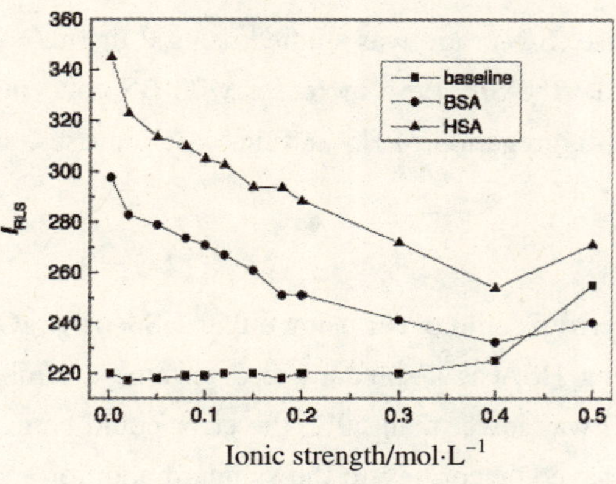

Fig. 6 Effect of ionic strength on the aggregation of BS in the presence of BSA and HSA. Concentration: BS, 2 × 10^{-5} mol·L^{-1}; all the proteins are 2 μg·mL^{-1}, pH 2.21.

Table 1 Effects of foreign substances on the RLS method for BSA determination

Substance	Concentration*	Change in RLS intensity
Na^+	100000	-9.53
K^+	20000	3.51
NH_4^+	20000	-6.16
Citric acid	5000	5.00
PO_4^{3-}	4000	1.59
Urea	1869	6.21
Gly	553.5	2.88
L-Lys	512	5.11
Ca^{2+}	500	8.05
Zn^{2+}	204.725	9.067
Mg^{2+}	200	6.12
Pb^{2+}	54.25	8.62
L-Ser	50	-1.44
Glu	10	9.14
Hg^{2+}	5.03	8.74
Fe^{3+}	5.02	-1.78
Lac	5	7.79
Cu^{2+}	2	4.11
Mn^{2+}	1.1	3.68
F^-	1	-3.66
y-RNA	0.1 μg·mL^{-1}	4.36
CT-DNA	0.05 μg·mL^{-1}	9.17

*Concentrations of non-protein substances are expressed as ×10^{-6} mol·L^{-1}. Concentrations: BS, 2 × 10^{-5} mol·L^{-1}; BSA, 2μg·mL^{-1}; ionic strength, 0.0018 mol·L^{-1}; pH 2.21; λ = 286.0 nm

3.5.3.3 Tolerance of foreign substances

The interference of foreign substances, such as metal ions, amino acids, glucose, nucleic acid and urea, was tested. As can be seen in Table 1, common components in fluids such as Na^+, Ca^{2+}, K^+, NH_4^+, PO_4^{3-}, urea and citric acid could be allowed at high concentrations, whereas Hg^{2+}, Cu^{2+} and Mn^{2+} could be allowed only at lower concentration levels without significant interference. However, diluting with water can minimize all interferences in the analysis of fluids, such as human serum samples.

3.5.3.4 Analytical parameters for the determination

Using the optimized flow injection scheme, a calibration graph was obtained for protein. The analytical parameters for the determination are shown in Table 2. The linear ranges extended with an increase of the concentration of BS. Since the enhanced RLS signals depend on the feature of charges and the size of the components [11], different proteins have different RLS responses.

The effect of BS concentration on the signal/noise (S/N) ratio was studied using 2 $\mu g \cdot mL^{-1}$ BSA, according to the above FI–RLS procedures. The results show that the S/N ratio increases with BS concentration. Unfortunately, high BS concentration generally results in self-aggregation of BS and the baseline rises, and the optimum BS concentration was 2.0×10^{-5} $mol \cdot L^{-1}$ in the carrier.

3.5.3.5 Sample determination

Since HSA and γ-IgG have different responses, errors could occur using either HSA or γ-IgG as the standard for the determination of human serum samples. Using HSA as a standard to determine the mixture containing HSA and γ-IgG, we found that if the content of γ-IgG was lower than 50%, the error could be neglected, given a determination error of 10%[20]. Two samples were assayed, according to the standard addition method procedure using HSA as a standard, and the results were compared with the Coomassie brilliant blue (CBB) method[1], which is widely used in clinical applications (Table 3).

Table 2 Analytical parameters for the determination of different proteins

BS ($\times 10^{-5}$ $mol \cdot L^{-1}$)	Protein	Linear range ($\mu g \cdot mL^{-1}$)	Linear regression Equation (c, $\mu g \cdot mL^{-1}$)	Limit of determination (3σ, $ng \cdot mL^{-1}$)	Correlation coefficient (r)
1.0	BSA	0.007～12	ΔI = -47.02 + 94.11 c	6.12	0.9968
2.0	BSA	0.008～16	ΔI = -76.67 + 108.65c	7.80	0.9984
1.0	HSA	0.015～12	ΔI = -5.836 + 97.72c	8.14	0.9989
2.0	HSA	0.005～18	ΔI = -33.48 + 108.0c	5.00	0.9975

Ionic strength, 0.0018 $mol \cdot L^{-1}$; pH 2.21; λ = 286.0 nm.

Table 3 Total content of proteins in human serum samples

Sample	Linear regression equation ($\mu g \cdot mL^{-1}$)	Correlation coefficient (r)	Found ($mg \cdot mL^{-1}$, n=5)	
			BS assay	CBB assay
1	ΔI = 69.85 + 101.6c	0.9993	75.76	77.09
2	ΔI = 77.95 + 100.2c	0.9983	80.29	78.98

Concentration: BS, 2.0×10^{-5} $mol \cdot L^{-1}$; ionic strength, 0.0018 $mol \cdot L^{-1}$; pH 2.21; λ = 286.0 nm.

3.5.4 Conclusion

The present assay for protein is sensitive and reliable, indicating the practical potential of the method for clinical tests. Automatic resonance light scattering detection techniques established with flow injection avoid the poor reproducibility of unstable systems, simplify the detection procedure and facilitate on-line detection of proteins. It is reasonable to expect that FI–RLS should be widely applicable and worthy of further exploration, considering that RLS could serve as a new principle to construct a sensitive liquid phase scattering detector, adaptable to methods such as HPLC or even capillary electrophoresis (CE). Further studies revealed that the FI–RLS was also adaptable to HPLC or CE as a postcolumn detector.

Acknowledgements

This work has been supported by the National Natural Science Foundation of China (NSFC, No: 20275032), Chun Hui Program (No: [2004] 7–24) directed under the Ministry of Education of the People's Republic of China, and the Municipal Science and Technology Committee of Chongqing, People's Republic of China.

References

[1] Bradford MM. A rapid and sensitive method for the quantitation of microgram quantities of protein utilizing the principle of protein–dye binding. Anal. Biochem. 1976; 72: 248～254.

[2] Lowry OH, Roseborough NJ, Farr AL, Randall RJ. Protein measurement with the Folin phenol reagent. J. Biol. Chem. 1951; 193: 265～275.

[3] Soedjak HS. Colorimetric micromethod for protein determination with erythrosin B. Anal. Biochem. 1994; 220: 142～148.

[4] Capitan-Vallvey LF, Duque O, Miron GG, Checa MR. Determination of protein content using a solid phase spectrophotometricprocedure. Anal. Chim. Acta 2001; 433: 155～163.

[5] Li N, Li KA, Tong SY. Fluorometric determination for microamounts of albumin and globulin fractions without separation by using α,β,γ,δ-tetra(4~-carboxyphenyl)porphin. Anal. Biochem. 1996; 233: 151～155.

[6] Li DH, Yang HH, Zhen H et al. Fluorimetric determination of albumin and globulin in human serum using tetra-substituted sulfonated aluminum phthalocyanine. Anal. Chim. Acta 1999; 401: 185～189.

[7] Tsukagoshi K, Tanaka A, Nakajima R, Hara T. On-line capillary zone electrophoretic separation-chemiluminescence detection of proteins labeled with fluorescamine. Anal. Sci. 1996; 12: 525～528.

[8] Li BX, Zhang ZJ, Zhao LX. Flow-injection chemiluminescence detection for studying protein binding for drug with ultrafiltration sampling. Anal. Chim. Acta 2002; 468: 65～70.

[9] Banks JF Jr, Dresch T. Detection of fast capillary electrophoresis peptide and protein separations using electrospray ionization with a time-of-flight mass spectrometer. Anal. Chem. 1996; 68: 1480～1485.

[10] Zhang HM, Zhu ZW, Li NQ. Electrochemical studies of the interaction of tetraphenylporphyrin tetrasulfonate (TPPS) with albumin. Fresenius J. Anal. Chem. 1999; 363: 408～412.

[11] Pasternack RF, Bustamante C, Collings PJ, Giannetteo A, Gibbs EJ. Porphyrin assemblies on DNA as studied by a resonance light-scattering technique. J. Am. Chem. Soc. 1993; 115: 5393～5399.

[12] Huang CZ, Li KA, Tong SY. Determination of nucleic acids by resonance light-scattering technique with α,β,γ,δ-tetrakis[4-(trimethylammoniumyl)phenyl]porphine. Anal. Chem. 1996; 68: 2259～2263.

[13] Huang CZ, Li YF, Mao JG, Tan DG. Determination of proteins by their enhancement effects on the preresonance light-scattering of α,β,γ,δ-tetrakis (5-sulfothienyl) porphine. Analyst 1998; 123: 1401～1406.

[14] Feng P, Shu WQ, Huang CZ, Li YF. Total internal reflected resonance light scattering determination of chlortetracycline in body fluid with the complex cation of chlortetracyclineeuropium-trioctyl phosphine oxide at water/tetrachloromethane interface. Anal. Chem. 2001; 73: 4307～4312.

[15] Liu SP, Zhou GM, Liu ZF. Resonance Rayleigh scattering for the determination of cationic surfactants with eosin Y. Fresenius J. Anal. Chem. 1999; 363: 651～654.

[16] Liu SP, Zhou GM, Liu ZF, Li M. Resonance Rayleigh scattering method for the determination of trace amounts of molybdenum with thiocyanate-basic triphenylmethane dye systems. Chem. J. Chinese Univ. 1998; 19: 1040～1044.

[17] Huang CZ, Liu Y, Wang YH, Guo HP. Resonance light scattering imaging detection of proteins with *α*, *β*, *γ*, *δ*-tetrakis (psulfophenyl)porphyrin. Anal. Biochem. 2003; 321: 236～243.

[18] Vidal E, Palomeque ME, Lista AG, Fernández Band BS. Flow injection analysis: Rayleigh light scattering technique for total protein determination. Anal. Bioanal. Chem. 2003; 376: 38～41.

[19] Chen ZX, Liu J, Luo D. Biochemistry Experiments. Chinese University Press of Science and Technology: Hefei, 1994.

[20] Tan KJ, Li YF, Huang CZ. Determination of proteins with Biebrich scarlet by a resonance light scattering technique. J. SW China Normal Univ. (Nat. Sci.) 2003; 28: 715～720.

(Kejun Tan, Yuanfang Li and Chengzhi Huang, published in *Luminescence*, 2005, 20, 176～180)

3.6 Resonance Light Scattering Imaging Detection of Proteins with α, β, γ, δ-tetrakis(p-sulfophenyl) Porphyrin

Abstract: A resonance light scattering (RLS) imaging technique was introduced to measure the light scattering of aggregation species induced by proteins, and thus a method of detecting proteins in the range of picograms was proposed. In acidic medium, *J*-aggregation of α, β, γ, δ-tetrakis (*p*-sulfophenyl) porphyrin ($TPPS_4$) in the presence of proteins occurs, resulting in strong RLS signals characterized at 490 nm. Under the excitation of a 488-nm light beam of argon ion laser source, the scattered light of single *J*-aggregation species could be observed with a common microscope, and the images could be captured with a cooled charge-coupled device camera. Data analysis for the digital images showed that the counts of aggregate species in the detection focus plane are proportional to the concentration of proteins in picograms. When 1.0×10^{-7} mol·L^{-1} $TPPS_4$ was employed, 0.01～210 ng·mL^{-1} bovine serum albumin and human serum albumin could be detected with limits of detection lower than 10 pg·mL^{-1} (3σ). Three human blood serum samples were satisfactorily detected with relative standard deviations lower than 3.04%.

Keywords: Protein; α, β, γ, δ-Tetrakis(p-sulfophenyl)porphyrin; Resonance light scattering imaging technique; Laser

The resonance light scattering (RLS)[1] technique has found wide applications in the designation of bioassemblies and aggregation species[1～7] in the past decade. In principle, when bio-assemblies or aggregation species were excited by a light beam with a wavelength close to the region of their absorption bands, enhanced RLS signals could be measured by coupling and scanning simultaneously both the excitation and the emission monochromators of a common spectrofluorometer[1]. For analytical purposes, we have applied this technique to establish sensitive methods of determination of proteins[8,9], nucleic acids[10～12], drugs[13], and surfactants[14] in real and artificial samples. Other researchers have also proposed RLS methods of detection of these biomolecules[15～19], saccharides[20,21], metallic ions[22,23], and nanoparticles[24]. Due to its simplicity, the RLS technique has been extensively used and numerous applications have been proposed [25]. These RLS measurements, however, are limited since they reflect only average light scattering features of the aggregation species in bulk solution, failing to disclose more information such as the identity of a single scatterer, even if the light-producing power of the scatterer is ten thousands times stronger than that of fluorescein and can act as fluorescent analogue tracers used for ultrasensitive immuno- and DNA probe assays[26～28]. In this study, we set up an optical system using a common microscope by introducing a laser beam to excite the bulk solution and directly observe the image of a single scatterer in situ.

Water-soluble porphyrins have been shown to form a variety of molecular complexes in aqueous solution through noncovalent interactions, and those bearing charged groups could be induced to aggregate by simply screening the repulsive interactions between side groups with the same charge [29,30]. The dimers or higher ag-

[1] Abbreviations used: RLS, resonance light scattering; $TPPS_4$, α, β, γ, δ-tetrakis(p-sulfophenyl)porphyrin; BSA, bovine serum albumin; HSA, human serum albumin; γ-IgG, γ-globulin; CBB, Coomassie brilliant blue; CCD, charge-coupled device; PTFE, polytetrafluoroethylene.

gregates of anion porphyrins such as α, β, γ, δ-tetrakis(p-sulfophenyl)porphyrin ($TPPS_4$) formed in aqueous media generally displayed enhanced RLS signals around the absorption bands of the *J*- and *H*- aggregate species[31,32]. Proteins, surfactants, and inorganic ions in acidic medium have been reported to induce the aggregation of anion porphyrins since they can change the charge state of the charge-bearing groups, resulting in enhanced RLS bands corresponding to the molecular absorption bands of *J*- and *H*-aggregation[33~36]. Thus, RLS methods of detection of proteins based on the aggregation of porphyrins have been established with sensitivity at nanogram levels in a milliliter[35~38]. Using our present optical system, however, we can further improve the detection sensitivity of proteins to picogram levels in a milliliter based on imaging $TPPS_4$ aggregation species induced by proteins.

3.6.1 Experimental

3.6.1.1 Apparatus

The RLS spectrum and intensity were measured with a Hitachi F-2500 spectrofluorometer (Tokyo, Japan) by simultaneously scanning both excitation and emission monochromators with $\Delta\lambda = 0$ nm according to the literature [1,2]. Absorption measurements were made by using a Techcomp UV-8500 spectrophotometer (Hong Kong, China). An S-10A digital pH meter (Xiaoshan Scientific Instruments Plant, Zhejiang, China) was used to measure the pH values of the solutions, and an MVS-1 vortex mixer (Beide Scientific Instrumental, Beijing, China) was employed to blend the solutions in 1.5-mL vials.

3.6.1.2 Optical system for image observations

Fig. 1 displays the optical setup for imaging detection. The 488-nm light beam emitted from an argon ion laser source (Ion Laser Technology, Shanghai, China) was guided by coupling to one end of a total reflected quartz optical fiber (0.6 mm inner diameter; Laser Institute of Physics, Southwest Normal University, Chongqing).

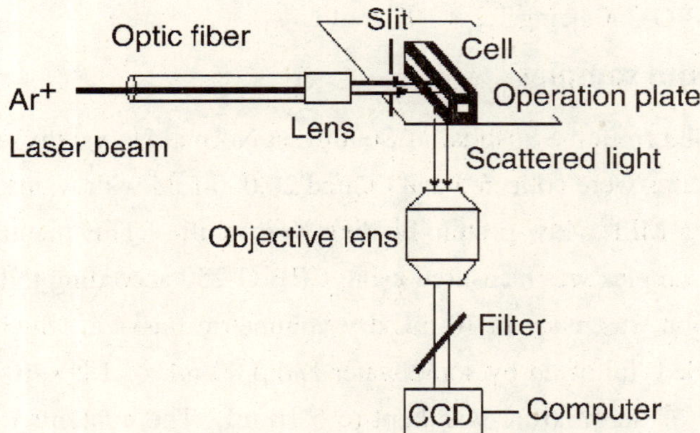

Fig. 1 Optical setup for RLS imaging detection of the aggregation species of $TPPS_4$. Quartz cell (5mm×2mm×43 mm).

The other end of the optical fiber was coupled to a quartz lens (f = 12 mm) so that the light beam transmitted from the optical fiber could be focused; the light spot of the laser beam at the sample cell was about 5 mm in diameter. The output power of the laser source was calibrated and monitored in every measurement with a WL-4 Power Meter (Laser Institute of Physics) to ensure that the power supply was stable. A magnetic film cut from a floppy disk, on which the aperture or slit were drilled or cut, was attached to the sidewall of the sample cell using glue tape, so that the luminous flux to excite the solution could be adjusted. An Olympus IX70 inverted microscope system, equipped with a BV mirror cube unit with barrier filter of 475～800 nm, a dichroic mirror of DM 455 nm (Olympus, Tokyo, Japan), and a 4 × objective (N.A. 0.10), was used to observe the light scattering of aggregation species solution filled in a transparent square quartz sample cell (5mm × 2mm × 43mm, Hitachi, Tokyo, Japan) at a right angle to the excitation laser beam. To capture the observed RLS images, a Cohu 4910 Series cooled CCD camera (Cohu, CA, USA), which was coupled with Scion Image software package for Windows 98, was employed. The Origin 5.0 software package was used for the linear regression.

3.6.1.3 Reagents

Proteins in this work included bovine serum albumin (BSA, Baitai Biochemicals, Chinese Academy of Sciences, Beijing, China), human serum albumin (HSA; Shanghai Biochemical Institute, Shanghai, China), and γ-globulin (γ-IgG; Serva, Heidelberg, Germany). The stock solutions were prepared by directly dissolving proteins into doubly distilled water, except that of γ-IgG, which was prepared with the aid of a small volume of 0.1 $mol{\cdot}L^{-1}$ NaCl solution. Working solutions of the three proteins were 10.0 $\mu g{\cdot}mL^{-1}$.

Water-soluble free-base porphyrin, α, β, γ, δ-tetrakis (*p*-sulfophenyl)porphyrin, was commercially available (Aldrich, Milwaukee, WI, USA), and its concentration of aqueous solution was determined according to its absorbance at 413.0 nm (the Soret maxima) by using $\varepsilon = 5.1 \times 10^5\ M^{-1}{\cdot}cm^{-1}$ in a medium of pH higher than 6.0[39].

Polybead–carboxylate microspheres 0.11 μm in diameter (2.5% solids–latex; Polysciences, Warrington, PA, USA) and polystyrene latex particles 0.30 and 0.46 lm in diameter (10%, Aldrich) were used to estimate the size of the aggregation species after appropriate dilution. HCl–KCl (pH 1.84) buffer solution was used to moderate the acidity, while 0.5 $mol{\cdot}L^{-1}$ KCl solution was used to control the ionic strength of the solution.

All the reagents were of analytical grade and used without further purification. Doubly distilled water was used throughout. All solutions, including water used for dilution, were filtered through a Millex low-proteinbinding hydrophilic PTFE membrane (0.45 μm, Millipore, Bedford, MA, USA) prior to use.

For comparison, Coomassie brilliant blue (CBB G-250, Fluka, Switzerland) was used for the detection of practical protein samples[40]. Its working solution was prepared by dissolving 0.1000 g CBB G-250 crystals in 50 ml 95% ethanol and then mixing with 100 mL 85% phosphoric acid. The mixture was diluted to 1000 mL with doubly distilled water with the final working CBB G-250 being $1.2 \times 10^{-5}\ mol{\cdot}L^{-1}$.

3.6.1.4 Pretreatment of human serum samples

Three human serum samples (freshly sampled from the hospital of Southwest Normal University) were centrifuged about 10 min at 1000 rpm. The supernatants were collected and diluted 20,000-fold with water; 25 μL of the diluted solution after being filtered through a Millex low-protein-binding hydrophilic PTFE membrane was transferred for analysis. Reference value for the samples was measured using CBB G-250 according to the procedures in clinical tests[40]. Briefly, the determination was made in 10-mL dry volumetric flasks in which 0~0.10 mL of standard HSA or sample solution was added, followed by some water and 5.00 mL of $1.2 \times 10^{-5}\ mol{\cdot}L^{-1}$ CBB G-250 working solution. The total volume of the mixture was kept to 5.10 mL. The contents of proteins were determined by measuring the absorbance at 595 nm against the reagent blank.

3.6.1.5 Procedures

Into a 1.5 mL vial was pipetted 10.0 μL: $TPPS_4$ and appropriate protein working solution. After the vial was vortexed, 10.0 μL HCl–KCl buffer solution was added; the vial was vortexed again and then diluted to 0.1 mL. The vial was then transferred into a 50 °C water bath for 20 min. After the vial was cooled down with flowing tap water, 0.4 mL HCl–KCl buffer and 0.5 mL water were added and the vial was again vortexed. The mixture finally was transferred to quartz cell (5mm × 2mm × 43 mm) for imaging detection.

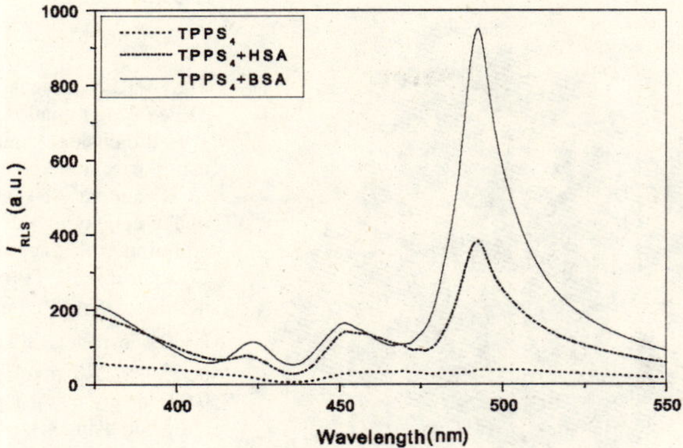

Fig. 2 RLS spectra of the aggregation of TPPS4 induced by proteins: TPPS4, 1.0×10^{-6} mol·L^{-1}; pH 1.84; I = 0.055 mol·L^{-1}. Concentration of proteins: BSA, 0.9 μg·mL^{-1}; HSA, 0.6 μg·mL^{-1}.

3.6.2 Results and discussion

3.6.2.1 RLS spectra of $TPPS_4$ aggregation in the presence of proteins

Proteins can induce the J- and H-aggregation of $TPPS_4$ through intermolecular electrostatic and hydrogen-bonding interactions between the anionic sulfonato groups and the positively charged porphyrin rings[33~35]. Since the absorptions of the *J*- and *H*-aggregation species are strong at 490 and 422 nm, respectively, induced RLS spectra corresponding to the molecular absorption bands of aggregation species were generally observed [31,32]. Fig. 2 displays typical RLS spectra of the *J*-aggregation species of $TPPS_4$ in the presence of BSA and HSA. The resonance band of the J-aggregation is located at 490 nm, confirming our earlier studies[33~36] and the studies of *J*-aggregation of $TPPS_4$ induced by H^+ or Na^+ by other authors[31,32,41,42]. Condition optimization tests showed that the aggregation of $TPPS_4$ in the presence of proteins should be completed in a medium of pH lower than 2.5, ionic strength lower than 0.12 mol·L^{-1} at 50 ℃ for 18~25 min.

3.6.2.2 Imaging of $TPPS_4$ aggregation species

By introducing an argon ion laser to excite the aggregation species of $TPPS_4$ induced by proteins, we can observe the RLS signals at a right angle to the excitation beam and, using a cooled CCD, could catch their RLS images in situ. Fig. 3 displays images of the aggregation species of $TPPS_4$ induced by BSA; similar images of the aggregation species of $TPPS_4$ induced by HSA could be obtained also. The observation depends on the features of the aggregation species and the instrumental conditions. For a single aggregation species with size in the Rayleigh range, the scattered light depends on the size of the aggregation species and the refractive indexes of the aggregation species and its environments [26];

$$I = \frac{16\pi^2 a^6 n_{med}^4 I_0}{r^2 \lambda_0^4} \left| \frac{m^2 - 1}{m^2 + 2} \right|$$

where I is the scattered light intensity, a is the size of the scatterer, n_{med} is the refractive index of the medium, I_0 is the intensity of the excitation beam, r is the distance between the scatterer and the detector, λ_0 is the wave- length in vacuum, and m is the relative refractive index of the scatterer at the excitation wavelength. When the extreme case at a wavelength that the denominator term in Eq. (1) of $m^2 + 2$ becomes zero occurs, strong enhanced RLS signals will be observed. In the present case, the *J*-aggregation species has a molecular absorption band at 490 nm; thus when excited with a 488-nm argon ion laser beam, strong RLS signals could be obtained. As Yguerabide and Yguerabide reported[27], particles with size in the range of Rayleigh scattering could have the light productivity ten thousands times stronger than that of fluorescein molecules as fluorescent analogues.

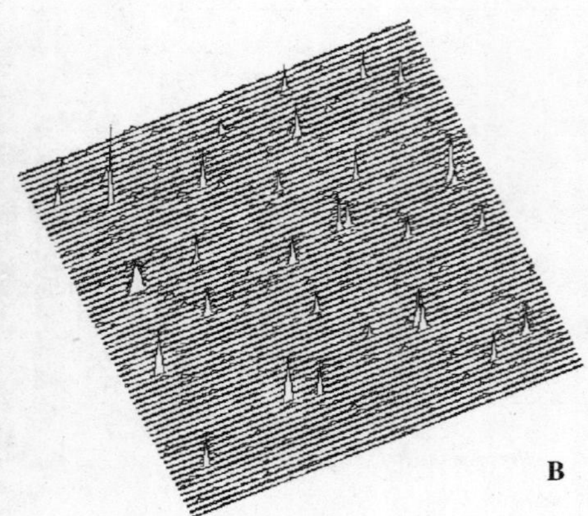

Fig. 3 RLS images of BSA-induced $TPPS_4$ aggregation species. (A) Two-dimensional image observed by using 4 × objective and caught by CCD camera. (B) Three-dimensional image displaying the intensity of RLS emission of aggregation species. Concentration: $TPPS_4$, 1.0×10^{-7} $mol \cdot L^{-1}$; BSA, 40.0 $ng \cdot mL^{-1}$. pH 1.84; I = 0.055 $mol \cdot L^{-1}$. The subframe area is 320 × 280 pixels; and it is about 0.02 cm^2 by using 1 pixel= 4.8×10^{-4} cm when using 4 × objective.

The pixel size in our optical system is about 4.8 μm when using a 4×objective, and most of the aggregation species induced by proteins occupy two to five pixels; thus the aggregation species seems to have the size of about 10～24 μm. That size, however, possibly due to lateral diffusion[43], is much larger than itself in reality, since we found that when roughly estimating the size of the aggregation species by using standard 0.11-, 0.3-, and 0.46-μm latex particles under the same optical setup, single latex particles of both 0.11 and 0.30 μm in size occupy two to four pixels, while those of 0.46 μm in size occupy four to six pixels. Thus, we roughly estimated that our aggregation species have a size in the range of 0.2～0.3 μm. In such a case, the scattered light should be described by Mie theory and cannot be calculated simply using Rayleigh theory[26]. However, their light productivities are also very strong [27]. Thus, we could easily observe single aggregation species of $TPPS_4$ induced by proteins even when using a common microscope.

3.6.2.3 Optical factors affecting the imaging detection

Fig. 4 shows the imaging of $TPPS_4$ aggregation species both in the presence and in the absence of proteins. There were only a few bright squares displayed in the imaging obtained from $TPPS_4$ solutionwithout proteins and from the protein solution without $TPPS_4$. However, the counts of the bright squares of the BSA-induced $TPPS_4$ aggregation species increased with increasing BSA concentration. The measured counts of the bright squares in Fig. 4 depend on the setup of the threshold value. Herein we set the threshold value at 40 according to the photoelectron count distribution obtained from these images. This threshold was chosen at a value of three times the standard above the photoelectron count distribution obtained from these images[43]. We also tried different threshold values and found that there were too many bright squares representing the aggregation species to be counted since some aggregation species out of the focus plane could be measured when small threshold values are set up. In addition, we cannot exclude the possibility that some aggregation species, even if they are in the focus plane, have very weak scattered light due to small size according to Eq. (1). In fact, it is not necessary to set the threshold so small since it will lead to large counting errors, and more than 99.7% of the pixels have lower intensity counts than the threshold value if there are no aggregation species in the solution [44]. Thus, the counts of the bright squares in Fig. 4 indeed represent the aggregation species of $TPPS_4$ induced by proteins. In following measurements, all the counts are measured with the threshold at 40.

The observations are also dependent on the instrumental conditions. As Eq. (1) shows, the scattered light intensity depends on the intensity of the excitation light beam (I_0). Fig. 5 displays the dependence of counts of the bright squares on the luminous flux controlled with different aperture diameters and slit widths. It can be seen that the counts of bright squares are identical when the aperture diameter or the slit width is larger than 1.5 mm. The identical counts of bright squares are possibly because power density is stable, and we measured the counts per square centimeter (N, counts/cm^2), not the integrated RLS intensity. Thus when the luminous flux is large enough to excite the aggregation species, the aperture diameter or slit width is not an important factor to the measurements. When the aperture diameter or slit width is less than 1.5 mm, however, the measured counts of bright squares are reduced following different curves.

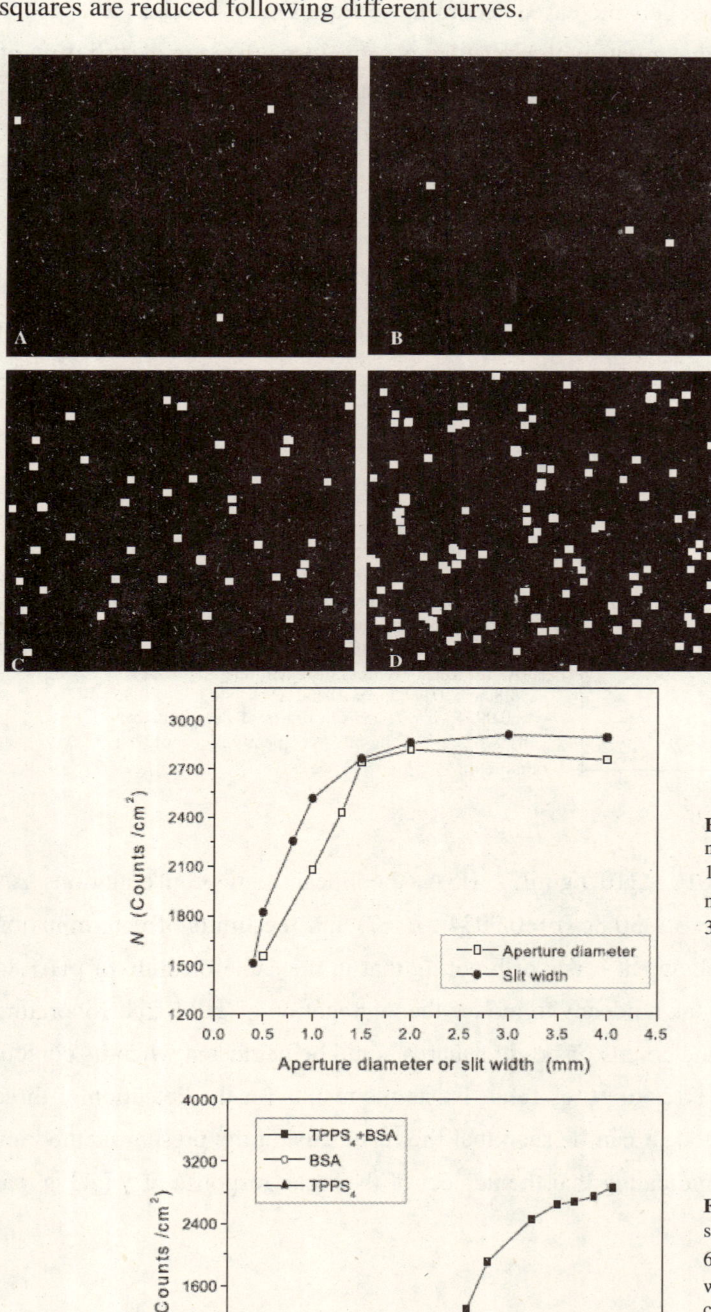

Fig. 4 Counts of $TPPS_4$ aggregation species induced by BSA at different concentrations. Concentration of $TPPS_4$ is 1.0×10^{-7} mol·L^{-1} for (A), (C), and (D); no $TPPS_4$ was added in (B). BSA (ng·mL): (A) 0; (B) 2000.0; (C) 60.0; (D) 180.0. pH 1.84; I = 0.055 mol·L^{-1}. The sub-frame area used for counts is 320×280 pixels (ca. 0.02cm^2). Threshold, 40; rank filters, 3.

Fig. 5 Dependence of the counts in unit area on the luminous flux of the excitation beam. Concentration: $TPPS_4$, 1.0×10^{-7} mol·L^{-1}; BSA, 60.0 ng·mL. pH 1.84; I = 0.055 mol·L^{-1}. The frame area used for count measurements is 320×280 pixels (ca. 0.02 cm^2). Threshold, 40.

Fig. 6 Dependence of the count density on the power supply. Concentration: $TPPS_4$, 1.0×10^{-7} mol·L^{-1}; BSA, 60.0 ng·mL^{-1}. pH 1.84; I = 0.055 mol·L^{-1}. Power density was calculated by dividing laser power by spot area, 0.20 $cm^{2!}$, with a 5-mm diameter. The frame area used for counts measurements is 320 × 280 pixels (ca. 0.02 cm^2). Threshold, 40.

The possible reason is that the luminous flux is too low and it is difficult to excite the aggregation species due to increasing light diffraction of the incident beam. In this study, a 1.5-mm aperture was used for measurements. Fig.

6 displays the dependence of the measured counts of bright squares on the power supply. It can be seen that the stronger the power, the larger are the measured counts, and they are stable when the power supply is in the range of 23～25 mW (or 115～125 mW·cm^2). The increasing trend of the counts with power density is because the scattered light intensity of small aggregation species gets increased according to Eq. (1) and reaches or exceeds the setup threshold of 40. In addition, the increasing counts with power supply discloses the size distribution of the aggregation species, and the stability of the counts within the power supply range 23～25 mW indicates that most of the aggregation species of $TPPS_4$ induced by proteins are in the range 0.2～0.3 μm. Our measurements were made in the power supply range 23～25 mW and stability monitoring of the power supply was made in every measurement.

3.6.2.4 Calibrations and protein determinations in human serum samples

Under the above-described optimal conditions, calibration curves were constructed according to the general procedure. Fig. 7 displays the linear responses of the counts per square centimeter with the BSA and HSA concentrations.

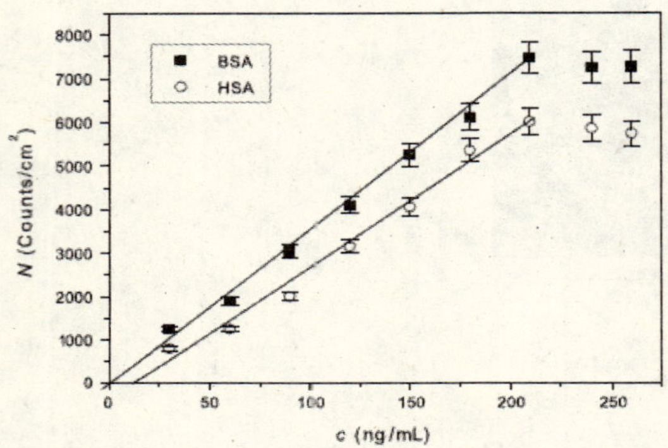

Fig. 7 Calibration curves for the determination of BSA and HSA. Concentration: $TPPS_4$, 1.0×10^{-7} mol·L^{-1}. pH 1.84; $I = 0.055$ mol·L^{-1}. Threshold, 40. The subframe area used for counts measurements is 320 × 280 pixels (ca. 0.02 cm^2). In the ranges 0.009–210 ng·mL^{-1} BSA and 0.010～210 ng·mL^{-1} HSA, the linear regression equations ΔN = - 14.3 + 34.8c ($r = 0.9978$, $n = 7$) and ΔN = - 463.3 + 30.8c ($r = 0.9934$, $n = 7$) and the limits of determination (3σ) 8.6 and 9.7 pg·mL^{-1}, respectively, could be obtained.

In the ranges 0.009～210 ng·mL^{-1} BSA and 0.010～210 ng·mL^{-1} HSA, the linear regression equations ΔN = - 14.3 + 34.8c ($r = 0.9978$, $n = 7$) and ΔN = - 463.3 + 30.8c ($r = 0.9934$, $n = 7$) and the limits of determination (3σ) 8.6 and 9.7 pg·mL^{-1}, respectively, could be obtained. It is worth noting that in the same medium of pH 1.84 and ionic strength of 0.055 mol·L^{-1}, γ-IgG has a weak tendency to induce the aggregation of $TPPS_4$, corroborating our previous reports [33,35], and its contribution to the counts of bright squares could be neglected when its content is lower than 20% with an allowed determination error of 10%. Table 1 lists the results for the detection of three fresh human serum samples with the present method. It can be seen that the results using the present method are identical to the reference method of CBB G-250, indicating that the neglect of the weak response of γ-IgG is reasonable.

3.6.3 Conclusions

Due to the strong RLS signals at a right angle to the excitation beam, single aggregation species of $TPPS_4$ induced by proteins could be observed by using a common microscope. Using a CCD camera enabled capturing the resulting images in situ. Measured counts of aggregation species in these images are proportional to the concentrations of BSA and HSA in the range of nanograms with the limits of determination at picogram levels, indicating that the present technique is sensitive and reliable. Unlike fluorescent labels, the RLS signals generated by aggregations are not prone to quenching and do not photobleach with repeated or continuous exposure to light.

Considering that the aggregation of chromophores is a very common phenomenon and small spheres, particularly nanometer-sized particles, are extensively applied when functionalized with proteins, nucleic acids, and other biomolecules using a variety of attachment and bioconjugate chemistries to impart specific binding of labels, we believe that the laser-induced RLS image technique will find wide applications in both analytical chemistry and biochemistry.

Table 1 Determination of proteins in human serum samples

Sample	Found by present method ($mg·mL^{-1}$, n = 5)	RSD (%)	Recovery range (n = 5, %)	Found by CBB G-250 method ($mg·mL^{-1}$, n = 3)
1	65.38	2.53	97.1–103.5	65.96
2	61.00	2.17	95.5–102.5	61.53
3	72.14	3.04	97.5–104.2	71.65

Concentration: TPPS4, 1.0×10^{-7} $mol·L^{-1}$; pH 1.84, I = 0.055 $mol·L^{-1}$. Subframe area 320 ×280 pixels; threshold, 40. CBB G-250 method followed [40].

Acknowledgments

All authors herein are grateful to the support of the National Natural Science Foundation of China (No. 20275032). We thank the suggestions and adjustment of the optical setup from Professor Fu Ren Zhang of the Laser Institute of Physics, Southwest Normal University.

References

[1] R.F. Pasternack, C. Bustamane, P.J. Collings, A. Giannetteo, E.J. Gibbs, Porphyrin assemblies on DNA as studied by a resonance light-scatteringtechnique, J. Am. Chem. Soc.115 (1993) 5393～5399.

[2] L.M. Scolaro, M. Castriciano, A. Romeo, S. Patane, E. Cefali, M. Allegrini, Aggregation behavior of protoporphyrin IX in aqueous solutions: clear evidence of vesicle formation, J. Phys. Chem. B 106 (2002) 2453～2459.

[3] M.Y. Choi, J.A. Pollard, M.A. Webb, J.L. McHale, Counteriondependent excitonic spectra of tetra (*p*-carboxyphenyl) porphyrin aggregates in acidic aqueous solution, J. Am. Chem. Soc. 125 (2003) 810～820.

[4] K. Kano, K. Fukuda, H. Wakami, R. Nishiyabu, R.F. Pasternack, Factors influencing self-aggregation tendencies of cationic porphyrins in aqueous solution, J. Am. Chem. Soc. 122 (2000) 7494～7502.

[5] N. Micali, F. Mallamace, A. Romeo, R. Purrello, L. Monsu Scolaro, Mesoscopic structure of meso-tetrakis (4-sulfonatophenyl) porphine J-aggregates, J. Phys. Chem. B 104 (2000) 5897～5904.

[6] A.S.R. Koti, N. Periasamy, Cyanine induced aggregation in mesotetrakis (4-sulfonatophenyl) porphyrin anions, J. Mater. Chem. 12 (2002) 2312～2317.

[7] R.F. Pasternack, E.J. Gibbs, D. Bruzewicz, D. Stewart, K.S. Engstrom, Kinetics of disassembly of a DNA-bound porphyrin supramolecular array, J. Am. Chem. Soc. 124 (2002) 3533～3539.

[8] C.Z. Huang, Y.F. Li, J.G. Mao, D.G. Tan, Determination of protein concentration by enhancement of the preresonance lightscattering of α, β, γ, δ-tetrakis(5-sulfothienyl)porphine, Analyst 123 (1998) 1401～1406.

[9] P. Feng, Y.F. Li, C.Z. Huang, Direct quantification of human serum albumin in human blood serum without separation of γglobulin by the total internal reflected resonance light scattering of thorium–sodium dodecylbenzene sulfonate at water/tetrachloromethane interface, Anal. Biochem. 308 (2002) 83～89.

[10] C.Z. Huang, K.A. Li, S.Y. Tong, Determination of nucleic acids by a resonance light-scattering technique with α, β, γ, δ-tetrakis[4-(trimethylammoniumyl)phenyl]porphine, Anal. Chem. 68 (1996) 2259～2263.

[11] C.Z. Huang, K.A. Li, S.Y. Tong, Determination of nanograms of nucleic acids by their enhancement effect on the resonance light scattering of the cobalt(II)/4-[(5-chloro-2-pyridyl)azo]-1,3-diaminobenzene complex, Anal. Chem. 69 (1997)

514～520.

[12] C.Z. Huang, Y.F. Li, X.D. Liu, Determination of nucleic acids at nanogram levels with safranine T by a resonance light-scattering technique, Anal. Chim. Acta 375 (1998) 89～97.

[13] P. Feng, W.Q. Shu, C.Z. Huang, Y.F. Li, Total internal reflected resonance light scattering determination of chlortetracycline in body fluid with the complex cation of chlortetracycline–europium–trioctyl phosphine oxide at the water/tetrachloromethane interface, Anal. Chem. 73 (2001) 4307～4312.

[14] C.X. Yang, Y.F. Li, C.Z. Huang, Determination of cationic surfactants in water samples by their enhanced resonance light scattering with azoviolet, Anal. Bioanal. Chem. 374 (2002) 868～872.

[15] B.S. Liu, H.Y. Zhang, H.L. Zhang, Y. Zhao, The high-sensitivity determination of protein concentration by the enhancement of resonance light scattering of chlorophenol red, Spectrosc. Spect. Anal. 23 (2003) 229～231.

[16] H.L. Wu, W.Y. Li, X.W. He, Interactions of night blue with nucleic acids and determination of nucleic acids using resonance light scattering technique, Chin. J. Chem. 21 (2003) 305～310.

[17] Y.J. Chen, J.H. Yang, X. Wu, T. Wu, Y.X. Luan, Resonance light scattering technique for the determination of proteins with resorcinol yellow and OP, Talanta 58 (2002) 869～874.

[18] H.L. Wu, W.Y. Li, X.W. He, Study of ethanol sensitizing effect on the interaction of titan yellow and proteins by resonance light scattering technology and its analytical application, Acta. Chim. Sin. 60 (2002) 1822～1827.

[19] L.J. Dong, J. He, Q.F. Li, X.G. Chen, Z.D. Hu, Study of the reaction of proteins with 3-hydroxy-4-(2-hydroxy-4-sulfo-1-naphthalenyl) azo (Cal-Red) by Rayleigh light scattering technique, Anal. Biochem. 315 (2003) 22～28.

[20] S.P. Liu, H.Q. Luo, N.B. Li, Z.F. Liu, W.X. Zheng, Resonance Rayleigh scattering study of the interaction of heparin with some basic diphenyl naphthylmethane dyes, Anal. Chem. 73 (2001) 3907～3914.

[21] S.Z. Zhang, N. Li, F.L. Zhao, K.A. Li, S.Y. Tong, Molecular spectroscopic studies on the interaction of glycosaminoglycans with brilliant cresol blue and its analytical application, Spectrochim. Acta A 58 (2002) 273～280.

[22] S.P. Liu, Z.F. Liu, M. Li, N.B. Li, H.Q. Luo, Resonance Rayleigh scattering method for the determination of trace amounts of cadmium with iodide-basic triphenylmethane dye systems, Fresenius J. Anal. Chem. 368 (2000) 848～852.

[23] X. Wu, L. Li, J.H. Yang, Y.B. Wang, S.N. Sun, N.X. Wang, Determination of yttrium by resonance light scattering technique, Microchim. Acta 141 (2003) 165～168.

[24] Z.L. Jiang, S.P. Liu, B.G. Zhao, S. Chen, J.A. Li, Studies on the resonance nonlinear scattering of aqueous CoFe2O4 nanoparticle, Spectrosc. Spect. Anal. 22 (2002) 615～618.

[25] C.Z. Huang, W. Lu, Y.F. Li, Analytical applications of resonance light-scattering signals totally reflected at liquid/liquid interface, Rev. Anal. Chem. 21 (2002) 267～278.

[26] J. Yguerabide, E.E. Yguerabide, Light-scattering submicroscopic particles as highly fluorescent analogs and their use as tracer labels in clinical and biological applications: I. Theory, Anal. Biochem. 262 (1998) 137～156.

[27] J. Yguerabide, E.E. Yguerabide, Light-scattering submicroscopic particles as highly fluorescent analogs and their use as tracer labels in clinical and biological applications: II. Experimental characterization, Anal. Biochem. 262 (1998) 157～176.

[28] P. Bao, A.G. Frutos, C. Greef, J. Lahiri, U. Muller, T.C. Peterson, L. Warden, X.Y. Xie, High-sensitivity detection of DNA hybridization on microarrays using resonance light scattering, Anal. Chem. 74 (2002) 1792～1797.

[29] O. Ohno, Y. Kaizu, H. Kobayashi, J-Aggregate formation of a water-soluble porphyrin in acidic aqueous media, J. Chem. Phys. 99 (1993) 4128～4139.

[30] D.L. Akins, H.R. Zhu, C. Guo, Absorption and raman scattering by aggregated meso-tetrakis(*p*-sulfonatophenyl)porphine, J. Phys. Chem. 98 (1994) 3612～3618.

[31] R.F. Pasternack, P.J. Collings, Resonance light scattering—a new technique for studying chromophore aggregation, Science 269 (1995) 935～939.

[32] R.F. Pasternack, K.F. Schaefer, P. Hambright, Resonance lightscattering studies of porphyrin diacid aggregates, Inorg. Chem. 33 (1994) 2062～2065.

[33] C.Z. Huang, Y.F. Li, N. Li, K.A. Li, S.Y. Tong, Spectral characteristics of the aggregation of α, β, γ, δ-tetrakis (p-sulfophenyl) porphyrin in the presence of proteins, Bull. Chem. Soc. Jpn. 71 (1998) 1791～1797.

[34] N. Li, S.Y. Tong, Spectrophotometric study of the interaction of tetraphenylporphyrin tetrasulfonate (TPPS4) with proteins, Talanta 41 (1994) 1657～1662.

[35] C.Z. Huang, J.X. Zhu, K.A. Li, S.Y. Tong, Determination of albumin and globulin at nanogram levels by a resonance lightscattering technique with α, β, γ, δ-tetrakis(4-sulfophenyl)porphine, Anal. Sci. 13 (1997) 263～268.

[36] C.Z. Huang, Y.F. Li, X.H. Huang, S.P. Liu, Spectral study on the aggregation of α, β, γ, δ-tetrakis(4-sulfophenyl) porphine in the presence of cation surfactants, Acta Phys. Chim.14 (1998) 731～736.

[37] Y.J. Wei, Molecular absorption and scattering spectroscopic probes of proteins. Ph.D. Dissertation of Peking University, Beijing, 1997, p. 108.

[38] C.Z. Huang, Y.F. Li, P. Feng, Determination of proteins with α, β, γ, δ-tetrakis(4-sulfophenyl)porphine by measuring the enhanced resonance light scattering at the air/liquid interface, Anal. Chim. Acta 443 (2001) 73～80.

[39] Y.E. Zeng, H.S. Zhang, Z.H. Chen, in: Handbook of Modern Chemical Reagents, vol. 4, Chemical Industry Press, Beijing, 1989, p. 435.

[40] D.A. Zhang, Experimental Handbook of Biological Molecules, Jilin University Press, Changchun, 1991, p. 327.

[41] J.M. Ribo, J. Crusats, F. Sagues, J. Claret, R. Rubires, Chiral sign induction by vortices during the formation of mesophases in stirred solutions, Science 292 (2001) 2063～2066.

[42] R. Rubires, J. Crusats, Z. El-Hachemi, T. Jaramillo, M. Lopez, E. Valls, J.A. Farrera, J.M. Ribo, Self-assembly in water of the sodium salts of meso-sulfonatophenyl substituted porphyrins, New J. Chem. 23 (1999) 189～198.

[43] X.H. Fang, W.H. Tan, Imaging single fluorescent molecules at the interface of an optical fiber probe by evanescent wave excitation, Anal. Chem. 71 (1999) 3101～3105.

[44] D. Skoog, F.J. Holler, T.A. Nieman, Principles of Instrumental Analysis, fifth ed., Saunders Brace, Philadelphia, PA, 1998, p. A9.

(Cheng Zhi Huang, Ying Liu, Yong Hong Wang, and Hong Ping Guo, published in *Analytical Biochemistry*,2003, 321, 236～243)

Chapter 4

Analytical Applications in Organic Micromolecles and Medicines Detection of Light Scattering Technique

4.1 Enhanced Plasmon Resonance Light Scattering Signals of Colloidal Gold Resulted from its Interactions with Organic Small Molecules Using Captopril as an Example

Abstract: Gold nanoparticles are known for their plasmon resonance absorption (PRA) depending on their size. Our this investigation shows that plasma resonance light scattering (PRLS) signals in the corresponding PRA region could be measured using a common spectrofluorometer, and be enhanced when aggregation of gold nanoparticles occurs due to their interaction with organic small molecules (OSMs). Using captopril (Cap) as an example, we investigated the interactions of gold nanoparticles with OSMs in order to propose a general method of OSMs such as typical clinic organic drugs. In aqueous medium of pH 2.09, there are about 2.2×10^3 Cap molecules covalently binding to the surface of a 10-nm diameter gold nanoparticle through the thiol functional group of Cap, and thus forms a core-shell assembly of [(Au)31000]@[(Cap)2200], displaying strong enhanced PRLS signals in the PRA region of gold colloid. The PRLS intensities characterized at 553.0 nm were found to be proportional to the concentration of Cap over the range of $0.1\sim1.7$ $mg\cdot L^{-1}$ with the determination limit (3σ) of 32.0 $\mu g\cdot L^{-1}$. With that, Cap in pharmaceutical preparations could be determined with the recovery of 97.0%～104.5% and RSD of less than 2.4%.

Keywords: Gold colloid; Organic small molecules (OSMs); Captopril (Cap); Plasmon resonance absorption (PRA); Resonance light scattering (RLS); Plasma resonance light scattering (PRLS)

4.1.1 Introduction

Light scattering is a very common phenomenon, and enhanced resonance light scattering (RLS) signals in the absorption region of bioassemblies or aggregation species could be detected by coupling and scanning simultaneously both the excitation and the emission monochromators of a common spectrofluorometer[1～7]. With taneously both the excitation and the emission monochromators of a common spectrofluorometer[1~7]. With this enhanced RLS signals, analytical purposes have been reached in quantifying proteins[3~5], nucleic acids[6~9], pharmaceutical drugs[10], sugars[11,12], surfactants[13] andmetalions[14] in artificial andreal samples. All these investigations have sufficiently shown that RLS technique is a favorite, powerful and promising tool due to its con venient manipulation and high sensitivity concerning the investigations of aggregate systems in which the analytes generally interact with corresponding organic small molecules (OSMs) through electrostatic attraction. Gold nanoparticles display interesting properties, and one of them is color size-dependent due to its plasmon resonance absorption (PRA). However, the investigations of combining the PRA of colloidal gold aggregation with RLS technique remain an unexplored area, particularly the area concerning assemblies of OSMs with aggregation of the colloidal gold, which could supply the possibility of preparing new materials for pharmaceutical and medical purposes.

Plasmons, which are charged density waves, are commonly generated either on a flat metal surface or within metal nanoparticles. When a gold nanoparticle is exposed to an electromagnetic wave, plasmon resonance occurs with the characteristic of the electrons in the nanoparticle oscillating at the same frequency as the incident wave[15]. Subsequently, the oscillating electrons radiate electromagnetic radiation with the same frequency as the oscillating electrons.

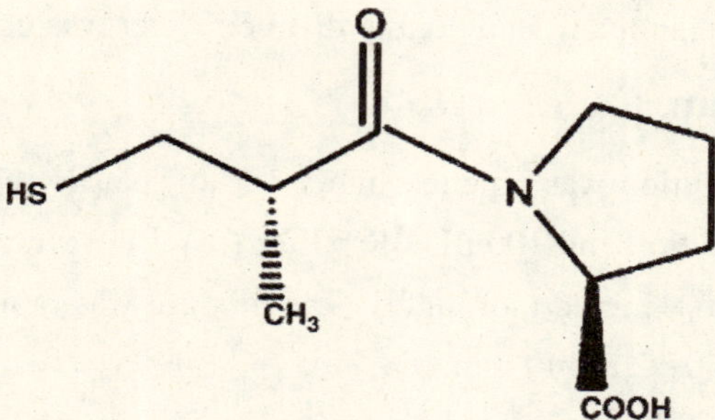

Fig. 1. Chemical structure of Cap.

It is this reradiation of light at the same incident frequency that is often referred to as plasmon resonance light scattering (PRLS)[16]. Thus, the PRLS signals of gold nanoparticles could be measured using a common spectrofluorometer, and be ascribed to RLS signals. Considering that the light scattering properties of a nanoparticle depend on their size, shape, composition, and the refractive index of the suspending medium, we expect that significant differences in PRLS between the aggregates and monodispersed gold nanoparticles could be observed, and could be applied for analytical purposes.

(2*S*)-1-[(2*S*)-3-Mercapto-2-methylpropanoyl] pyrrolidine-2-carboxylic acid (Cap, Fig. 1 shows its molecular structure) is an orally active inhibitor of the angiotensine converting enzyme and widely used for the treatment of hypertensive diseases on its own or in combination with other drugs[17]. This drug can also be used to treat congestive heart failure[18]. Several methods of Cap quantitative analysis in pharmaceutical preparations have been reported including iodometric titration[19], liquid chromatography (LC)[20], differential pulse polarography[21], chemiluminescence[22] also in connection with LC [23] or flow injection systems[24,25], fluorimetry[26], voltammetry [27], colorimetry and potentiometry[28] or biosensors[29]. In this contribution, combining with the PRA induced light scattering of colloidal gold, we apply the RLS technique to investigate colloidal gold aggregation, which is induced by trace amounts of Cap. With the aids of TEM and absorbance spectroscopy, this investigation could show that light scattering technique is effective to detect thiol-functioned substances, such as amino acid or proteins using colloidal gold as RLS probes.

4.1.2 Experimental

4.1.2.1 Apparatus

RLS spectra and intensities were obtained with a Hitachi F-4500 spectrofluorometer (Tokyo, Japan), the absorption spectra were measured by a Hitachi 3010 spectrophotometer (Tokyo, Japan), and TEM was performed on a Hitachi H-600 electron microscope (Tokyo, Japan). An MVS-1 vortex mixer (Beide Scientific Instrumental Ltd., Beijing, China) and a galvanothermy constant temperature water bath (Shanghai Apparatus Company, Shanghai, China) were used to blend the mixtures and control the temperature, respectively.

4.1.2.2 Reagents

Colloidal gold nanoparticles (10nm, 2.4×10^{-4} $mol{\cdot}L^{-1}$) was commercially purchased from the Sino-American Biotechnology Company (Beijing, China). Cap standard (Material Medical and Biologic Product Verification Institution of China, Beijing) was directly dissolved in water to prepare stock solution of 4.0×10^{-4} $mol{\cdot}L^{-1}$ and stored at 0～4 °C. The working solutions were then prepared by appropriate dilution of this stock solution. Britton Robinson buffer (BR, pH 2.09) was prepared and used to control the acidity. All other reagents were of analytical reagent grade or pharmacopoeial purity, and doubly distilled water was used throughout.

4.1.2.3 General procedure

About 250 μL gold colloid solution was pipetted into a 1.5-mL plastic tube, then an appropriate volume of Cap working solution or sample solution and 100 μL BR buffer (pH 2.09) were subsequently added. The mixture was then diluted to 500 μL and vortex-mixed thoroughly. The mixture was rapidly used for RLS, absorbance and TEM detection, after incubation at 40 °C for 40 min.

The RLS spectrum was obtained by scanning simultaneously ($\Delta\lambda = 0$ nm) the excitation and emission monochromators of the spectroflurometer from 250.0 to 700.0 nm, during which the spectral bandwidths of the excitation and emission monochromators were both kept at 5.0 nm. RLS intensity was measured at 553.0 nm.

4.1.2.4 Procedure for pharmaceuticals

For the analysis of Cap sample, we use three groups of 20 tablets with each tablet containing 25.0 mg of active pharmaceutical ingredients (commercially purchased from three company including Chongqing Kerui Pharmacy Ltd. with batch no. 050501, Chongqing, China; Zhejiang De'ende Pharmacy Ltd. with batch no. 0505102, Hangzhou, China; Shanxi Jinhua Pharmacy Ltd. with batch no. 050307, Hejin, China). Every group was precisely weighed and then ground in a mortar. Subsequently, a proportionate amount of resultant powder equivalent to 21.7 mg of active pharmaceutical ingredients was precisely weighed and completely dissolved in water. The sample solution was then filtered, diluted and detected according to the general procedure with five replicates for each sample. In order to evaluate the accuracy of method, other quantities of Cap standard were added to the sample solution and dissolved for recovery tests.

4.1.3 Results and discussion

4.1.3.1 Characteristics of the RLS spectra

Fig. 2 shows that the RLS spectra of the interaction between gold colloid and Cap at pH 2.09. Both the light scattering signals of Cap solution and the PRLS of gold colloid solution are very faint over the scanning wavelength range of 250.0～700.0 nm.

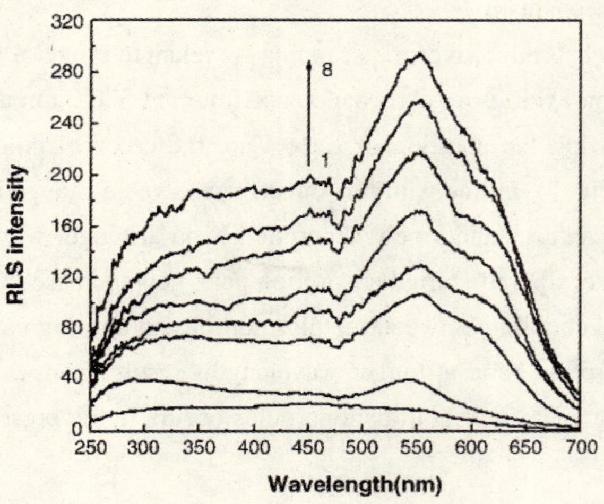

Fig. 2 RLS spectra of the interaction of gold colloid and Cap. Curve 1, Cap; curve 2, colloidal gold; curves 3～8, the mixture of colloidal gold and Cap. Concentrations: colloidal gold, 1.2×10^{-4} mol·L^{-1} except that of curve 1 in which no any addition of colloidal gold was made; Cap ($\times 10^{-6}$ mol·L^{-1})—from curves 1～8: 40.0, 0, 0.5, 1.0, 2.0, 4.0, 6.0, 8.0; pH 2.09.

even though gold colloid solution displays an obvious PRLS peak at about 544.0 nm close to its PRA band, which characterized at 520.0 nm for the 10-nm diameter gold colloid. Experiments have shown that PRLS intensity of gold colloid solutions get slightly enhanced with increasing its concentration over the range of $0.5 \sim 1.7 \times 10^{-4}$ mol·L^{-1}.However, the RLS characteristics of the interacting systems of gold colloid and Cap are quite different from those of gold colloid and Cap in the whole scanning region, obviously displaying that Cap has interacted with gold colloid. Firstly, strong PRLS signals could be observed with the characteristic peak at 553.0 nm. Secondly, it has also been found that the enhanced PRLS signals of the interacting system increase proportionally with increasing Cap concentration, indicating that Cap acts as a ligand to induce aggregation of the gold nanoparticles and the extent of aggregation depends upon the concentration of Cap. The following UV–vis, TEM, and color changes show that significant cross-linking of the gold nanoparticles occurs *via* hydrogen bonding between the Cap molecules located on different gold nanoparticles.

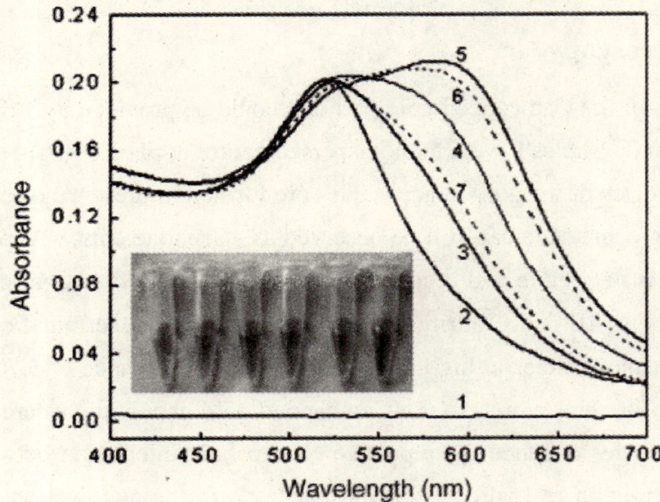

Fig. 3 Optical spectra against buffer solutions of the interaction of gold colloid and Cap. Curve 1, Cap; curve 2, colloidal gold; curves 3～5, the mixture of colloidal gold and Cap. Concentrations: colloidal gold, 1.2×10^{-4} mol·L^{-1} except that of curve 1 in which no any addition of colloidal gold was made; Cap ($\times 10^{-6}$ mol·L^{-1})—from curves 1～5: 40.0, 0,1.0, 4.0, 6.0; pH, 2.09. In addition, curves 6 and 7 are the optical spectrum of redispersed aggregates corresponding to curve 5, after ultrasonic vibration for 15 min and ultrasonic vibration after adjusting pH of the medium to 3.78 with NaOH for the same time, respectively. The inserted picture from left to right displays the changes in color corresponding to curves 2～7.

4.1.3.2 Characteristics of the PRA of colloidal gold

Enhanced RLS signals are always associated with a strong electronic coupling between adjacent chromophores, the size and the geometry of the resulting aggregate, and intense molar absorbance of the monomeric constituents [14]. Therefore, it is important to observe the molecular absorption spectra of the interaction between gold colloid and Cap to understand the interaction mechanism.

As shown in Fig. 3, Cap almost has no absorption over the scanning wavelength range of 400.0~700.0 nm, while UV–vis spectrum of gold colloid solution exhibits an absorbance maximum at 520.0 nm as a result of resonant excitation of surface plasma [15]. Following the addition of trace Cap, the color of gold colloid solution gradually changes from red to blue (inset in Fig. 3). In line with this directly observable change in appearance, the extent of the plasma absorbance at 520.0 nm reduces and a new absorption band at longer wavelengths appears. With increasing Cap concentration, the extent of the red-shifted absorption peak gets increased (curves 3~5) as a result of electric dipole–dipole interaction and coupling between the plasmon of neighboring nanoparticles [30]. In other words, the appearance of the new absorption band at longer wavelengths results from the close contact of gold nanoparticles, demonstrating that the aggregation of gold nanoparticles occurs in the presence of Cap at pH 2.09.

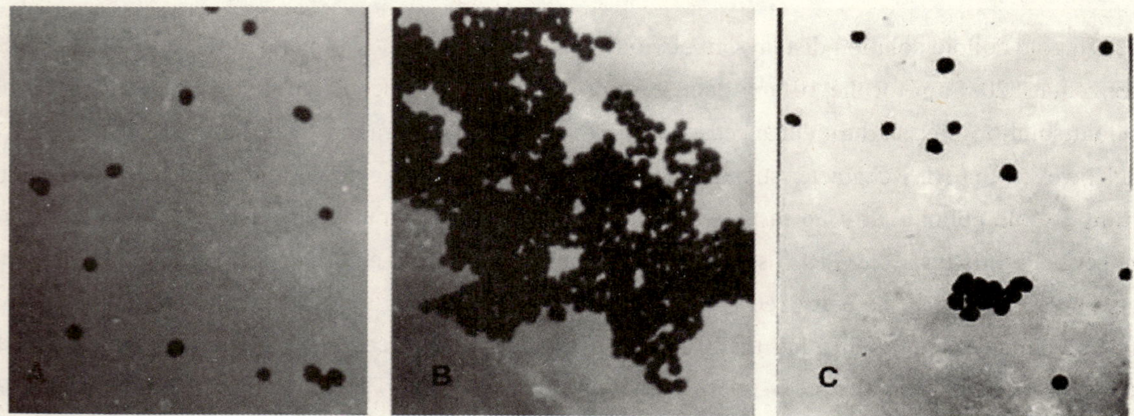

Fig. 4 TEM image (100,000×) of: (A) colloidal gold, at pH 2.09; (B) colloidal gold + 4.0×10^{-6} mol·L^{-1} Cap, at pH 2.09; (C) colloidal gold + 4.0×10^{-6} mol·L^{-1} Cap, at pH 3.78; all of the concentrations of gold colloid solutions were 1.2×10^{-4} mol·L^{-1}.

4.1.3.3 Transmission electron microscopy

Direct evidence for the state of aggregation of the Cap-capped gold particles could be provided by TEM studies (Fig. 4). It could be observed that the gold nanoparticles have a monodispersed nature at pH 2.09 in absence of Cap (Fig. 4A). On the contrary, the aggregate species of the gold nanoparticles are formed in presence of captopril at pH 2.09 (Fig. 4B), even if each particle in aggregate state can still be observed as a separate entity. At pH 3.78, however, the aggregation of gold nanoparticles is negligible and it can still keep well-dispersed state in presence of captopril (Fig. 4C). The differences between Fig. 4B and C attribute to the ionization of the terminal carboxyl in the Cap molecules located on different gold nanoparticles at high pH-value. Cap has pK_{a1}-value of 3.70 due to its carboxyl group and pK_{a2}-value of 9.80 due to its thiol group, so the Cap-capped gold nanoparticles are mainly negatively charged at pH 3.78. The negative charges enhance the repulsive electrostatic interaction between the colloidal particles and thereby hold back the formation of hydrogen bonds that leads to the aggregation of gold nanoparticles.

4.1.3.4 Optimization of the general procedures

In order to verify the important role of hydrogen bonds in the aggregation process, we could also adjust the pH of the medium that decides the charge status of the Cap molecules anchored on different gold nanoparticles and thereby affect the formation of hydrogen bonds. As Fig. 5 shows, with the variation of pH-values, the blank PRLS intensities of gold colloid solution are weak and stable, whereas those of gold colloid solution containing Cap present different traits. That is, the RLS intensities of the systems of gold colloid and Cap are strong and keep stable in the pH range of 1.81～2.56 as a result of aggregate formation, and lessen distinctly with increasing pH-value so that they nearly approach to the blank level of gold colloid solution when the pH-value reaches 3.78. The reason is that they are negatively charged at high pH-value and could not aggregate *via* hydrogen bonding among the Cap molecules because of the repulsive electrostatic interaction. In other words, the extent of ionization of the terminal carboxyl in the Cap molecules is weak at low pH-value, which is in favor of the formation of hydrogen bonds, resulting in the aggregation of gold colloidal particles.

The result of RLS measurements at different pH-values is perfectly consistent with that of the TEM detection presented in Fig. 4, supporting the contention that hydrogen bonding is responsible for the gold nanoparticles aggregation. As we know, the free thiol groups in Cap molecules can covalently bind to the surface of the gold nanoparticles [31,32]. So, we infer that the aggregation of the gold nanoparticles of this study could occur *via* hydrogen bonding between the Cap molecules on the surface of the gold nanoparticles at low pH-value.

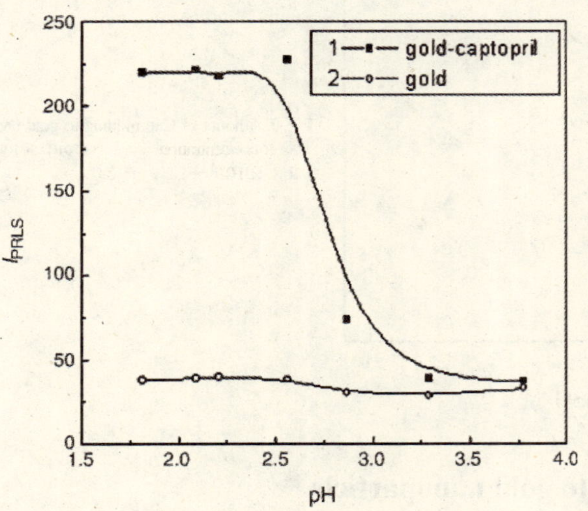

Fig. 5 Dependence of the RLS intensity on the pH of the system. (1) 1.2×10^{-4} mol·L^{-1} colloidal gold + 4×10^{-6} mol·L^{-1} Cap; (2) 1.2×10^{-4} mol·L^{-1} colloidal gold.

Additionally, curves 6 and 7 and the corresponding color changes in Fig. 3 indicate that the particles in aggregation state can disaggregate again to a certain degree by ultrasonic vibration at the pH of 3.78 for a given time, 15 min, for instance. It should be ascribed to the negatively charged carboxylic acid groups of the surface-bound Cap molecules at high pH-value, which can destroy the formed hydrogen bond. The reversibility of the aggregation of the gold particles upon varying the pH of the medium also highlights the role of hydrogen bonds in the aggregation process.

Fig. 6 shows the ΔI_{RLS} of the interacting systems of gold colloid and Cap as a function of time at different temperature. It is clear that the strongest ΔI_{RLS} of the systems can be obtained in the shortest time at 50℃, but the time of its stability is also the shortest. At room temperature, in spite of the long time of its stability, it takes the longest time to reach the balance and the ΔI_{RLS} of the systems is also the minimum. So, incubated at 40℃ water for 40 min is suitable for the determination of Cap.

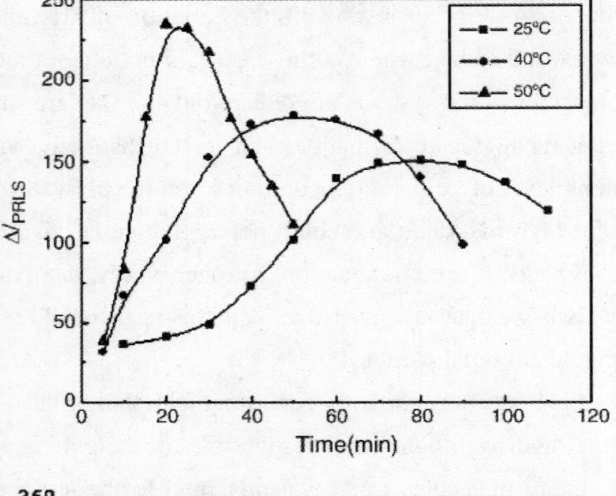

Fig. 6 Effect of time on the RLS intensity of 1.2×10^{-4} mol·L^{-1} gold colloid solution + 4.0 $\times 10^{-6}$ mol·L^{-1} Cap; pH 2.09.

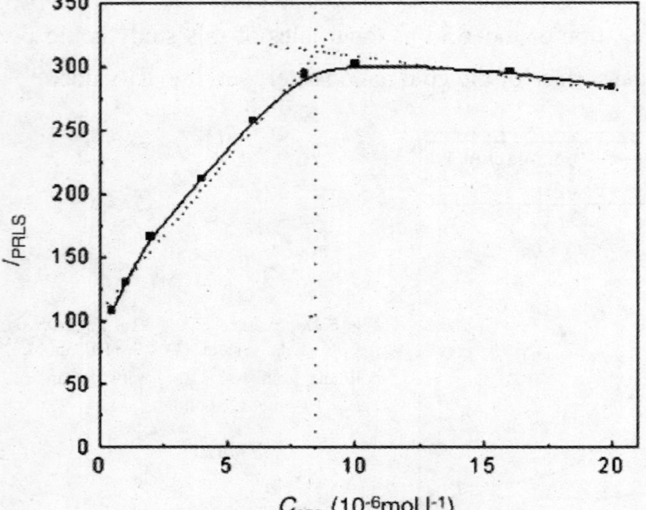

Fig. 7 Amount of Cap binding to gold nanoparticle. The concentration of gold colloid solution was 1.2×10^{-4} mol·L^{-1}; pH 2.09.

4.1.3.5 Amount of Cap binding to gold nanoparticle

A 10 nm-diameter gold nanoparticle consists of 3.1×10^4 gold atoms [33], Therefore, the 500 μL of 1.2×10^{-4} mol·L^{-1} concentrated gold colloid solution is comprised of 3.6×10^{16} gold atoms, and has 1.2×10^{12} gold nanoparticles with a diameter of 10 nm. As Fig. 7 shows, the saturated Cap concentration is 8.6×10^{-6} mol·L^{-1} when it binds to the surface of the 1.2×10^{12} gold nanoparticles at pH 2.09. So, the density of Cap molecule binding to the surface of gold nanoparticle can be expressed as follows:

$$d = \frac{C_{cap} V N_0}{\pi n_p D^2}$$

where C_{cap} is the Cap concentration, $V$the volume of the sample, n_p the number of gold nanoparticle in the sample, D the diameter of gold nanoparticle and N_0 is the Avogadro constant. We could deduce that the value of d is 6.9 nm^{-2}. At the same time, we could also calculate that there are about 2.2×10^3 Cap molecules binding to the surface of a 10-nm diameter gold nanoparticle, which is equivalent to the amount of mercaptoundecanol selfassembling to the surface of gold nanoparticle reported by Yin et al.[34]

Table 1 Interferences of foreign substances

Substance	Concentration ($\mu g \cdot L^{-1}$)	Change of I_{RLS} (%)
l-Lys	50.0	4.5
l-Try	50.0	2.3
Maize starch	150.0	-4.3
CMC-Na	70	3.4
Magnesium stearate	40	3.9
Lactose	72.0	-3.6
Sucrose	68.6	4.8
Glucose	66.0	2.8
Vitamin C	88.0	4.5
Triton X-100	25.0	2.3
EDTA	49.6	1.7
Na^+, Cl^-	46.0	-4.5
NH_4^+, Cl^-	40.0	2.3
Ca^{2+}, Cl^-	16.0	-6.2
Mg^{2+}, Cl^-	12.1	-6.8
Ba^{2+}, Cl^-	13.7	2.8
Al^{3+}, Cl^-	8.1	-4.5
Cu^{2+}, SO_4^{2-}	4.0*	3.4
Pb^{2+}, Cl^-	6.0*	-1.7
Fe^{3+}, Cl^-	6.2*	-6.2

Notes: *coexisting Cu(II), Pb(II) and Fe(III) show interference, but could be reduced if adding the 30 $\mu g \cdot mL^{-1}$ concentrated EDTA. Concentrations: gold colloid, 1.2×10^{-4} $mol \cdot L^{-1}$; Cap, 4.0×10^{-6} $mol \cdot L^{-1}$, respectively.

The thiol portion of Cap covalently binds to the surface of the gold nanoparticle and hence forms the core-shell super assembly of [(Au)31000]@[(Cap)2200], which destabilizes the gold nanoparticles and leads to the aggregation of Cap-capped gold nanoparticles interconnected *via* hydrogen bonds between supermolecules at pH 2.09.

4.1.3.6 Calibration curves and sample determinations

According to the above standard procedures, different concentrations of Cap were used to construct the calibration curves. The RLS intensity was obtained at 553.0 nm for all measurements of Cap. There is linear relationship between the intensities and the Cap concentrations. The linear response can be fitted as the equation of $\Delta I = 68.4 + 112.40c$ (Cap, $mg \cdot L^{-1}$) over the range of $0.1 \sim 1.7$ $mg \cdot L^{-1}$. The correlation coefficient is 0.9932 with the detection limit (3σ) of 32.0 $\mu g \cdot L^{-1}$.

In order to identify this method, the effects of coexisting substances and practical samples were detected. It has been found that foreign coexisting substances, including common excipients, amino acids, carbohydrates, Vitamin C, Triton X-100, EDTA, Na^+, $NH4^+$ can be allowed with high concentration, whereas those ions such as Cu^{2+}, Pb^{2+} and Fe^{3+} cause to a certain extent interference in the determination of Cap (Table 1). Even though, additionally adding 30 $\mu g \cdot mL^{-1}$ of EDTA could diminish their interferences and improve the selectivity of the method. Thus, this proposed method could be satisfactorily applied to the Cap analyses in the pharmaceutical preparations. The results and recoveries resulting from the average of five determinations were summarized in Table 2. They are in agreement with the nominal content and the precision is quite satisfactory, which is consistent with the absence of interference substances.

Table 2 Determination results of Cap content in Cap samples (n = 5)

Sample	Found (mg·tablet^{-1})	R.S.D. (%)	Original (mg·L^{-1})	Added (mg·L^{-1})	Total found (mg·L^{-1})	R S D (%)	Recovery (%)
050501	25.8	2.1	0.22	0.44	0.68	3.1	104.5
0505102	24.6	2.4	0.43	0.58	0.99	2.9	97.0
050307	25.6	1.8	0.43	0.87	1.33	2.6	103.4

Notes: all of the nominal content of Cap samples is 25 mg·tablet^{-1}. Columns 2 and 3 show the determination results of three batch of the commercial drug commercially purchased from Chongqing Kerui Pharmacy Ltd. with batch no. 050501 (Chongqing, China), Zhejiang De'ende Pharmacy Ltd. with batch no. 0505102 (Hangzhou, China) and Shanxi Jinhua Pharmacy Ltd. with batch no. 050307. Columns 4~8 from left to right show the results for recovery detection. Concentration of gold colloid, 1.2×10^{-4} mol·L^{-1}; pH 2.09; λ = 553.0 nm.

4.1.4 Conclusion

RLS spectroscopy was successfully used to investigate the process of colloidal gold aggregation induced by a kind of thiolcontaining pharmaceutical Cap. As a special RLS signals, PRLS resulting from the aggregation of gold nanoparticles could be used to detect a minimum of 32.0 μg L^{-1} of Cap under certain conditions. Therefore, when combining with colloidal goldbased assay, RLS technique may have potential applications in determining thiol-containing substances. On the other hand, the mechanism of colloidal gold aggregation is that the presence of the carboxylic acid functional groups on the surface of the gold nanoparticles leads to hydrogen bond formation and thereby cross-linking of the colloidal gold particles at pH 2.09. The process may be reversible, and the dispersion of the particles from the aggregates can be accomplished by adjusting pH of the medium to the alkaline condition and ultrasonic vibration. The protocol based on Cap derivatized gold nanoparticles may be extended to controlled cross-linking and is currently being pursued.

Acknowledgements

All authors herein are grateful to the supports from the National Natural Science Foundation of China (NSFC, no. 20425517), and the Municipal Science and Technology Committee of Chongqing.

References

[1] R.F. Pasternack, P.J. Collings, Science 269 (1995) 935.
[2] R.F. Pasternack, C. Bustamante, P.J. Collings, A. Giannetto, E.J. Gibbs, J. Am. Chem. Soc. 115 (1993) 5393.
[3] C.Z. Huang, Y.F. Li, J.G. Mao, D.G. Tan, Analyst 123 (1998) 1401.
[4] R.P. Jia, L.J. Dong, Q.F. Li, X.G. Chen, Z.D. Hu, Y. Nagaosa, Anal. Chim. Acta 442 (2001) 249.
[5] W. Lu, P. Feng, Y.F. Li, C.Z. Huang, Anal. Lett. 35 (2002) 227.
[6] C.Z. Huang, K.A. Li, S.Y. Tong, Anal. Chem. 68 (1996) 2259.
[7] C.Z. Huang, K.A. Li, S.Y. Tong, Anal. Chem. 69 (1997) 514.
[8] P. Bao, A.G. Frutos, C. Greef, J. Lahiri, U. Muller, T.C. Peterson, L. Warden, X.Y. Xie, Anal. Chem. 74 (2002) 1792.
[9] W. Lu, C.Z. Huang, Y.F. Li, Analyst 127 (2002) 1392.
[10] P. Feng, W.Q. Shu, C.Z. Huang, Y.F. Li, Anal. Chem. 73 (2001) 4307.
[11] S.P. Liu, H.Q. Luo, N.B. Li, Z.F. Liu, W.X. Zheng, Anal. Chem. 73 (2001) 3907.
[12] S.Z. Zhang, F.L. Zhao, K.A. Li, S.Y. Tong, Anal. Chim. Acta 431 (2001) 133.
[13] S.P. Liu, G.M. Zhou, Z.F. Liu, Fresen. J. Anal. Chem. 363 (1999) 651.
[14] Y.K. Zhao, Q.E. Cao, Z.D. Hu, Q.H. Xu, Anal. Chim. Acta 388 (1999) 45.
[15] K.L. Kelly, E. Coronado, L.L. Zhao, G.C. Schatz, J. Phys. Chem. B 107 (2003) 668.
[16] K. Aslan, P. Holley, L. Davies, J.R. Lakowicz, C.D. Geddes, J. Am. Chem. Soc. 127 (2005) 12115.

[17] B.F. Yang (Ed.), Pharmacology, 6th ed., People's Medical Publishing House, Beijing, 2005, 247 pp.
[18] R.G. Ye, Z.Y. Lu (Eds.), Medicine, 5th ed., People's Medical Publishing House, Beijing, 2002, 155 pp.
[19] Editorial Committee of Pharmacopoeia of People's Republic of China, The Pharmacopoeia of People's Republic of China (Part II), Chemical Industry Press, Beijing, 2000, p. 131.
[20] G. Favaro, M. Fiorani, Anal. Chim. Acta 332 (1996) 249.
[21] J.M.G. Fraga, A.I.J. Abizanda, F.J. Moreno, J.J.A. Leon, Talanta 46 (1998) 75.
[22] X.R. Zhang, W.R.G. Baeyens, G. Van der Weken, A.C. Calokerinos, K. Nakashima, Anal. Chim. Acta 303 (1995) 121.
[23] J. Ouyang, W.R.G. Baeyens, J. Delanghe, G. Van der Weken, W. Van Daele, D. De Keukeleire, A.M. Garcia Campana, Anal. Chim. Acta 386 (1999) 57.
[24] D.G. Economou, G. Themelis, P.D. Theodoridis, Tzanavaras, Anal. Chim. Acta 463 (2002) 249.
[25] Li, Z. Zhang, M. Wu, Microchim. J. 70 (2001) 85.
[26] S.M. Al-Ghannam, A.M. El-Brashy, B.S. Al-Farhan, Farmaco 57 (2002) 625.
[27] X. Ioannides, A. Economou, A. Voulgaropoulos, J. Pharm. Biomed. Anal. 33 (2003) 309.
[28] A.M. Pimenta, A.N. Araujo, M.C.B.S.M. Montenegro, Anal. Chim. Acta 438 (2001) 31.
[29] R.I. Stefan, J.F. Van Staden, H.Y. Aboul-Enein, Anal. Chim. Acta 411 (2000) 51.
[30] S. Mandal, A. Gole, N. Lala, R. Gonnade, V. Ganvir, M. Sastry, Langmuir 17 (2001) 6262.
[31] N.T.K. Thanh, Z. Rosenzweig, Anal. Chem. 74 (2002) 1624.
[32] X.H. Huang, H.Z. Huang, N.Z. Wu, R.S. Hu, T. Zhu, Z.F. Liu, Surf. Sci. 459 (2000) 183.
[33] Z.L. Jiang, Z.W. Feng, T.S. Li, Sci. Chin. B 44 (2001) 175.
[34] H. Yin, H. Liu, Y. Li, Acta Chim. Sinica 63 (2005) 734.

(Zhong De Liu ,Cheng Zhi Huang , Yuan Fang Li, Yun Fei Long,
published in *Analytica Chimica Acta*, 2006, 577, 244～249)

4.2 Total Internal Reflected Resonance Light Scattering Determination of Chlortetracycline in Body Fluid with the Complex Cation of Chlortetracycline-Europium-Trioctyl Phosphine Oxide at the Water/ Tetrachloromethane Interface

A highly selective method of chlortetracycline (CTC) is proposed on the basis of the measurements of total internal reflected resonance light scattering (TIR-RLS) at water/tetrachloromethane (H_2O/CCl_4) interfaces. In the pH range of 7.54～8.14, the interaction of the binary complex ofEu(III)/CTC in the presence oftrioctyl phosphine oxide (TOPO) occurs at the H_2O/CCl_4 interface, resulting in greatly enhanced TIR-RLS signals with the maximum peak located at 340 nm. The enhanced TIRRLS intensity is in proportion to the CTC concentration in the range $0.98 \sim 20.0 \times 10^{-7}$ $mol \cdot L^{-1}$. The limit of detection is 9.8×10^{-9} $mol \cdot L^{-1}$. Synthetic samples and body fluid samples including human urine, human serum, and fresh milk were determined with the recovery of 95.4%～106.4% and RSD of 2.9%～3.9%.

The quantification of chlortetracycline (CTC) is of importance, because it has been employed extensively as a bacteriostatic and antibiotic drug in clinical medicine and food science. Spectrophotometric methods have been reported on the basis of the oxidation of CTC by ammonium vanadate,[1] sodium cobaltinitrite,[2] sodium molybdate,[3] and uranyl acetate[4] and on its chelate complex with tungstate.[5] These methods, however, have suffered from drawbacks such as instability, complicated reaction conditions and low sensitivity. CTC has weak intrinsic fluorescence, but it can be degraded into strongly fluorescent products (anhydro- or isotetracyclines) in acidic or alkaline solutions.[6,7] In addition, spectrofluorometric methods also can be established by chelating with di- or trivalent cations such as calcium,[8] aluminum,[9] europium,[10,11] and lanthanum.[12] To improve the sensitivity of the spectrofluorometric method, surfactants have been employed.[13～15] These spectrofluorometric methods, however, have suffered from difficulties in the CTC determination in body fluids because of the interference of other components and the strong background fluorescence. Therefore, it is necessary to develop a simple assay method for CTC that has high sensitivity, accuracy, and selectivity.

Adsorption and reaction at the liquid/liquid interfaces have recently become attractive subjects in the fundamental studies of solvent extraction of metal ions, the detection of liquid separation, ion-selective electrodes, optical sensors, and counter current chromatography.[16] When a light beam passes through a liquid/ liquid interfaces and is totally reflected from the interfaces between the optically rarer and denser phase, it develops an evanescent field on the side of an optically rarer phase at the interface.[17] Because the refractive index plays a very important role in the formation of the evanescent field at the liquid/ liquid interfaces, it occurred to us that the total internal reflection of light could be coupled with the resonance light scattering (RLS) technique. The RLS technique was constructed on the basis of the fluctuations of the refractive index in an aqueous solution in which the steep change of the refractive indexes of the inner scattered particle and that of its outer atmosphere occurs.[18,19] It has been proved that the RLS signals resulting from the supermolecular interaction of stacked dyes with nucleic acids or proteins in an absorption medium can be used to the sensitive determination of these biological molecules.[20～24] Because the extent to which a particle absorbs and determination of these biological molecules.[20~24] Because the extent to which a particle absorbs and scatters depends on its size, shape and refractive index as compared to the surrounding medium, and the refractive index of the particle itself is different from that of its outer atmosphere,[18] the difference of the indexes between the particle itself and that of the outer atmosphere builds up a mini-interface. As a result, we suppose that the combination of total internal reflection of light with RLS measurements can produce extraordinary results and can be used to study the molecular recognition and assembly at the interfaces. Herein we present our first try with the total internal reflected resonance light scattering (TIR-RLS) technique to establish a new sensitive and highly selective method of CTC detection in body fluids.

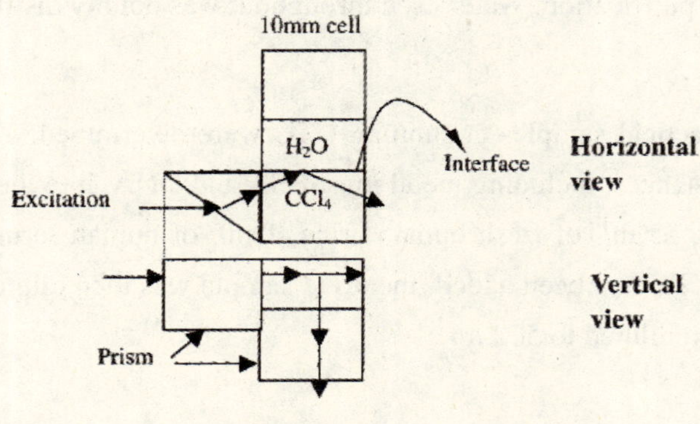

Fig. 1 Optical arrangement of the liquid/liquid interface formed by H_2O/CCl_4. Right-angle prism, 10mm × 10 mm × 10 mm.

4.2.1 Experimental Section

4.2.1.1 Apparatus

TIR-RLS spectra and intensities were measured with a Hitachi F -2500 spectrofluorometer (Tokyo, Japan). The under inside of an optical quartz cell (10 mm) was treated with dichlorodimethylsilane in benzene so as to make the inside wall hydrophobic and afford a flat H_2O/CCl_4 interface. Fig. 1 illustrates the optical arrangement in the sample compartment of the spectrophotometer. Two right-angle quartz prisms were attached to the cell walls facing the excitation light source and the fluorescence detector, respectively, so that the excitation light beam passing through the prism and the cell wall was impinged upon the H_2O/CCl_4 interfaces in the cell. According to the Snell law, the incidence angle is 72.6°(see Supporting Information), which is sufficiently greater than the critical angle of 65.6°for the total internal reflection of H_2O/CCl_4 system. As a result, the penetration depth can be calculated at the H_2O/CCl_4 interfaces for an incidence light beam according to following equation:[25]

$$d_p = \frac{\lambda}{2\pi\left[\sin^2\theta - (n_2/n_1)^2\right]^{1/2}}$$

where θ and λ are the angle and wavelength of the incidence light beam and n_1 and n_2 are the refractive index of CCl_4 (1.460 at 25 ℃) and H_2O (1.333 at 25 ℃), respectively. For an incidence light beam of 340 nm, the penetration depth is 194 nm at the H_2O/CCl_4 interfaces.

4.2.1.2 Reagents

Chlortetracycline (CTC) solution was prepared by dissolving 0.0479 g of its hydrochlorides (Sino

-American Biotech. Co., China) in 100 mL of distilled water. The working solutions were freshly prepared before use by diluting the 1.0×10^{-3} mol·L^{-1} stock solution with doubly distilled water.

The stock solution of Eu(III) was prepared by dissolving Eu_2O_3 (99.85%, Chemical Plant of Peking University, Beijing, China) in diluted HCl. The working solution was obtained by diluting the stock solution to 1.0×10^{-5} mol·L^{-1} with water. A 1.0×10^{-2} mol·L^{-1} triocyctyl phosphine oxide (TOPO, E. Merck, Darmstadt) solution was prepared by dissolving 0.3867 g of the commercial product in 100 mL of tetrachloromethane. A 1.0×10^{-3} mol·L^{-1} working solution was prepared by diluting the stock solution with tetrachloromethane.

Tris-HCl buffer solution (0.05mol·L^{-1}, pH 7.77) was used to control the acidity of the aqueous medium. All reagents were of analytical grade without further purification. Water used throughout was doubly distilled.

4.2.1.3 Pretreatment of Samples

To test the present assay, synthetic and practical samples containing CTC were determined. The synthetic samples were constructed by adding foreign substances, including metal ions, BSA and DNA, into the appropriate working solution of CTC. For practical samples, 25 mL of fresh human urine, 1 mL of human serum, and fresh milk were employed. After a series of standard CTC had been added, the urine sample was then diluted to 50 mL, and the human serum and milk samples were each diluted to 500 mL.

4.2.1.4 Standard Procedure

An appropriate volume of the CTC working solution or sample solution was placed in a 10-mL volumetric flask so as to keep the interaction system at 0.98-20.00 × 10^{-7} mol·L^{-1} of CTC, then 5 mL of Eu(III) working solution and 1 mL of buffer solution were added. The mixture was then diluted to 10 mL with doubly distilled water and mixed thoroughly. A 1 mL of TOPO working solution was pipetted into a dry optical quartz cell, along with 1 mL of the Eu(III)-CTC mixture, was mixed thoroughly, and then allow to stand for 30 min. The TIR-RLS spectra and the intensities were measured against the blank treated in the same way without CTC.

The TIR-RLS spectra were obtained by scanning simultaneously the excitation and emission monochromators of the F-2500 spectrofluorometer from 220 to 700 nm with $\lambda_{ex} = \lambda_{em}$. The RIT-RLS intensities were measured at 340 nm using a slit width of 5.0 nm for both excitation and emission. The fluorescence measurements in aqueous medium were made at 619 nm using 397-nm excitation.

4.2.2 Results and Discussion

4.2.2.1 Spectral Characteristics

In the optical arrangement illustrated in Fig. 1, the aqueous phase was the aqueous solutionof the binary complex of Eu(III)-CTC, and the organic phase was the CCl_4 solution of TOPO. As Fig. 2 shows, without any addition of CTC, the TIR-RLS intensity of the system was very faint in the region 280～620 nm. If a trace amount of CTC was added to form the binary complex in the aqueous phase, however, strong TIR-RLS signals extended into the region of 340～370 nm can be observed, and the TIR-RLS intensity increases with increasing CTC concentration.

Under the experimental conditions, Eu(III) can combine with CTC to form a complex of Eu(III)-CTC in the aqueous phase,[10～13,15,26] but the coordination number of Eu(III) is unsaturated. In such a case, the water molecules will occupy the coordination sites of Eu(III). If a synergistic ligand, such as TOPO, is added, the synergistic ligand will replace the coordinated water molecules to meet the requirements of the saturated coordination of the central Eu(III) ion, which acts as a bridge between the TOPO and CTC. Because the TOPO and Eu(III)-CTC binary complexes dissolve in CCl_4 and the aqueous phase, respectively, the interfacial region in H_2O/CCl_4 system is amphipathic. It has been proved that the RLS signals of the Eu(III)-CTC binary complex in aqueous solution and the TIR-RLS signals of the binary complex at the H_2O/CCl_4 interfaces are very weak; therefore, the greatly enhanced TIR-RLS signals at the H_2O/CCl_4 interfaces are obviously ascribed to the formation of the complex cation of Eu-(III)-CTC-TOPO, in which TOPO acts as a synergistic ligand. Therefore, the TIR-RLS signals disclose the information of the complex at the H_2O/CCl_4 interfaces.

The formation of the ternary complex at the H_2O/CCl_4 interfaces encourages the movement of TOPO and Eu(III)-CTC molecules in bulk solution both in aqueous and organic phases toward the interfaces, displaying adsorption properties. In such cases, more of the ternary complex can be concentrated at the H_2O/CCl_4 interfaces. The TIR-RLS intensities of the complex were found to be proportional to the concentration of CTC, indicating that the determination of CTC with the TIR-RLS data at the H_2O/CCl_4 interfaces is possible.

4.2.2.2 Optimization of the General Procedures

It was found that the TIR-RLS intensity depends on the pH of the aqueous medium. As Figure 3 shows, the strongest enhanced TIR-RLS intensity can be found in the range of pH 7.54~8.14, and the intensity decreases at any pH outside this range. This pH range is in agreement with the disassociation of the second proton (pK_{a2} =7.4) in a phenolic diketone system of CTC molecular structure[27]. That means the disassociation of the second proton of CTC is of benefit to the formation of the complex cation at the interfaces. The decrease of the enhanced TIR-RLS intensity above pH 8.1 is probably due to the increase in the solubility of CTC[27] that is unfavorable for its movement toward the interface. In this work, the aqueous solution was controlled with a Tris-HCl buffer solution pH 7.77.

Emulsification at the interfaces will increase the TIR-RLS intensity and even makes the intensity unstable. Allowing the mixture to standing without agitation for some time can solve this problem. We found that the suitable standing time is 25 min. The TIR-RLS data of the multibasic complex at the interfaces will then stay constant for 60 min.

4.2.2.3 Molar Ratio of Eu(III)-CTC at H_2O/CCl_4 Interfaces

As the center of the complex, Eu(III) plays a critical role; therefore, the effect of the Eu(III) concentration should be considered first. Fig. 4 shows that the role of both Eu(III) and CTC played in the complex cation at H_2O/CCl_4 interfaces. When $c_{Eu(III)}$ and c_{CTC} are equal, the complex cation is formed at a molar ratio of 1:1 at the interfaces, and the enhanced TIR-RLS data does not show significant changes. The 1:1 molar ratio of Eu(III)-CTC can be proved also by keeping the total concentration of Eu(III) and CTC as 4.0×10^{-6} mol·L^{-1} while the concentrations of the two components are changed simultaneously (Fig. 5). The results from both Fig. 4 and Fig. 5 indicate that the complex cation in the interfaces was formed as $[Eu(CTC)(TOPO)_x]^{2+}$. In the same way, the molar ratio of the Eu(III)-CTC complex in aqueous solution can be determined through spectrofluometric measurements with the aqueous solution; 1:1 can also be obtained (Fig. 5); therefore, the complex in water should be $[Eu(CTC)(H_2O)_y]^{2+}$. This 1:1 molar ratio is in agreement with the results of other reports;[12,13,15,26] however, in a practical situation, the concentration of CTC acting as an analyte is unknown, and an excess of Eu(III) must be used. In this assay, 5.0×10^{-6} mol·L^{-1} Eu(III) was used for the determination of synthetic and body fluid samples.

4.2.2.4 Selection of the Synergistic Ligand

Because ofthe introduction of hydrophobic synergistic ligands, the water molecules of $[Eu(CTC)(H_2O)_y]^{2+}$ in the aqueous phase are replaced so as to make the complex cation $[Eu(CTC)(TOPO)_x]^{2+}$ like an amphipathic molecule at the interfaces. In addition, the introduction of the synergistic ligands can meet the requirements ofthe saturation coordination of the central Eu(III) ion; therefore, the selection of the synergic ligand is very important. A series of synergistic ligands has been tested (Table 1). It can be seen that TOPO is the most suitable synergistic ligand. When the concentrations of CTC and Eu(III) were kept fixed, the effect of the concentration of TOPO was tested. Figure 6 shows that the TIR-RLS data at the H_2O/CCl_4 interfaces were stable in the TOPO concentration range of $0.75 \sim 1.0\times10^{-3}$mol·L^{-1}.

4.2.2.5 Interferences of Coexisting Foreign Substances

The influences of foreign coexisting substances such as proteins, DNA and metal ions were tested. We found that the common ions in fluids, such as Ca(II), Mn(II), Cu(II), Ni(II), Fe(III), and Cr(III), and Mg(II), Pb(II), Zn(II), Al(III), and PO_4^{3-}, can be allowed at very high concentrations under the tolerance level of 10% (larger than 1.0×10^{-4} mol·L^{-1} for the former six ions and 1.0×10^{-3} mol·L^{-1} for the latter five ions, respectively). These ions, however, can only be allowed at the concentration levels of 1.0×10^{-5} to 1.0×10^{-8} mol·L^{-1} in the spectrofluorometry of CTC in aqueous phase, where surfactants such as sodium dodecylsulfonate (SDS) should be used.[14] Substances including K^+, Na^+, NH_4^+, and urea do not display any effect for the present TIR-RLS method, even if they are at high concentration levels (larger than 1.0×10^{-2} mol·L^{-1}). Biological molecules such as bovine serum albumin (BSA) and calfthymus DNA (ctDNA) can be allowed at 15 μg·mL^{-1} and 5.0 μg·mL^{-1}, respectively, which supplies a good permission for the assay of CTC in body fluid samples; therefore, it is obvious that this method has fair selectivity and can be applied to the direct determination of trace amounts of CTC in biological materials without separating the interfering materials, even though we found the present method cannot distinguish CTC from other tetracyclines, such as tetracycline and oxytetracycline.

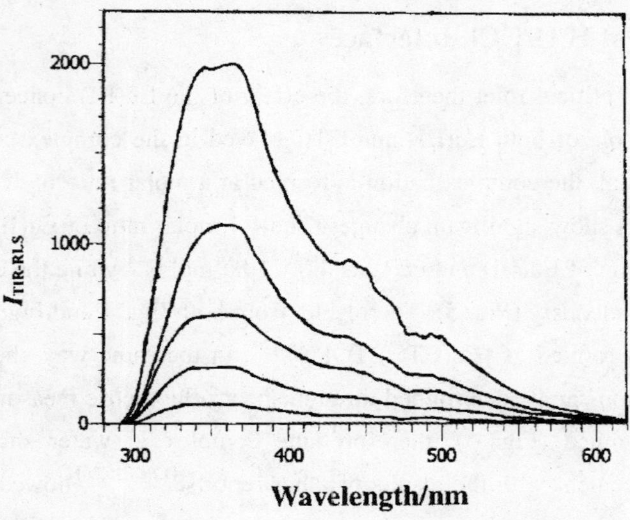

Fig. 2 TIR-RLS spectra of the interaction of Eu(III)-CTC-TOPO at the H_2O/CCl_4 interface. Concentrations: TOPO, 1×10^{-3} mol·L^{-1}; Eu(III), 5×10^{-6} mol·L^{-1}; CTC (from top to bottom, $\times10^{-6}$ mol·L^{-1}), 2.0,1.0, 0.5, 0.25, 0; pH 7.77.

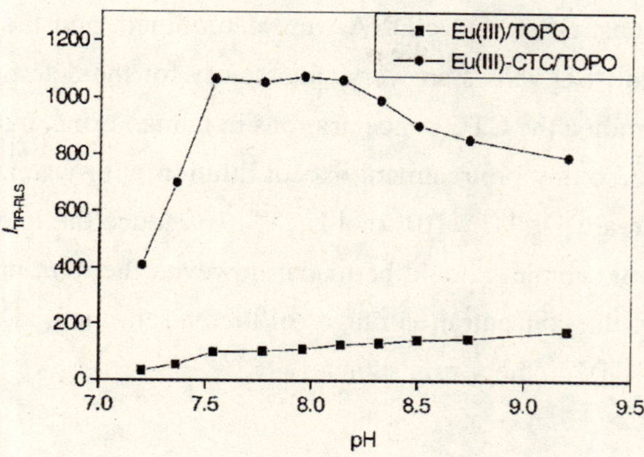

Fig. 3 Effect of pH on TIR-RLS intensity. Concentration: CTC, 1×10^{-6} mol·L^{-1}; Eu(III), 5×10^{-6} mol·L^{-1}; TOPO, 1×10^{-3} mol·L^{-1}.

4.2.2.6 Calibration Curves and Sample Determinations

According to the general procedures, the relationship of the intensity of RLS at the interface and the concentration of CTC was constructed (Fig. 7). A linear relationship range of $0.98 \sim 20.0 \times 10^{-7}$ mol·L^{-1} could be established using the equation $\Delta I = 919.5\ c + 9.6$ (c, 10^{-6} mol·L^{-1}; $r = 0.9978$; $n=8$) if 5.0×10^{-6} mol·L^{-1} Eu(III) was used. The limit of detection is 9.8×10^{-9} mol·L^{-1}(3σ). According to the 1:1 molar ratio of Eu(III)-CTC, the linear range should be, theoretically, up to 5.0×10^{-6} mol·L^{-1} when using 5.0×10^{-6} mol·L^{-1} Eu(III) for the CTC determination in Fig. 7; however, the linear range is $0.98 \sim 20.0 \times 10^{-6}$. The reason, we think, is that the complex at the interface is saturated, and the interface cannot accept much more Eu(III)-CTC complex, so the TIR-RLS intensity will not increase again even if 5.0×10^{-6} mol·L^{-1} Eu(III) is employed.

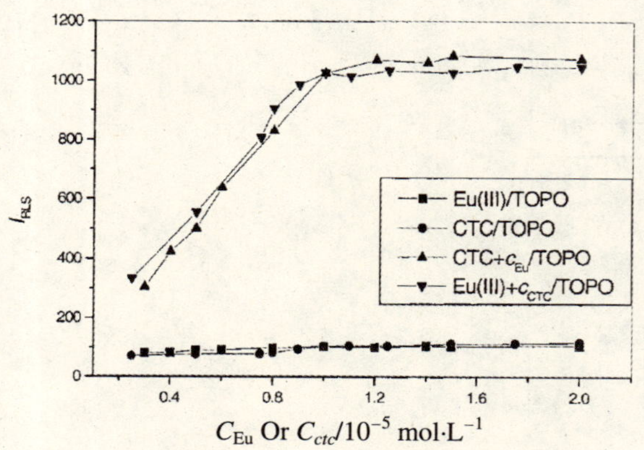

Fig. 4 Effects of Eu(III) and CTC concentration on TIR-RLS intensity. Concentration: CTC or Eu(III), 1.0×10^{-6} mol·L^{-1}; TOPO, 1.0×10^{-3} mol·L^{-1}; pH 7.77. As the Figure can be seen that the molar ratio is 1:1 for Eu(III)-CTC in the complex of Eu(III)-CTCTOPO.

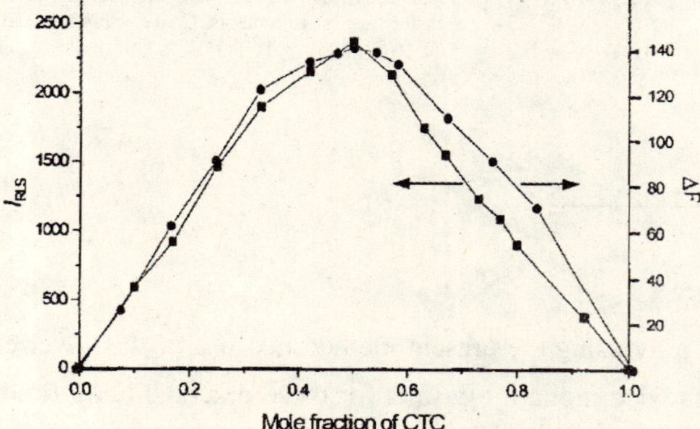

Fig. 5 Molar ratio of Eu(III)-CTC, both in the aqueous phase (●) and at the H_2O/CCl_4 interfaces (■). Concentration, TOPO, 1.0×10^{-3} mol·L^{-1}; pH 7.77. ΔF is the fluorescence intensity difference between the Eu(III)-CTC complex in the aqueous solution and the aqueous blank solution (Eu(III) + buffer solution). In aqueous solution, both the CTC and Eu(III) concentrations were changed simultaneously by keeping the total concentration of CTC and Eu(III) at 4.0×10^{-6}mol·L^{-1}. Determination of the fluorescence intensity Eu(III)- CTC complex and the blank solution was at 619 nm with 397-nm excitation.

Synthetic samples for CTC containing metal ions, BSA, and ctDNA were determined, and the results are given in Table 2. It can be seen that the recovery and RSD values are very satisfactory for the determinations of synthetic samples. To test the present assay, we determined the CTC concentrations in human urine, human serum, and fresh milk samples. These samples did not undergo any pretreatment except dilution with water. The maximum levels of tetracyclines in human serum or urine are $1\sim1.7\times10^{-5}$ mol·L^{-1}.[28] To reduce the interference of protein in human serum samples, a dilution of the real samples should be made; however, the dilution will make the CTC concentration lower than the linear range of the concentration ranges of the present method, so we used the standard addition method of determination of the CTC in the serum sample.

Table 1 Effect of Synergistic Ligands

synergistic ligands[a]	BA	DPPhen	Phen	DPG	TOPO
$\lambda_{ex}=\lambda_{em}$/nm	370	367	349	347	340
ΔI_{RLS}	750.6	509.5	279.5	693.8	1003

[a] 1×10^{-3}mol·L^{-1}. BA, benzoylacetone; DPPhen, 4,7-diphenyl-1,10- phenantholine; Phen, 1,10-phenanthroline; DPG, diphenyl guanidine; TOPO, trioctylphosphine oxide.

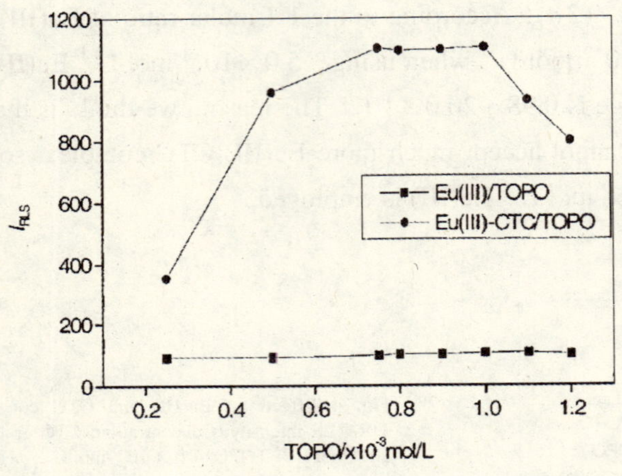

Fig. 6 Effect of TOPO concentration on RLS intensity. Concentration: CTC, 1×10^{-6} mol·L^{-1}; Eu(III), 5×10^{-6} mol·L^{-1}; pH 7.77.

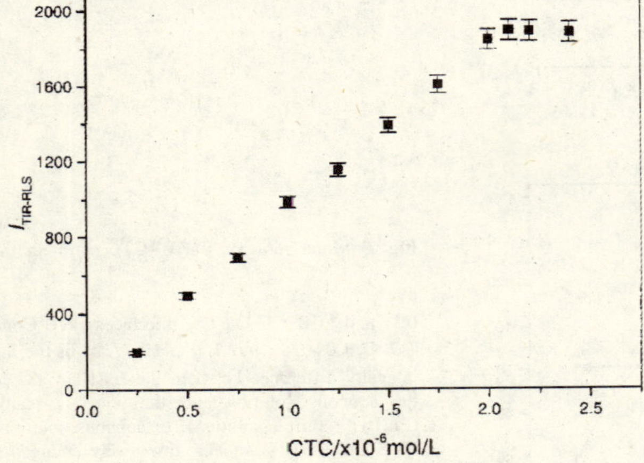

Fig. 7 Calibration graph for CTC detected by TIR-RLS. Error bars represent one standard deviation for four measurements. Concentration: Eu(III), 5×10^{-6} mol·L^{-1}; TOPO, 1×10^{-3} mol·L^{-1}. pH 7.77.

The determination of CTC in urine sample is very easy using the present method because of the lower content of proteins in the urine samples. As Table 3 shows, the determination results for these practical body fluid samples are very satisfactory also. All of the determinations can be made at a recovery of 95.4%～106.4% and RSD of 2.9%～3.9%.

4.2.3 Conclusion

Generally, the synergistic ligands listed as Table 1 are hardly soluble in aqueous medium, so surfactants should be used to increase the solubility of the synergetic ligands into the aqueous medium.[13,14] To establish spectrophotometric or spetrofluorometric methods of CTC in samples through synergistic ligands, Yang et al.[14] employed sodium dodecylsulfonate (SDS) to sensitize the fluorescence of the complex of Eu(III)-CTC-TOPO.

Table 2 Determination Results for Synthetic Samples

CTC in samples ($\times10^{-5}$ mol·L^{-1})	main interferences[a]	found ($\times10^{-5}$ mol·L^{-1})	recovery (%, n= 5)	RSD (%, n=5)
0.50	BSA, Ca(II), Al(III), Mn(II)	0.51	~98.2-103.8	3.9
0.75	ctDNA, Mg(II), Cr(III), Ni(II)	0.74	~96.3-101.6	3.4
1.00	$PO4^{3-}$, Cu(II), Zn(II), Fe(III)	0.97	~95.4-100.1	2.9

[a]Concentrations: BSA, 5.0μg·mL; ctDNA, 2.0μg·mL; Ca(II), 2×10^{-4}mol·L^{-1}; Al(III), 1.5 $\times10^{-4}$mol·L^{-1}; Mn(II), 3×10^{-4}mol·L^{-1}; Mg(II), 20×10^{-4} mol·L^{-1};Cr(III), 2×10^{-4}mol·L^{-1}; Ni(II), 2×10^{-4}mol·L^{-1}; PO_4^{3-}, 20×10^{-4}mol·L^{-1}; Cu(II), 2×10^{-4}mol·L^{-1}; Zn(II), 10×10^{-4}mol·L^{-1}; Fe(III),1×10^{-4} mol·L^{-1}; TOPO, 1×10^{-3}mol·L^{-1}; Eu(III), 5×10^{-6}mol·L^{-1}. pH, 7.77.

Table 3 Determination Results for Body Fluid Samples[a]

sample	added CTC[b] ($\times10^{-6}$mol·L^{-1})	CTC found ($\times10^{-6}$ mol·L^{-1}, n=5)	recovery (%)
human urine	1.00	1.00 ± 0.044	100.2
	2.00	1.99 ± 0.054	99.5
	3.00	3.01 ± 0.067	100.5
human serum	0.50	0.50 ± 0.026	100.4
	0.75	0.75 ± 0.044	100.3
	1.00	1.02 ± 0.027	102.0
fresh milk	0.25	0.27 ± 0.011	106.4
	0.50	0.53 ± 0.015	105.6
	1.50	1.51 ± 0.036	100.8

[a] Concentration: TOPO, 1×10^{-3}mol·L^{-1}; Eu(III), 5×10^{-6}mol·L^{-1}; pH 7.77. [b]Concentration of added CTC in the samples after dilution. Urine samples were diluted 2-fold, while human serum and fresh milk samples were diluted 500-fold.

Besides increasing the solubility of TOPO in aqueous medium, SDS acts as the negative ion to form an ion associate. It is obvious that the introduction of SDS makes the determination system much more complicated. The enhanced RLS signals at the liquid/liquid interfaces (namely, the TIR-RLS signals), resulting from the amphipathic adsorption species in the interfacial region of the 194-nm penetration depth when 340-nm incident light beam was used, is a very common phenomenon and may provide important applications in a wide range of areas. In addition, disuse of surfactants simplifies the procedures of the assay.

As for the tolerance of foreign substances, the TIR-RLS technique supplies a high selectivity for the determinations of body fluid; therefore, it is obvious that the TIR-RLS technique plays an important role in decreasing the interference of foreign components and can find wide applications in the determinations of samples in which the contents of coexisting substances are very high. Therefore, this technique is suitable for the determination of biological samples in which the interference of coexisting substances is serious. In addition, the present technique can be not only used to the determination of ion-association with high sensitivity, accuracy and selectivity, but also used to study the distribution equilibrium of liquid/liquid.

Acknowledgments

The authors acknowledge financial supports from the Excellent Young University Teachers Foundation directed under the Ministry of China (no. 2000-11-123), the National Natural Science Foundation of China (NSFC, no. 29875019), and the Municipal Science Foundation of Chongqing.

Supporting Information Available

Calculation of the angle at the CCl/H_2O interface. This material is available free of charge via the Internet at http://pubs.acs.org.

References

[1] Abdel-Khalek, M. M.; Mahrous, M. S. Talanta 1983, 30, 792～794.
[2] Mahrous, M. S.; Abdel-Khalek, M. M. Talanta 1984, 31, 289～291.
[3] Salah, M. S. Analyst 1986, 111, 97～99.
[4] Saha, U.; Sen, A. K.; Das, T. K. Talanta 1990, 37, 1193～1196.
[5] Al-Tamrah, S. A.; Alwarthan, A. A. Anal. Lett. 1992, 25, 1865～1876.
[6] Kelly, R. G.; Peets, L.; Lucia, M.; Hoyt, K. D. Anal. Biochem. 1969, 28,222～229.
[7] Katz, S. E.; Fassbender, C. A.; Hackett, A. J.; Mitchell, R. G. J. Assoc. Of. Anal. Chem. 1973, 56, 706～712.
[8] Van Den Bogert, C.; Kroon, A. M. J. Pharm. Sci. 1981, 70, 186～189
[9] Abdel-Hady Elsayed, M.; Barary, M. H.; Mahgoub, H. Talanta 1985, 32, 1153～1155.
[10] Rakicioglu, Y.; Perrin, J. H.; Schulman, S. G. J. Pharm. Biomed. Anal.1999, 20, 397～399.
[11] Milofsky, R. E.; Greer, B. Abstr. Pap. Am. Chem. Soc.. 1997, 213, 307 Ched Part 1.
[12] Hirschy, L. M.; Hirschy, E. M.; Dose, E. V.; Winefordner, J. D. Anal. Chim. Acta 1983, 147, 311～316.
[13] Georges, J.; Ghazarian, S. Anal. Chim. Acta 1993, 276, 401～409.
[14] Yang, J. H.; Tong, C. L.; Jie, N. Q.; Wu, X.; Zhang, G. L.; Ye, H. Z. J. Pharm. Biomed. Anal. 1997, 15, 1833～1838.
[15] Jee, R. D. Analyst 1995, 120, 2867～2872.
[16] Gracia -Fadrique, J. Langmuir 1999, 15, 3279～3282.
[17] Okumura, R.; Hinoue, T.; Watarai, H. Anal. Sci. 1996, 12, 393～397.
[18] Pasternack, R. F.; Bustamante, C.; Collings, P. J.; Giannetteo, A.; Gibbs, E. J. J. Am. Chem. Soc. 1993, 115, 5393～5399
[19] Pasternack, R. F.; Collings, P. J. Science (Washington, DC) 1995, 269, 935～939
[20] Huang, C. Z.; Li, K. A.; Tong, S. Y. Anal. Chem. 1996, 6, 2259～2263.
[21] Huang, C. Z.; Li, K. A.; Tong, S. Y. Anal. Chem. 1997,6, 514～520
[22] Huang, C. Z.; Li, Y. F.; Liu, X. D. Anal. Chim. Acta 1998, 375, 89～97.
[23] Huang, C. Z.; Li, Y. F.; Mao, J. G.; Tan, D. G. Analyst 1998, 123, 1401～1406.
[24] Huang, C. Z.; Zhu, J. X.; Li, K. A.; Tong, S. Y. Anal. Sci. 1997, 13, 263～268.
[25] Xue, Q. Spectral Techniques in the Studies of Polymer Structures; High Education Press: Beijing, 1995; p 102.
[26] Liu, X. J.; Li, Y. Z.; Ci, Y. X. Anal. Chim. Acta 1997, 345, 213～21
[27] An, D. K. Pharmaceutical Analysis, 3rd ed.; People's Health Press: Beijing, 1996; p 244
[28] Liu, C. X. Pharmacokinetics; Hunan Science and Technology Press: Changsha, 1980; p 17

(Ping Feng, Wei Qun Shu, Cheng Zhi Huang, and Yuan Fang Li, published in *Analytical Chemistry*, 2001, 73, 4307～4312)

4.3 Novel Assay of Thiamine Based on its Enhancement of Total Internal Reflected Resonance Light Scattering Signals of Sodium Dodecylbenzene Sulfonate at the Water/Tetrachloromethane Interface

Abstract: A new assay of thiamine (Vitamin B_1) is proposed by use of total internal reflected resonance light scattering (TIR-RLS) with high selectivity and sensitivity. At pH 3.29 and ionic strength 0.003, the adsorption of thiamine with anionic surfactants, such as sodium dodecylbenzene sulfonate (SDBS), sodium dodecylsulfonate (SDS) and sodium lauryl sulfate (SLS), occurs at the water/tetrachloromethane interface, giving rise to greatly enhanced TIR-RLS signals characterized at 375.0 nm. The enhanced TIR-RLS intensity at 375.0 nm is proportional to the concentration of thiamine in the range 0.12～850 ng·mL^{-1} and its limit of detection (3σ) is 120 pg·mL^{-1}. The results of analysis of artificial samples are in agreement with the specified values, and those ones for Vitamin B_1 tablets and injection solutions are identical with those obtained according to the method of the Chinese Pharmacopoeia.

Keywords: Thiamine; Sodium dodecylbenzene sulfonate; Total internal reflected resonance light scattering

4.3.1 Introduction

Thiamine (Vitamin B1, Fig. 1), is present in the bran coat of grains, in yeast and in meat. It is an important natural nutrient since it is necessary for carbohydrate metabolism, maintenance of normal neural activity and prevention and treatment of beriberi, neuralgia, etc. Since the discovery and isolation of thiamine, biological, microbiological and chemical methods have been established and applied to determine thiamine[1], in which chemical quantification is widely accepted for routine assays[2]. Of these chemical methods, the thiochrome method is most commonly employed[3]. The classical thiochrome method, first used by Jansen, involves the reaction between thiamine and potassium hexacyanoferrate(III) in an alkaline solution and the extraction of thiochrome formed from the aqueous phase into butan-2-ol[4] and then the detection of its fluorescence. However, this method suffers from several disadvantages[5]: (1) the addition of the amount of potassium hexacyanoferrate(III) is very hard to control; (2) the addition of the oxidant, the mixture of the oxidant with thiamine, and the extraction of thiochrome with butan-2-ol must be performed rapidly and standardized carefully in order to keep this method reproducible; and (3) the yield of thiochrome is only about 67%. To better the classical thiochrome method, two main approaches have been practiced. One is to utilize other oxidants such as Hg(II)[6], BrCN[7], Co(II)[8], Cu(II)[3], V(V)[9] and H_2O_2[10]. However, these improvements are still not satisfactory[11]. The other is to employ flow-injection analysis (FIA) [12]. It is a pity that this also makes determination of thiamine more complicated. Therefore, it is necessary to develop a new assay method of thiamine.

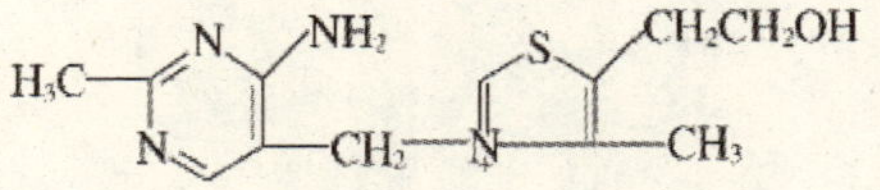

H_3C, N, NH_2, S, CH_2CH_2OH, N, CH_2, N, CH_3

Fig. 1 Molecular structure of thiamine.

Total internal reflection occurs on the side of the optically rarer medium of the interface of two immiscible mediums when a beam of light is incident from the medium of high refractive index to that of low refractive index at an angle beyond the critical angle θc, with which an evanescent field is coupled [13]. Because the intensity of the evanescent wave decays exponentially with increasing distance from the interface, falling to undetectable levels within less than one wavelength [14], the chemical species in the interfacial region can be highly selectively excited[15]. Accordingly a series of microscopic techniques, including total internal reflection aqueous fluorescence (TIRAF) microscopy, total internal reflection fluorescence (TIRF) microscopy and total internal reflection microscopy (TIRM), has been established [2]. Recently, we successfully coupled resonance light scattering with total internal reflected light at liquid/liquid interfaces, and proposed a total internal reflected resonance light scattering (TIR-RLS) technique[16], whose RLS signals derive from the chemical species at liquid/liquid interfaces with the excitation of the evanescent wave. Compared with RLS based on bulk solutions, TIR-RLS has at least four advantages: (1) it can reduce the interferences of coexisting foreign substances very effectively owing to the extraction of analytes into liquid/liquid interfaces by the formation of corresponding amphiphilic species; (2) assays with high sensitivity can also be expected as a result of the enrichment of analytes at the liquid/liquid interfaces; (3) TIR-RLS is very appropriate to investigate recognition between hosts and guests with an immiscible property free from surfactants as emulsifiers because they can encounter and interact at liquid/liquid interfaces; (4) it is possible to study orientation of molecules at liquid/liquid interfaces with polarized TIR-RLS on account of the relative simplex light scattering components at liquid/liquid interfaces. Consequently, TIR-RLS is a very promising, new spectroscopic technique.

In aqueous solutions, thiamine exists as a type of cation of large size. Through electrostatic attraction, it can interact with hydrophilic part of an anionic surfactant such as dodecylbenzene sulfonate (SDBS), sodium dodecylsulfonate (SDS) and sodium lauryl sulfate (SLS) to form an ion associate. In an oil/water system, due to ion associate adsorption thiamine will come into the oil/water interface region with the anionic surfactant. We have discovered that when thiamine is present in the aqueous medium, the TIR-RLS intensity of the water/tetrachloromethane interface is greatly enhanced in the presence of anionic surfactant, and the enhanced TIR-RLS intensity is proportional to the concentration of thiamine. This method does not involve oxidizing thiamine to thiochrome and, under the optimum conditions, thiamine can interact with SDBS easily and fully and the adsorption progresses very quickly, so the troubles mentioned above can be averted. Besides, the adsorption and uptake of drugs into their target cells are essentially relevant to the membrane of these cells[17] and a liquid/liquid interface is just considered to be a model of a cell membrane[18]. As a consequence, studies of drugs at a liquid/liquid interface are of much significance. Therefore, in this communication, we present the application of TIR-RLS to the determination of trace thiamine at the H_2O/CCl_4 interface.

4.3.2 Experimental

4.3.2.1 Apparatus

Total internal reflected resonance light scattering spectra and intensities were measured with a Hitachi F-2500 spectrofluorometer (Tokyo), whose sample compartment was modified as the displayed optical arrangement in Fig. 2. Two right-angled quartz prisms

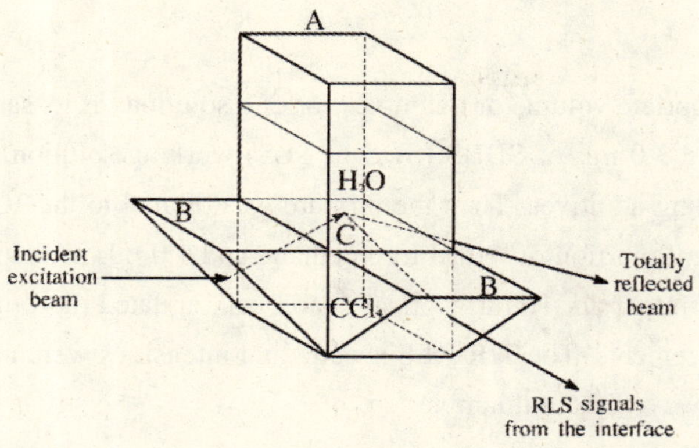

Fig. 2 Schematic drawing of the optical cell arrangement for TIR-RLS measurements: (A) 10 mm optical quartz cell, (B) right-angled quartz prism, (C) the H_2O/CCl_4 interface.

(10 mm × 10 mm × 10 mm, Huaguang Optics Co., Chongqing, China) were fastened to the two sides of the cell holder, facing the excitation light source and the fluorescence detector, respectively. Then the excitation light beam passing through the prism and the cell wall was introduced into the organic medium and impinged upon the H_2O/CCl_4 interface at an angle of incidence of 72.6°, calculated according to the Snell equation[19] with the refractive index of CCl_4 and H_2O being 1.460 and 1.333 at 25 °C, respectively. Obviously, the incidence angle of 72.6° is sufficiently greater than the critical angle of 65.6° for total internal reflection at the H_2O/CCl_4 interface.

In order to prepare a flat H_2O/CCl_4 interface, the lower interior of the optical quartz cell (10 mm) was treated with a toluene solution of 2% dichlorodimethylsilane to make it hydrophobic.

A PHS-3CA digital pH meter (Shanghai Dazhong Analytical Instruments Factory, Shanghai, China) was used to measure the pH values of the aqueous solutions, and an MVS-1 vortex mixer (Beide Scientific Instrumental Ltd., Beijing, China) was utilized to mix the solutions in volumetric flasks.

4.3.2.2 Reagents

A standard stock solution of thiamine (337 $mg \cdot L^{-1}$, 1×10^{-3} $mol \cdot L^{-1}$) was prepared by dissolving 0.0337 g of its hydrochloride (biochemical-reagent grade, Shanghai Chemical Reagents Co., China) with100 mL of water. The working solution (3.37 $mg \cdot L^{-1}$, 1×10^{-5} $mol \cdot L^{-1}$) was obtained by diluting the standard stock solution with water.

Three anionic surfactants, sodium lauryl sulfate (Sino-American Biotech. Co., Henan, China), sodium dodecylsulfonate (Shanghai Chemical Reagents Co.) and sodium dodecylbenzene sulfonate (Shanghai Chemical Reagents Co.) were employed; their working concentrations were all 1.0×10^{-5} $mol \cdot L^{-1}$.

Tetrachloromethane (Chongqing Jiyuan Chemistry Ltd. Co.) was used directly as the organic phase. Britton–Robinson buffer solutions were utilized to control the acidity of the interacting system, and 0.1 $mol \cdot L^{-1}$ NaCl was used to adjust the ionic strength of the aqueous solutions. All other reagents were of analytical-reagent grade, and used without further purification. Doubly distilled water was used throughout.

4.3.2.3 Pretreatment of samples

Ten commercial Vitamin B_1 tablets (Beijing Pharmaceutical Factory, Beijing, China) were ground into a fine powder, dissolved in ca. 30 ml of water in a 100-mL beaker and filtered. The filtrate was transferred to a 1000 mL volumetric flask and diluted to the mark with water. The sample solution was obtained by diluting 1.0 mL of the solution with 100 mL of water, which was analyzed according to the general procedure.

For clinical injection solution (purchased from Shanghai Tenth Pharmaceutical Factory, Shanghai, China), these was no special treatment except dilution with water.

4.3.2.4 General procedure

Into a 10 mL volumetric flask were added an appropriate volume of thiamine working solution, or its sample solution, 1 mL of Britton–Robinson buffer solution, and 3.0 mL of SDBS (SDS or SLS) working solution. The mixture was vortexed after each addition of the interacting additives. Then the mixture was diluted to the 10 mL mark with water and finally blended thoroughly. A 1.0 mL portion of tetrachloromethane and 1.0 mL of the mixture of thiamine and SDBS (SDS or SLS) were pipetted into a dry 10 mm optical quartz cell, agitated thoroughly, and allowed to stand for 15 min before TIR-RLS measurements. The TIR-RLS spectra and intensities were measured against parallel blank solutions treated in the same way without thiamine.

4.3.3 Results and discussion

4.3.3.1 Features of TIR-RLS spectra at the H_2O/CCl_4 interface

As Fig. 3 shows, the TIR-RLS intensities of the H_2O/CCl_4 interface in the absence of thiamine are very weak over the whole scanning region, and it is hard to identify TIR-RLS intensity changes with increasing SDBS concentration. When a trace of thiamine is present in the aqueous medium, however, a wide and greatly enhanced TIR-RLS band in the range 350～550 nm with the maximum scattering peak located at 375.0 nm appears and shoulder peaks can also be observed in the range of 450～500 nm, which sufficiently indicates that a new chemical species has been formed and adsorbed at the interface. It has also been found that the enhanced extent of the TIR-RLS is proportional to the concentration of thiamine. Similar TIR-RLS spectra of the H_2O/CCl_4 interface can be obtained when SDS or SLS is used instead of SDBS, albeit with different intensities.

As an anionic surfactant, SDBS contains both a hydrophilic head and a hydrophobic tail, and is presumed to reside well at a liquid/liquid interface [20,21]. As a result, the weak TIR-RLS spectrum characterized by the peak at 350.0 nm in Fig. 3 illustrates the spectral characteristics of SDBS adsorbed and concentrated at the H_2O/CCl_4 interface. According to the ion association adsorption mechanism at liquid/liquid interfaces [22], when thiamine is added to the aqueous medium, thiamine can combine with SDBS through electrostatic attraction to form an ion associate which transfers to the H_2O/CCl_4 interfacial region, where the adsorption and enrichment of thiamine occur. The adsorption of SDBS and the ion associate at the H_2O/CCl_4 interface can explain the two different features of the TIR-RLS spectra illustrated in Fig. 3. One is that the dissimilarities of the scatterers adsorbed at the interface bring about TIR-RLS spectra shape variation. The other is that the different intensity of the TIR-RLS spectra in absence and presence of thiamine probably arises from the discrimination in size of the scatterers at the interface. According to Pasternack and coworkers [23,24] and Huang et al. [25,26] the RLS intensity is very sensitive to the size of the scatterer.

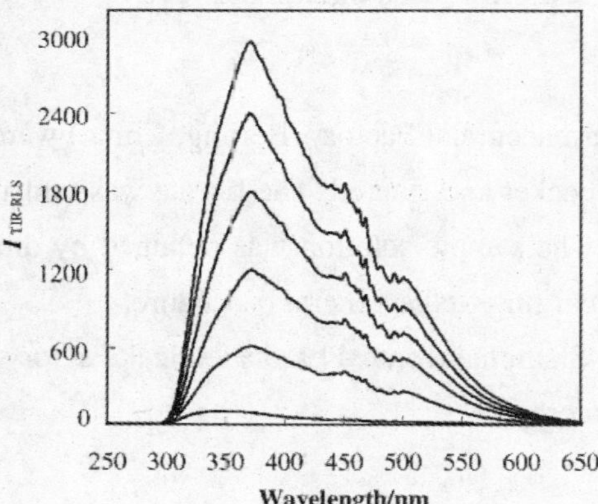

Fig. 3 TIR-RLS spectra of SDBS at the H_2O/CCl_4 interface in the absence and presence of thiamine. Concentrations: SDBS, 3×10^{-6} mol·L^{-1}; thiamine (from bottom to top, μg·mL^{-1}), 0, 0.17, 0.34, 0.51, 0.68, 0.85; pH of aqueous medium, 3.29. Ionic strength of aqueous medium, 0.003.

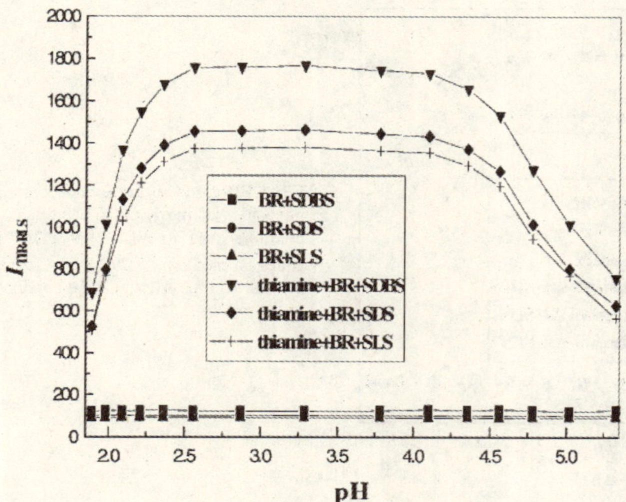

Fig. 4 Dependences of TIR-RLS intensities of the H_2O/CCl_4 interface on pH values of aqueous media. Concentrations: thiamine, 0.51 μg·mL^{-1} (1.5 × 10^{-6} mol·L^{-1}); surfactant, 3 × 10^{-6} mol·L^{-1}; pH of aqueous medium, 3.29. Ionic strength of aqueous medium, 0.005. All data were obtained at 375.0 nm.

4.3.3.2 Optimization of the general procedures

As stated above, the enhanced TIR-RLS signals of the H_2O/CCl_4 interface are due to the ion associate produced by the interaction of thiamine with anionic surfactants. Thus, any factor which could result in changes of state thiamine and anionic surfactant, would markedly affect the assay sensitivity. As Fig. 4 shows, the TIR-RLS intensities display different tendencies depending on the pH values of the aqueous media. It has been found that the enhanced TIR-RLS intensities are stable and maximal in the pH range 2.56～4.10, and decrease considerably at any pH value outside this range whether SDBS, SDS or SLS is employed. The optimum pH range is in good agreement with the pH range of a Vitamin B_1 injection solution[27] and Connors also thinks that thiamine is the most stable at pH values adjacent to 2[28]. Consequently, we consider that the distinct decrease of TIR-RLS intensities beyond the optimal pH range mostly results from the unstable state of thiamine. In addition, that the maximal TIR-RLS intensities do not appear below pH 2.56 is probably a result of an increasing shielding effect of hydrogen ion on the positively charged nitrogen atom, which blocks the electrostatic attraction between thiamine with an anionic surfactant. Moreover, it has been noticed that the three curves (coexistence of thiamine and surfactants) are almost the same except for different intensities, which further proves that the enhanced TIR-RLS intensities come from ion associates formed by the interaction of thiamine with anionic surfactants and are greatly influenced by the dimensions of the ion associates[23～26]. Under the same experimental conditions, the enhancement of TIR-RLS signals by use of anionic surfactants follows the sequence SDBS > SDS > SLS. For thiamine determination, the pH value of the aqueous medium should be controlled to 3.29 with 1.0 mL of Britton–Robinson buffer and SDBS was used as ion-pairing reagent.

Fig. 5 displays the role that anionic surfactants play in the enhanced TIR-RLS intensities of the H_2O/CCl_4 interface. It can be seen that the enhanced signal strongly depends on the concentration of anionic surfactant. Without anionic surfactants in the aqueous media, the signals of the H_2O/CCl_4 interface are very faint. This can be explained by the fact that thiamine is well soluble in the aqueous media and is surface-inactive, thus cannot be adsorbed and enriched at the interface. With a gradually increasing concentration of anionic surfactant, the TIR-RLS signals become correspondingly stronger, indicating that thiamine gradually accumulates at the interfacial region.

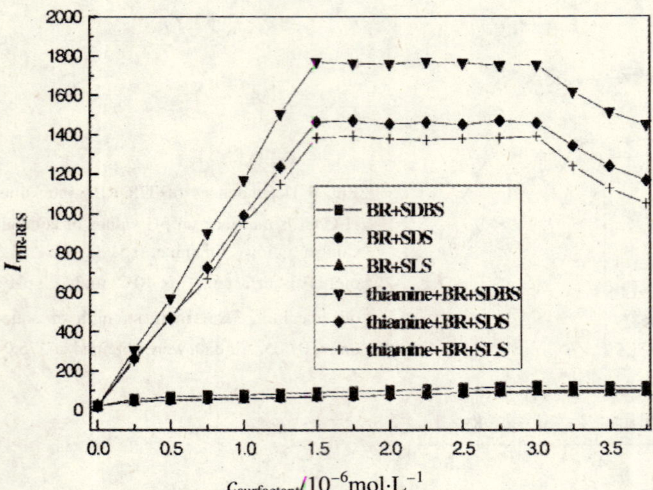

Fig. 5 Effects of surfactant concentration on TIR-RLS intensities of the H_2O/CCl_4 interface. Concentration: thiamine, 0.51 μg·mL^{-1} (1.5 × 10^{-6} mol·L^{-1}); pH of aqueous medium, 3.29. Ionic strength of aqueous medium, 0.003. All data were obtained at 375.0 nm.

When the surfactant concentration reaches 1.5×10^{-6} mol·L^{-1}, there is an inflection on each of the three curves, at which the mole ratio of thiamine to surfactant is 1:1. The mole ratio of thiamine to surfactants can also be identified by keeping the total concentration of thiamine and anionic surfactants as 3.0×10^{-6} mol·L^{-1} while changing the concentrations of the two components simultaneously. As Fig. 6 shows, when the fraction of anionic surfactants in the ion associate is 0.50, the enhanced TIR-RLS signals reach a maximum, again showing the mole ratio of thiamine to surfactants to be 1:1. While the concentration of surfactants is the range $1.5\times10^{-6}\sim3.0\times10^{-6}$ mol·L^{-1}, the TIR-RLS intensity is maximal and constant. Although in this range there is a excess of anionic surfactant and which can compete for space at the interface with the ion associate, it has been found to have little effect on the TIR-RLS signal. This may be due to the disordered array of anionic surfactants at the interface because of the electrostatic interaction between the charged head groups [19,29]. However, in the ion associate the charges of thiamine and surfactant are screened from each other as a result of their interaction. As a consequence, it is favorable for the ion associate to enter into the interfacial region and form closely packed layers. However, the TIR-RLS intensities begin to decrease with further increase in anionic surfactant concentration. This may arise because anionic surfactant in large excess will block the ion associate from the interfacial region. For thiamine determination, it is recommended that 3×10^{-6} mol·L^{-1} anionic surfactant be employed to five maximal sensitivity.

The ionic strength of the aqueous medium has a significant effect on the TIR-RLS signal of the H_2O/CCl_4 interface. As Fig. 7 shows, the signals of the ion associates decline sharply, which can possibly be ascribed to the encumbrance of adsorption of the thiamine-surfactant associate at the interface as a result of the gradual increase of the shielding effect of the charges on both thiamine and anionic surfactant. As a result, the ionic strength of the aqueous medium should be kept as 0.003 in the assay in order to obtain strong TIR-RLS signals.

It is noticeable that the aqueous and organic media in the optical cell should be agitated thoroughly so that the extraction of thiamine with anionic surfactants can be achieved in a short period of time. It has been found that stable TIR-RLS data can be obtained after the two media in the optical cell are mixed thoroughly and allowed to stand motionless for 15 min after the flat interface is constructed. The TIR-RLS signal remains constant for about 20 min.

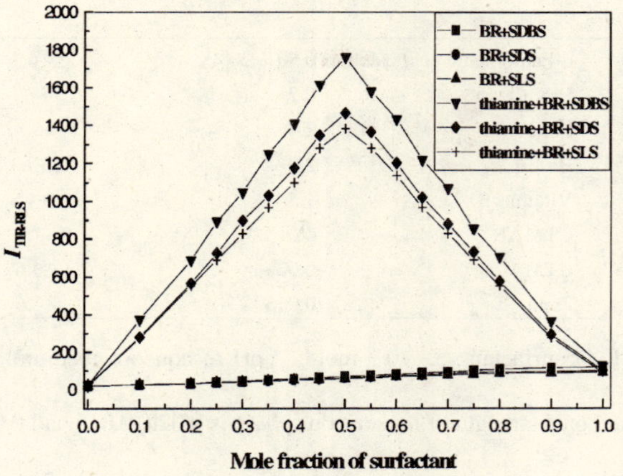

Fig. 6 Mole ratio of thiamine and anionic surfactant. The total concentration of thiamine and anionic surfactant was kept as 3.0×10^{-6} mol·L^{-1} by simultaneously changing the concentration of the two components; pH of aqueous medium, 3.29. Ionic strength of aqueous medium, 0.003. All data were obtained at 375.0 nm.

4.3.3.3 Tolerance of coexisting substances

The tolerance of this assay $\pm 10\%$ was investigated by use of 0.51 μg·mL^{-1} (1.5×10^{-6}mol·L^{-1}) thiamine in the general procedure by premixing it with potential interfering substances (common metal ions, sugars, amino acids, pharmaceuticals and surfactants).

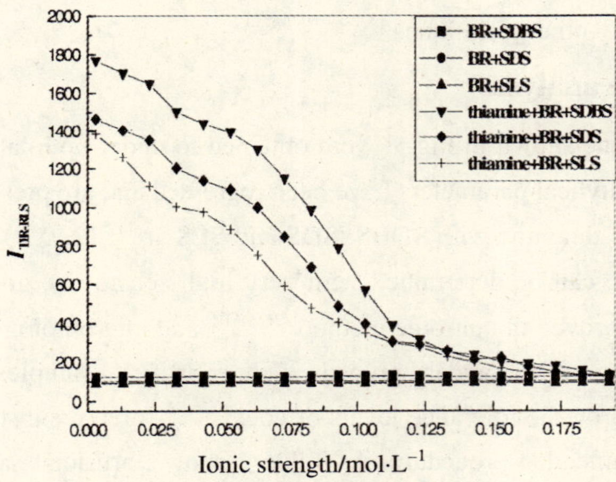

Fig. 7 Dependence of the TIR-RLS intensities on ionic strength of the aqueous medium. Concentrations: thiamine, 0.51 μg·mL^{-1} (1.5×10^{-6} mol·L^{-1}); surfactant, 3×10^{-6} mol·L^{-1}; pH of aqueous medium, 3.29. All data were obtained at 375.0 nm.

Table 1 Tolerance levels of coexisting substances

Coexisting substance	Concentration tolerated ($\times 10^{-4}$ mol·L^{-1})	Change in $I_{TIR\text{-}RLS}$ (%)	Coexisting substance	Concentration tolerated ($\times 10^{-4}$ mol·L^{-1})	Change in $I_{TIR\text{-}RLS}$ (%)
Ca(II), Cl$^-$	20	+5.6	L-Lysine	27	+8.2
Mn(II),Cl$^-$	15	+3.0	L-Phenylalanine	11.5	+9.1
Cu(II), Cl$^-$	10.5	+4.5	L-Glycine	15	+6.4
Ni(II), Cl$^-$	16	+7.2	L-Tryptophan	12	-4.8
Fe(III), Cl$^-$	22.5	-5.2	L-Histidine	35	+4.5
Cr(III), Cl$^-$	10	-6.3	Starch[b]	52.0	-8.2
Mg(II),Cl$^-$	70	+2.5	Ascorbic acid	12.5	-6.1
Pb(II), Cl$^-$	45	-4.2	Quinine sulfate	0.2	+9.5
Zn(II), Cl$^-$	75	+5.9	Brucine	1.5	+8.6
Al(III), Cl$^-$	40	-8.1	Niacin	1.1	-8.7
Hg(II), Cl$^-$	60	-6.9	Nicotinamide	1.2	-9.9
Co(II), Cl$^-$	50	-5.6	Pyridoxine hydrochloride	1.4	+3.6

Continued

Cd(II), Cl^-	35	+7.6	d-Pantothenic acid calcium	0.50	+6.1
$(K^+, Cl^-)^a$	200	-5.2	Riboflavin	0.2	+7.7
$(Na^+, Cl^-)^a$	150	+4.2	Folic acid	2.4	-6.3
$(NH4^+, Cl^-)^a$	120	+2.3	Biotin	2.0	+5.3
Glucose	15	-5.6	Vitamin B12	1.5	+4.8
Lactose	10	-6.2	CTMAB	0.01	-7.5
Maltose	27	+7.7	CTMAC	0.02	-6.6
Sucrose	12	+5.4	Zeph	0.015	-4.6

Concentrations: thiamine, 0.51 μg·mL^{-1} (1.5×10^{-6} mol·L^{-1}); surfactant, 3×10^{-6} mol·L^{-1}; pH of aqueous medium, 3.29. All data were obtained at 375.0nm.

[a] Ionic strength of the aqueous phase is 0.003 except that ionic strength of the aqueous phase is 0.020, 0.015 and 0.012 from top to bottom, respectively.

[b] Represented by mg·L^{-1}. CTMAB, cetyltrimethylammonium bromide; CTMAC, cetyltrimethylammonium chloride; Zeph, zephiramine.

As Table 1 shows, the common metal ions can be allowed at very high concentrations ($>1\times10^{-3}$ mol·L^{-1}), in which, especially, K^+, Na^+ and NH_4^+ can be tolerated at $>1.0\times10^{-2}$ mol·L^{-1}. Organic compounds (glucose, lactose, sucrose, maltose, l-lysine, l-phenylalanine, l-glycine, l-tryptophane, l-histidine, starch and ascorbic acid) did not interfere at high concentrations ($>1\times10^{-3}$ mol·L^{-1}), and quinine sulfate, brucinez, niacin,nicotinamide, pyridoxine hydrochloride, d-pantothenic acid calcium and riboflavin can be tolerated at 1×10^{-5} mol·L^{-1}. Thus, this method has good selectivity, better than many other techniques [3,4,6~10,30,31].

4.3.3.4 Calibration and sample analyses

The linear calibration graphs of thiamine shown in Fig. 8 were obtained to under optimal conditions andaccording to the general procedure. All the analytical parameters have been regressed and are presented in Table 2. It can be seen that the 3σ limits of detection of thiamine with SDBS, SDS and SLS are 0.12, 0.20 and 0.27 ng·mL^{-1}, respectively. These data show that thiamine can be determined with very high sensitivity, greater than UV-Vis. Asspectrophotometry[30,31], the classic or improved thiochrome method[3,4,6~10] and microbiological methods [32,33].

Under optimal conditions and according to the standard procedure, three artificial samples, in which a series of foreign substances had been added based on the tolerance levels of coexisting foreign substances displayed in Table 1, were analyzed according to recommended procedure. As Table 3 shows, artificial samples were determined with recovery ranging from 94.5% to 105.2%, and the RSD is <2.7%. The results for the artificial samples indicate that the assay of thiamine by this method is reliable and reproducible. This method was also applied to determine the thiamine in Vitamin B_1 tablets and Vitamin B_1 injection solutions.

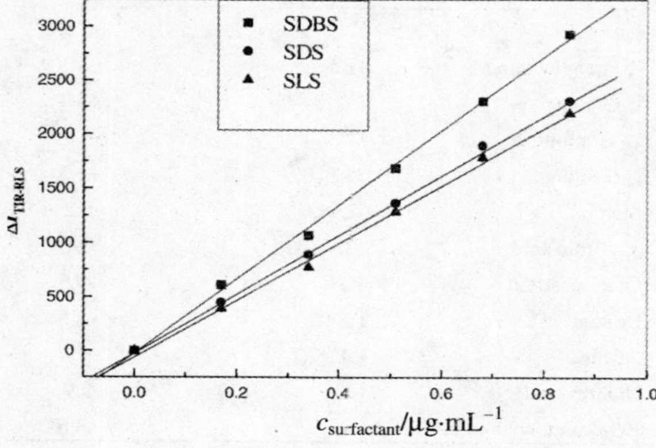

Fig. 8 Calibration graphs for thiamine when SDBS, SDS and SLS are employed. Concentrations: anionic surfactant, 3×10^{-6} mol·L^{-1}; pH of aqueous medium, 3.29. Ionic strength of aqueous medium, 0.003. All data were obtained at 375.0 nm.

Table 2 Analytical parameters for the determination of thiamine

Anionic surfactant	Linear range ($ng·mL^{-1}$)	Linear regression equation (c in $\mu g·mL^{-1}$)	LOD[a] ($pg·mL^{-1}$)	Correlation coefficient (r) (n = 5)
SDBS	0.12～850	$\Delta I_{TIR\text{-}RLS}$ =-23.2+ 3430c	12	0.9990
SDS	0.20～850	$\Delta I_{TIR\text{-}RLS}$ =-18.0+ 2750c	20	0.9996
SLS	0.27～850	$\Delta I_{TIR\text{-}RLS}$ =-48.7+ 2630c	27	0.9985

[a] 3σ limit of detection. Concentrations: anionic surfactants, 3×10^{-6} $mol·L^{-1}$; pH of aqueous medium, 3.29. Ionic strength of aqueous medium, 0.003. All data were obtained at 375.0 nm.

Table 3 Determination results for artificial samples

Thiamine in sample ($\mu g·mL^{-1}$)	Main additives[a]	Mean found value ($\mu g·mL^{-1}$, n = 5)	Recovery range (%, n = 5)	R S D (%)
0.51	Ca(II), Mg(II), Al(III), Cu(II), Co(II), Zn(II), Fe(III)	0.48	94.5～103.8	1.6
0.51	Ascorbic acid, quinine sulfate, brucinez, niacin, pyridoxine hydrochloride	0.50	96.3～105.2	2.0
0.51	Starch, glucose, lactose, l-lysine, l-phenylalanine	0.52	95.6～102.8	2.7

[a] Concentrations of additives: metal ions, 2×10^{-5} $mol·L^{-1}$; ascorbic acid, 1×10^{-5} $mol·L^{-1}$; quinine sulfate, 2×10^{-6} $mol·L^{-1}$; brucine, 1.0×10^{-5} $mol·L^{-1}$; niacin, 1.0×10^{-5} $mol·L^{-1}$; pyridoxine hydrochloride, 2×10^{-5} $mol·L^{-1}$; starch, 5 $mg·L^{-1}$; sugars, 5×10^{-5} $mol·L^{-1}$; amino acids, 1×10^{-4} $mol·L^{-1}$. Concentrations: SDBS, 3×10^{-6} $mol·L^{-1}$; pH of aqueous medium, 3.29. Ionic strength of aqueous medium, 0.003. All data were obtained at 375.0 nm.

Table 4 Determination results for real samples

Vitamin B1 tablet	Present method (n = 5)		Official CP[a] method (n = 5)		Vitamin B1 injection	Present method (n = 5)		Official CP[a] method (n = 5)	
	Recovery (%)	R S D (%)	Recovery (%)	R S D (%)		Recovery (%)	R S D (%)	Recovery (%)	R S D (%)
1	93.8	2.6	94.7	1.2	1	95.3	2.1	94.9	1.0
2	94.8	2.1	95.0	1.8	2	92.3	2.4	92.6	1.6
3	94.8	3.1	95.2	2.2	3	93.4	1.8	94.8	1.1

[a] Chinese Pharmacopoeia. Concentrations: SDBS, 3×10^{-6} $mol·L^{-1}$; pH of aqueous medium, 3.29. Ionic strength of aqueous medium, 0.003. All data were obtained at 375.0 nm.

The results obtained by the proposed method and the official method are compared in Table 4. A Student's t-test shows that the new method is accurate (95% confidence level).

4.3.4 Conclusions

TIR-RLS is a new spectroscopic technique based on coupling the RLS technique with total internal reflected light at a liquid/liquid interface. This paper shows that this technique is a powerful tool to study the liquid/liquid interface and has two typical advantages of separation and enrichment of analytes. Due to the analytes being separated from the bulk and enrichment at the interface, the analytes can be determined with high selectivity and sensitivity. Other spectroscopic techniques established in bulk solutions cannot have these benefits.

In this report, the assay of thiamine is carried out with anionic surfactants at the H_2O/CCl_4 interface with use of TIR-RLS. Compared with other methods mentioned above, this method is simple. Results for artificial and real samples show that this method is of high sensitivity, selectivity and good reproducibility.

Acknowledgements

This research was supported by the National Natural Science Foundation of China (No.: 20275032).

References

[1] R.B. Roy, J.K. Foreman, P.B. Stockwell, Topics in Automatic Chemical Analysis, Horwood, Chichester, 1979.
[2] N. Grekas, A.C. Calokerinos, Talanta 37 (1990) 1043.
[3] T. Perez-Ruiz, C. Martinez-Lozano, V. Tomas, I. Ibarra, Talanta 39 (1992) 907.
[4] B.C.P. Jansen, Rec. Trav. Chim. 55 (1936) 1046.
[5] M.A. Ryan, J.D. Ingle Jr., Anal. Chem. 52 (1980) 2177.
[6] Y. Yang, R.X. Cai, H.P. Huang, Chin. J. Anal. Chem. 21 (1993) 360.
[7] T. Kawasaki, Methods Enzymol. 122 (1986) 15.
[8] N.Q. Jie, J.H. Yang, Z.G. Zhan, Anal. Lett. 26 (1993) 2283.
[9] N.Q. Jie, J.H. Yang, W.D. Liu, J. Shi, Chin. J. Anal. Chem. 21 (1993) 333.
[10] N.Q. Jie, J.H. Yang, Z.G. Zhang, Chin. J. Anal. Chem. 20 (1992) 984.
[11] X.M. Chen, L.Z. Huang, S.Q. Li, S. Xia, Chin. J. Anal. Chem. 27 (1999) 1435.
[12] B. Karlberg, S. Thelander, Anal. Chim. Acta 114 (1980) 129.
[13] A.R. Clapp, R.B. Dickinson, Langmuir 17 (2001) 2182.
[14] M.A.S. Vigeant, M. Wagner, L.K. Tamm, R.M. Ford, Langmuir 17 (2001) 2235.
[15] R. Okumura, T. Hinoue, H. Watarai, Anal. Sci. 12 (1996) 393.
[16] P. Feng, W.Q. Shu, C.Z. Huang, Y.F. Li, Anal. Chem. 73 (2001) 4307.
[17] A. Mälkiä, P. Liljeroth, A.K. Kontturi, K. Kontturi, J. Phys. Chem. B 105 (2001) 10884.
[18] S. Tsukahara, H. Watarai, Langmuir 14 (1998) 7072.
[19] Q. Xue, Spectral Techniques in the Studies of Polymer Structures, High Education Press, Beijing, 1995, p. 102.
[20] R.R. Naujok, J.P. Hillary, R.M. Corn, J. Phys. Chem. 100 (1996) 10497.
[21] M.C. Messmer, J.C. Conboy, G.L. Richmond, J. Am. Chem. Soc. 117 (1995) 8039.
[22] H. Watarai, Y. Saitoh, Chem. Lett. 4(1995) 283.
[23] R.F. Pasternack, C. Bustamante, P.J. Collings, A. Giannetteo, E.J. Gibbs, J. Am. Chem. Soc. 115 (1993) 5393.
[24] R.F. Pasternack, P.J. Collings, Science (Washington, DC) 269(1995) 935.
[25] C.Z. Huang, K.A. Li, S.Y. Tong, Anal. Chem. 68 (1996) 2059.
[26] C.Z. Huang, K.A. Li, S.Y. Tong, Anal. Chem. 69 (1997) 514.
[27] Chinese Pharmacopoeia, 2nd ed., vol. 2, Chemical Industry Press, Beijing, 2000, p. 786.
[28] S.P. Liu, Z.Y. Zhang, H.Q. Luo, L. Kong, Anal. Sci. 18 (2002) 971.
[29] H.J. Paul, R.M. Corn, J. Phys. Chem. B 101 (1997) 4494.
[30] A.M. Wahbi, Analyst 106 (1981) 960.
[31] F.J. Bandelin, J.V. Tuschhoff, Anal. Chem. 25 (1953) 1198.
[32] R.F.M. Macias, Appl. Microbiol. 5(1957) 249.
[33] R.H. Diebel, J.B. Evans, C.F. Niven Jr., J. Bacteriol. 74 (1957) 818.

(Wei Lu, Cheng Zhi Huang, Yuan Fang Li, published in *Analytica Chimica Acta*, 2003, 475, 151～161.)

4.4 Adsorption of Penicillin–berberine Ion Associates at a Water/Tetrachloromethane Interface and Determination of Penicillin Based on Total Internal-reflected Resonance Light Scattering Measurements

Abstract: In aqueous medium of pH 5.33, penicillin, such as ampicillin (AmP), benzyl penicillin (BP), oxacillin (OA) and amoxycillin (AmO), interacts with berberine (BB), forming ion associates through electrostatic attraction of the polar head groups of penicillin and BB. The formed ion associates are then adsorbed into the amphiphilic H_2O/CCl_4 interfaces, displaying greatly enhanced total internal-reflected resonance light scattering (TIR-RLS) signals with the maximum peak at 370 nm. With the enhanced TIR-RLS data, thermodynamic parameters of adsorption of penicillin –BB ion associates into interfaces were measured. Mechanism studies show that the ion associates of penicillin with BB at H_2O/CCl_4 interfaces have 1:1 binding molar ratio, and the formation constants are in the range of $3.67\times10^4\sim5.48\times10^4$ $mol^{-1}\cdot dm^4$. It was found that the enhanced TIR-RLS intensity was directly proportional to the concentration of penicillin in the range of $0.98\times10^{-7}\sim10.0\times10^{-7}$ $mol\cdot L^{-1}$ for BP, $0.87\times10^{-7}\sim10.0\times10^{-7}$ $mol\cdot L^{-1}$ for OA,$1.1\times10^{-7}\sim12.0\times10^{-7}$ $mol\cdot L^{-1}$ for AmP and $1.2\times10^{-7}\sim12.0\times10^{-7}$ $mol\cdot L^{-1}$ for AmO with the corresponding limits of determination (3σ) being 3.48×10^{-8}, 3.85×10^{-8}, 4.22×10^{-8} and 4.86×10^{-8} $mol\cdot L^{-1}$, respectively.

Keywords: Water/tetrachloromethane interface; Total internal-reflected resonance light scattering; Penicillin; Berberine chloride

4.4.1 Introduction

The adsorption of pharmaceuticals at the liquid–liquid interface is of critical importance in biomedical and biophysical studies since the liquid–liquid interface could be used as a model interface to study the pharmacological activity of drugs, to study drug delivery, and as a simple analogue to study complex biomembranes [1,2]. Along these lines, much has been done mainly by spectroscopic techniques such as attenuated total reflection spectroscopy[3], Raman spectroscopy[4], ellipsometry [5], second harmonic generation (SHG)[6,7], sum-frequency generation (SFG)[8,9], neutron reflection[10] and atomic force microscopy [11]. These equipments, however, are complicated and not affordable for a common laboratory. Therefore, it is necessary to propose much more convenient methods to measure the properties at liquid–liquid interfaces and quantitate the molecular populations.

Resonance light scattering (RLS) technique is a recently developed one, constructed based on the steep change between the refractive index of the inner scattered particle and that of its outer atmosphere[12,13], and the RLS spectra are easily available by simultaneously scanning the excitation and emission monochromators of a common spectrofluorometer. This technique has successfully been employed for analytical purposes with high sensitivity and simplicity[14~18], but it has suffered from drawbacks such as poor selectivity and it is difficult to detect trace amount of analytes in complicated samples. In order to improve the selectivity, we have supposed a total internal-reflected resonance light scattering (TIR-RLS) technique based on the supramolecular interaction of host–guest at liquid–liquid interface [19~21].

It is known that total internal reflection of light occurs when an incident light beam penetrates from a medium of high refractive index to the one of lower refractive index with an angle above the critical angle (θ_c). Although all ofthe visible light is reflected from the interface, electromagnetic energy is carried across the interface in the form of an evanescent wave, which follows an exponential decay with depth from the interface, falling to undetectable levels within less than one wavelength [22]. Therefore, the chemical species in the interfacial region could be highly selectively excited [23]. Our coupling of the RLS technique with total internal-reflected light at liquid–liquid interface shows that the TIR-RLS technique, based on the molecular recognition and assembly at the interface [19], is suitable for the determination of samples, in which the interference of coexisting substances is serious, since the technique has the functions of enriching analyte and separating coexisting substances[19~21].

Penicillin is a widespread employed antibacterial drug family nowadays, containing the structure of 6-aminopenicillin-alkylation acid. It is very important to quantitate penicillin both in pharmaceutical preparations and biological samples (Fig. 1 displays the molecular structure of typical members ofpenicillin family). Methods have been reported for the determination of penicillin including microbiology[24], titrimetry[25], liquid chromatography (LC)[26], fluorimetry[27] and spectrophotometry[28]. Compared with the fluorimetric and LC ones, the microbiological methods lack specificity, while the titrimetric and spectrophotometric methods are less sensitive. Although fluorimetric and LC methods have higher sensitivity, pretreatments such as oxidation and hydrolysis with complicated reaction conditions and operation procedures are generally needed. It is well known that mixed cationic and anionic amphiphilic species were more concentrated at liquid/liquid interface due to electrostatic interactions of the polar head groups[29]. Since penicillin[30] and berberine[31] (BB) with amphiphilic structures are negatively and positively charged in the medium of appropriate pH, we reason that they could be coadsorbed at the H_2O/CCl_4 in the form of ion associates by electrostatic adsorption mechanism.

4.4.2 Experimental

4.4.2.1 Apparatus

RLS and TIR-RLS spectra and intensities were measured with a Hitachi F-2500 spectrofluorometer (Tokyo, Japan) equipped with a 150 W Xe lamp. For RLS measurements, 10 mm quartz optical cell was employed without any internal surface modification of the sample cell. In order to make a liquid/liquid interface for TIR-RLS measurements, the under inside of a 10 mm optical quartz cell was treated with dichlorodimethylsilane in benzene so as to make the inside wall hydrophobic and afford a flat H_2O/CCl_4 interfaces.

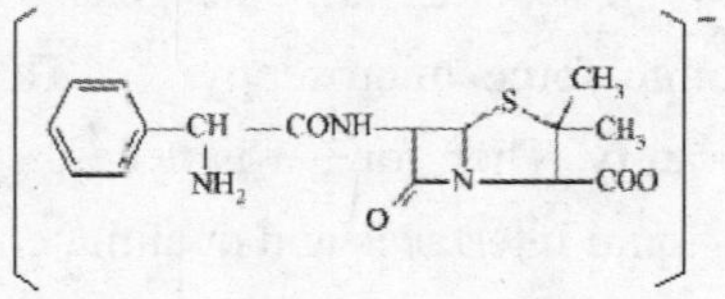

Ampicillin (AmP)

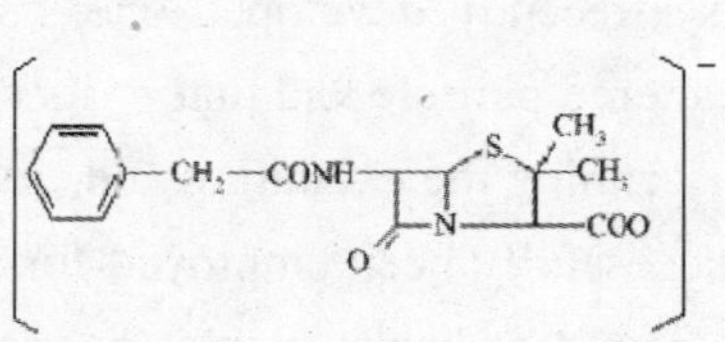

Benzylpenicillin (BP)

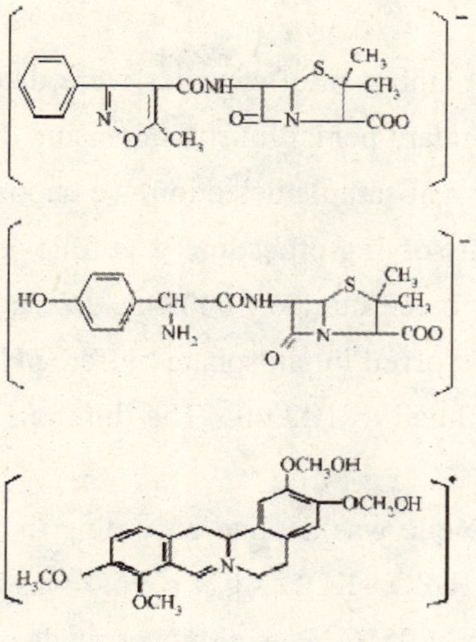

Oxacillin (OA)

Amoxycillin (AmO)

Berberine (BB)

Fig. 1 Molecular structures of ampicillin (AmP), benzyl penicillin (BP), oxacillin (OA), amoxycillin (AmO) and berberine (BB). p*K*a1-values are 2.5, 2.8, 2.8 and 2.4 for AmP, BP, OA and AmO, respectively [30].

An optical setup for TIR-RLS measurements as the same as our previous reports [19~21] was mounted in the sample compartment of the spectrofluorometer.

A Shimadzu LC system with two LC-10AVT pump assembly, SPD-10AVP UV detector, CTO-10ASVO column oven, and DGU-14A degasser, controlled with SCL-10AVP controller, and an Allsphere ODS-2 column (5 μm, 250 mm×4.6 mm, Alltech, Chicago, USA) were used for sample detection for comparison.

4.4.2.2 Reagents

1.0×10^{-3} mol·L^{-1} stock solutions of penicillin and berberine were prepared by dissolving ampicillin sodium, benzyl penicillin sodium, oxacillin sodium and amoxycillin sodium (Chongqing Institute of Pharmacology, China) and berberine chloride (BDH) in doubly distilled water, and the working solutions were prepared according to practical necessity by successive dilution with doubly distilled water. Britton–Robinson buffer solution was used to control the acidity of the aqueous system. All other reagents were of analytical-reagent grade, and doubly distilled water was used throughout.

4.4.2.3 General procedure

Add 1.0 mL tetrachlorometnane into the internal surfacemodified optical quartz cell, appropriate volume of penicillin solution, 0.1 mL BB (1.0×10^{-4} or 1.0×10^{-5} mol·L^{-1}) working solution, and 0.5 mL buffer solution (pH 5.33). The mixture of aqueous phase was diluted to 2.0 mL with doubly distilled water and mixed thoroughly. After standing motionlessly for 15 min, the mixture was then used for TIR-RLS measurements. The TIR-RLS spectra and the intensities were measured against the blank treated in the same way without penicillin. All these operation was kept at 25°C.

Both RLS and TIR-RLS spectra were obtained by scanning simultaneously the excitation and emission monochromators of the F-2500 spectrofluorometer from 220 to 700 nm with $\lambda_{ex} = \lambda_{em}$. The TIR-RLS intensities were measured at 370 nm with 5.0 nm of excitation and emission slit widths.

4.4.2.4 Sample detections

To identity the method, artificial samples and amoxycillin capsules were detected. Artificial samples were made through adding foreign substances into the standard penicillin solutions, and directly transferred to TIR-RLS measurements following the general procedure. For real sample detection, we choose amoxycillin capsules (Kerui Pharmaceutical Ltd., Chongqing, PR China). The dissolving procedure was followed according to Ref.[31]. Shortly, the inner solid contents of 10 amoxycillin capsules (batch number: 040943, 0.25 g for each capsule) were mixed completely, and 0.612 g of the solid mixture was dissolved in phosphate buffer (pH 5.01), and diluted to 1000 mL. After filtration, 4 mL of the filtrate was taken and diluted to 100 mL. The dilutions then transferred for TIR-RLS detection according to above general procedure.

For comparison, liquid chromatographic technique was applied according to Ref.[31] to detect the sample of the content of amoxycillin capsules. The pH 5.0 KH_2PO_4–KOH:ACN = 96:4 was used as flow carrier with flow rate 1.0 mL·min^{-1}. The column was kept in the oven of 25°C. Detection was made at 254.0 nm.

4.4.3 Results and discussion

4.4.3.1 Spectral characteristics of the interaction

Fig. 2 displays the RLS signals of BB, BP and the mixture of BP–BB, respectively. It could be seen that both BB and BP have weak RLS signals in aqueous medium, while BP–BB mixture has stronger RLS signals than both BB and BP with an increase factor about 3, characterized with two RLS peak at 310 and 370 nm, indicating interaction of BP and BB has occurred. However, using spectrophotometeric and spectrofluorometric methods, we failed to observe spectral changes during the interaction, indicating that the RLS method is much more sensitive to study the interaction than both spectrophotometric and spectrofluometric methods.

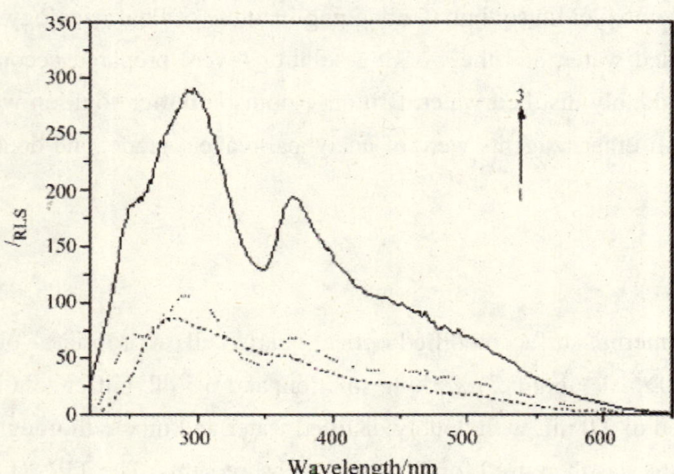

Fig. 2 RLS spectra of BP (curve 1, dashed), BB (curve 2, dotted) and BP–BB (curve 3, solid) in aqueous solution: BB 5.0 × 10^{-6} mol·L^{-1}; BP 2.0 × 10^{-6} mol·L^{-1}; pH 5.33.

On the other hand, if H_2O–CCl_4 interface is introduced, the TIR-RLS signals of BP–BB get much enhanced with an increase factor about 15 (Fig. 3). Curves 1 and 2 in Fig. 3 display the TIR-RLS features of BP and BB, respectively. It could be seen that the TIR-RLS signals of both BP and BB at the CCl_4/H_2O interfaces are weak in the whole scanning region. Greatly enhanced TIR-RLS signals could be observed when a trace amount of BP–BB mixture is present with the maximum peak at 370 nm. It was found that these TIR-RLS signals of CCl_4/H_2O interfaces are increased with increasing BP concentration.

Penicillin is negatively charged in the aqueous medium of pH 5.33 since the p*K*a1-values are 2.5, 2.8, 2.8 and 2.4 for ampicillin (AmP), benzyl penicillin (BP), oxacillin (OA) and amoxycillin (AmO), respectively[30], and these drugs would be fully ionized.

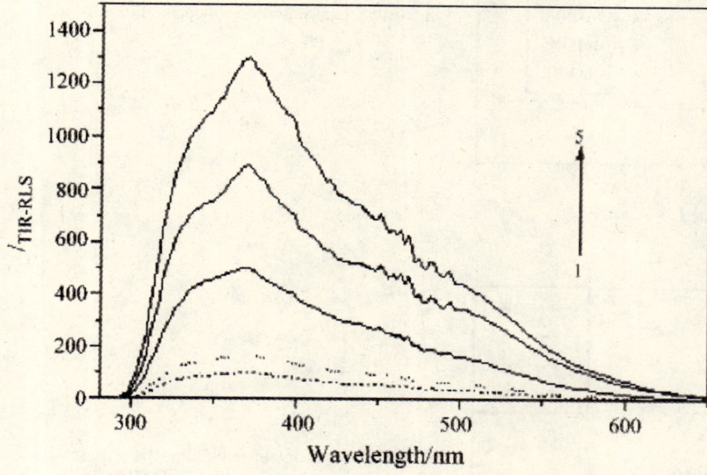

Fig. 3.TIR-RLS spectra of the BP (curve 1, dashed), BB (curve 2, dotted) and BP–BB (curves 3～5, solid) at H_2O/CCl_4 interface. Concentrations: BP (curves 3～5, × 10^{-6} mol·L^{-1}): 0.25, 0.50 and 0.75; BB 5.0 × 10^{-6} mol·L^{-1}; pH 5.33.

Thus, they could interact with positively charged amphiphilic BB through electrostatic interaction[31], forming ion associates, and then adsorbed into liquid/liquid interface due to electrostatic interactions of the polar head groups[29]. The electrostatic interaction between the penicillin and BB promotes the movement of penicillin in aqueous phase towards the H_2O/CCl_4 interfaces, displaying coadsorption properties. In such cases, the penicillin–BB complexes could be concentrated at the H_2O/CCl_4 interface, resulting in enhanced TIR-RLS signals.

4.4.3.2 Optimal conditions for the interaction

It was found that the TIR-RLS intensity of penicillin–BB ion associates varies greatly with the pH-values of the aqueous solution, while the TIR-RLS intensity of BB gets increased slowly with pH-change. Experiments showed that the TIR-RLS intensities of BP–BB, OA–BB, AmP–BB and AmO–BB reach the maximum and constant at pH 5.02～5.67, and decrease out of this pH range. In this work, the acidity of the aqueous medium was controlled with Britton–Robinson buffer solution of pH 5.33.

Fig. 4 shows that the effect of BB concentration on TIRRLS intensity. There is a turning point at 1:1 molar ratio of penicillin and BB occurred on each of the curves of BP–BB, OA–BB, AmP–BB and AmO–BB, indicating that the binding number of penicillin and BB is 1:1 for the ion associates at the interface. The 1:1 molar ratio of penicillin–BB could be identified also using mole-ratio method which was made by keeping the total concentration of penicillin and BB as 10.0×10^{-7} mol·L^{-1} (Fig. 5).

4.4.3.3 Adsorption equilibrium of ion-associates at H_2O/CCl_4 interface

According to the 1:1 binding ratio between penicillin and BB, we could establish a stoichiometric model for the enrichment of ion-association of penicillin (P) and BB (B) at the H_2O/CCl_4 interface from aqueous medium:

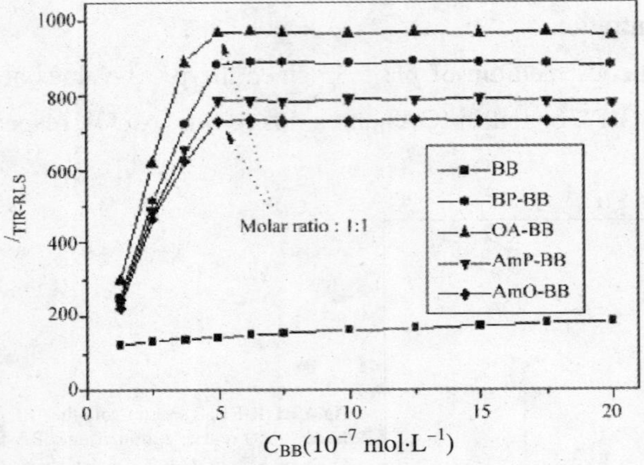

Fig. 4 Effect of BB-concentration on TIR-RLS intensity. Concentration of penicillin 5.0 × 10^{-7} mol·L^{-1}; pH 5.33.

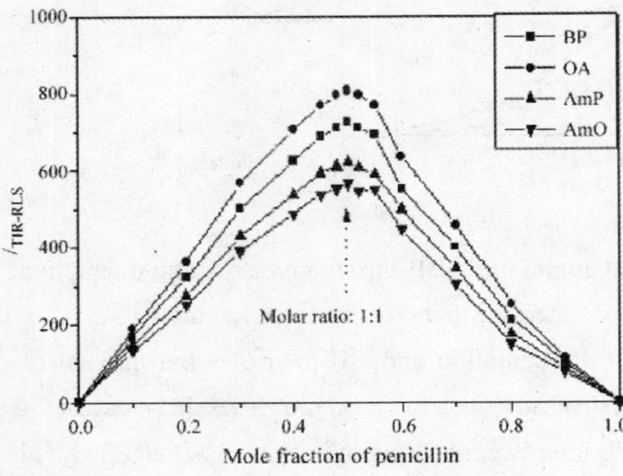

Fig. 5 Molar ratios of penicillin–BB ion associates co-adsorbed into the H_2O/CCl_4 interface. The total concentration was kept as 10.0 × 10^{-7} mol·L^{-1}; pH, 5.33.

$$P + B \rightleftharpoons PB \rightleftharpoons PB_i \qquad (1)$$

$$K_{PB} = \frac{PB}{[P][B]} \qquad K' = \frac{[PB]_i}{[PB]} \qquad (2)$$

where K_{PB} (mol·L^{-1}), [P], [B] and [PB] are the associate constant, free concentration of penicillin, BB and PB in aqueous medium, respectively, [PB]i is the concentration of PB in interface extracted from the aqueous phase. K' (dm) is a constant indicating the enrichment degree of PB through the interface extraction. Thus, a complex constant K(mol^{-1}·dm^{4}) could be obtained concerning the formation of PB and extraction of PB in interface:

$$K = K_{PB}\,K' = \frac{[PB]_i}{[P][B]} \qquad (3)$$

[PB]i refers to the equilibrium concentrations in interface (mol·dm^{-2}), and couldbe calculated from the following equation:

$$[PB]_i = \Gamma_I \frac{\Delta I}{\Delta I_{max}} \qquad (4)$$

where Γ_i is the adsorption quantity, and could be estimated from the decrements of BB concentrations in the aqueous phase until ΔI reaches the maximum (ΔI_{max}). ΔI was the enhanced TIR-RLS intensity when the equilibrated concentration of penicillin, [P], is approximated by the total initial concentration of penicillin, $[P]_t$, (i.e.,

$[P]_t V \geqslant [PB]_i S_i$) and ΔI_{max} was the maximum enhanced TIR-RLS intensity when [P] and the equilibrated concentration of berberine, [B], are approximated by $[P]_t$ and the total initial concentration of BB in aqueous phase, $[B]_t$ (i.e., $[P]_t V \geqslant [PB]_i S_i$ and $[B]_t V \geqslant [PB]_i S_i$).

Table 1 Thermodynamic parameters of coadsorption of penicillin and BB into interfaces

Penicillin	$\Gamma_i/\Delta I_{max}$ ($\times 10^{-13}$, $n = 5$)	Linear regression equation	r	K($\times 10^4$ mol$^{-1}\cdot$dm^4)
BP	2.36	$\log[BP]_i = -1.15 + 1.26 \log[B]_t$	0.995	5.48
OA	2.21	$\log[OA]_i = -1.27 + 1.17 \log[B]_t$	0.996	3.67
AmP	2.26	$\log[AmP]_i = -1.18 + 1.15 \log[B]_t$	0.996	4.93
AmO	2.52	$\log[AmO]_i = -1.22 + 1.27 \log[B]_t$	0.993	4.31

Concentration: penicillin 2.0×10^{-6} mol·L^{-1}; pH 5.33. The temperature was controlled at 25°C

In the case of interface extraction, the total BB quantity could be expressed as:

$$[B]_t V = [B]V + [PB]V + [PB]_i S_i + [B]_{org} V_{org} + [PB]_{org} V_{org} \tag{5}$$

where the V, S_i and V_{org} are the volume of aqueous phase (2.0×10^{-3} L), the interfacial area (1.0×10^{-2} dm^2) and thevolume of organic phase (1.0×10^{-3} L), respectively. Since the solubility of penicillin and BB in CCl_4 is very small, the partition equilibrium of both penicillin and BB could be neglected between the aqueous/organic phases, and it is not necessary to consider the contributions from both penicillin and BB again in organic phase. On the other hand, even if the interaction of BP and BB has occurred as shown in Fig. 2, we have proved that the interaction of penicillin and BB in aqueous medium is very weak using molecular spectrophotometry and spectrofluorometry, and the concentration [PB] in aqueous medium is very small. Neglecting penicillin–BB complex in aqueous medium, we have Eq. (6) from Eq. (5):

$$[B] = [B]_t - [PB]_i \frac{S_i}{V} \tag{6}$$

If penicillin is greatly excessive in aqueous medium,then we could get following linear equation according to Eqs. (3) and (6) by substituting the [P] with $[P]_t$:

$$\log [PB]_i = \log \left\{ \frac{K[P]_t}{1 + K[P]_t(S_i/V)} \right\} + \log[B]_t \tag{7}$$

Thus, a linear relationship between log[PB]i and $\log[B]_t$ could be constructed according to Eq. (7) and corresponding thermodynamic parameters ofpenicillin–BB in interfaces could be available (Table 1). It could be seen that the linear relationships of Eq. (7) are obeyed very well. From the intercept of the plots or the linear regression equations, applicable equations supposing b as the intercept in order to calculate K-values could be available by substituting the values of $V = 2.0 \times 10^{-3}$ L and $S_i = 1.0 \times 10^{-2}$ dm^2:

$$K = \frac{1}{(10^{-b} - 5)[P]_t} \tag{8}$$

Table 2 Effect of foreign substances

Foreign substance	Concentration tolerated ($\times 10^{-4}$ mol·L^{-1})	Foreign substance	Concentration tolerated ($\times 10^{-4}$ mol·L^{-1})	Foreign substance	Concentration tolerated ($\times 10^{-4}$ mol·L^{-1})
NH_4^+, Cl^-	350	Starch	50.8[a]	Ascorbic acid	14.5
Mg^{2+}, NO_3^-	210	Sucrose	120	Quinine sulfate	1.2
Ca^{2+}, Cl^-	160	Maltose	112	Brucine	1.8
Al^{3+}, Cl^-	15.5	Lactose	220	Thiamine hydrochloride	0.6
Cu^{2+}, Cl^-	10.4	Glucose	120	Niacin	1.5
Zn^{2+}, Cl^-	42.5	l-Lys	18.6	d-pantothenic acid calcium	0.8
Se(IV)	35.5	l-Phe	25.6	Nicotinamide	1.4
Fe^{3+}, Cl^-	24.6	l-Gly	15.6	Pyridoxine hydrochloride	1.1
Cd^{2+}, NO_3^-	21.3	l-Try	20.3	Urea	5000
Pb^{2+}, NO_3^-	26.5	l-His	21.5		

[a] mg·L^{-1}; concentration: BB 5.0×10^{-6} mol·L^{-1}; BP 5.0×10^{-7} mol·L^{-1}; pH 5.33; $\lambda_{ex}=\lambda_{em}=370$ nm.

Table 3 Analytical parameters of the determination

Penicillin	Linear regression equation (c, $\times 10^{-6}$ mol·L^{-1})	Linear range ($\times 10^{-6}$ mol·L^{-1})	Correlation coefficient (n=5, r)	Detection limit (3σ, 10^{-8} mol·L^{-1})
BP	ΔI =-66.4+ 1591.2 c	0.10～1.0	0.996	3.48
OA	ΔI =-48.9+ 1781.2 c	0.09～1.0	0.997	3.85
AmP	ΔI =-35.6+ 1367.6 c	0.11～1.2	0.996	4.22
AmO	ΔI =-40.9+ 1240.8 c	0.12～1.2	0.993	4.86

pH 5.33; concentration: BB 5.0×10^{-6} mol·L^{-1}; $\lambda_{ex}=\lambda_{em}$=370 nm.

Table 4 Determination results for synthetic samples

Penicillin in samples ($\times 10^{-6}$ mol·L^{-1})	Coexist substances ($\times 10^{-4}$ mol·L^{-1})	Founded ($\times 10^{-6}$ mol·L^{-1}, n= 5)	Recovery (%)	RSD (%)
OA 1.0	$Mg(NO_3)_2$, 15; $CuCl_2$, 5; $ZnCl_2$, 5; $Pb(NO_3)_2$, 5; $CaCl_2$, 10; $AlCl_3$, 2; $FeCl_3$, 4	1.03	103.2	3.2
BP 2.0	Nicotinamide, 0.2; ascorbic acid, 2.0; quinine sulfate, 0.1; thiamine chloride, 0.2	1.96	98.3	2.2
AmP 2.0	Starch[a], 25; maltose, 25; glucose, 25; l-phenylalanine, 10	2.04	102.1	2.1

[a] mg·L^{-1}; pH 5.33; concentration: BB 5.0×10^{-6} mol·L^{-1}; $\lambda ex = \lambda em$ =370nm.

Table 5 Determination results for amoxycillin each capsule

Founded (g)	Average founded (g)	R S D (%)	Recovery (%)	Average recovery (%)
Pharmacopoeia [31]				
0.2576	0.2443 (n=3)	5.35	96.3, 100.3, 90.3, 105.7,103.0	99.12 (n=5)
0.2488				
0.2265				
Present method				
0.2621	0.2541 (n = 5)	3.73	97.3, 103.3, 94.7, 100.7, 104.7	100.14 (n = 5)
0.2488				
0.2399				
0.2665				
0.2532				

Label content for each amoxycillin capsule is 0.25 g. Here are the average results for 10 amoxycillin capsules (Kerui Pharmaceutical Ltd., Chongqing). Pharmacopoeia reference method is using liquid chromatography technique [31]

Thus it is very easy to deduce the K-values for the interfacial interactions of BP, OA, AmP and AmO with BB. In the experimental conditions, the K-values are 5.48×10^4, 3.67×10^4, 4.93×10^4 and 4.31×10^4 mol^{-1} dm^4, respectively.

4.4.3.4 Interferences of coexisting foreign substances

The influences of foreign coexisting substances on the determination of 5.0×10^{-7} mol·L^{-1} BP were tested and the results were listed in Table 2. Common cation ions such as NH_4^+, Ca(II), Mg(II), Cu(II), Fe(III), Se(IV), Zn(II), Pb(II), Al(III) and Cd (II) could be allowed with the concentrations of higher than 1.0×10^{-3} mol·L^{-1}. Organic compounds, including glucose, lactose, sucrose, maltose, L-phenylalanine, L-glycine, L-tryptophane, L-histidine, glycine and ascorbic acid, do not interfere at the concentration of higher than 1.0×10^{-3} mol·L^{-1}, while brucine, theobromine, niacin, D-pantothenic acid calcium, thiamine hydrochloride nicotinamide, pyridoxine hydrochloride, quinine sulfate could be tolerated at the concentration level higher than 5.0×10^{-5} mol·L^{-1}. In addition, urea could be allowed at high concentration level up to 0.5 mol·L^{-1}. So, it is obvious that this method has good selectivity, and could be applied to the direct determination of trace amounts of penicillin in complicated materials without separation to remove interfering materials.

4.4.3.5 Calibration curves and sample determinations

According to the general procedures, the relationships between TIR-RLS intensity with penicillin concentration could be constructed. All analytical parameters are presented in Table 3. Among the penicillin investigated, BP and OA have the stronger enhanced TIR-RLS response, while AmP and AmO have weaker enhanced TIR-RLS response. According to pK_{a1}-values of penicillin, AmP and AmO carry one negative charge in pH 5.33 aqueous solution, while BP and OA carry one negative charge. Therefore, BP and OA are less hydrophilic than AmP and AmO are [32], which makes them in favor of the movement toward the interface, resulting in stronger enhanced TIR-RLS signals. The limits of detection (3σ) are 3.48×10^{-8}, 3.85×10^{-8}, 4.22×10^{-8} and 4.86×10^{-8} mol·L^{-1} for BP, OA, AmP and AmO, correspondingly.

Artificial samples for various penicillin containing metal ions, carbohydrates and organic compounds were determined, and the results are given in Table 4. It could be seen that penicillin in artificial samples could be determined with the recovery of 98.3%～103.2% and R.S.D. of 2.1%～3.2%. To further prove the method, the content of amoxycillin in capsule was detected and the results are identical with the label values (Table 5). In order to identify the results, liquid chromatographic method has been applied. Fig. 6 shows the liquid chromatogram, and the analytical parameters. Thus, comparison of the detection could be made from the results showed in Fig. 6 and Table 5. In terms of the analytical parameters, it is obviously that the present method has higher sensitivity. The results of both Tables 4 and 5 indicate that the present method is reliable and applicable.

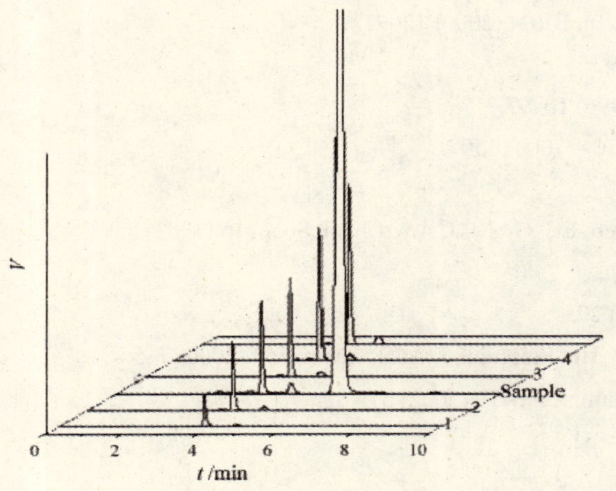

Fig. 6 Chromatogram of amoxycillin in sample detection. Concentration of standard ($\times10^{-4}$ mol·L^{-1}): 1, 1.0, 2, 2.0, 3, 3.0, 4, 4.0, 5 and 5.0. Linear regression, $A=3445+7.5\times10^{8}c$(where A is the peak area, c the concentration of amoxycillin in mol·L^{-1}), could be found in the range from 1.0×10^{-6} to 5.0×10^{-4} mol·L^{-1} with correlation coefficient of 0.9997 (n=11), and limits of detection of 4.5×10^{7} mol·L^{-1}(3σ). From the standard curve, the content of amoxycillin in capsule could be calculated

4.4.4 Conclusions

Since penicillin [30] and berberine [31] with amphiphilic structures are negatively and positively charged, respectively, in the studied medium, interaction between positive charged BB and negatively charged penicillin molecules could occur, resulting in higher hydrophobic complex of penicillin–BB in aqueous medium due to the decrease of charges, which was then coadsorbed into H_2O/CCl_4 interface. In fact, clinic practice has shown that coalescence of penicillin with BB has more effective to cure aspiratory affected disease [33].

The coadsorption of penicillin with BB results in strongly enhanced TIR-RLS signals. With the enhanced TIR-RLS, we studied the ion-associate adsorption equilibrium at H_2O/CCl_4 and found the coadsorption of penicillin and BB in the form of ion associates at H_2O/CCl_4 interfaces with molar ratio of 1:1, and the formation constants of ion associates in the range of 3.67×10^4 to 5.48×10^4 $mol^{-1} \cdot dm^4$. Since the enhanced TIR-RLS intensity is proportional to the concentration of penicillin about the ranges about 0.1×10^{-6} to 1.0×10^{-6} $mol \cdot L^{-1}$ shown in Table 3, a sensitive assay for penicillin could be established with the limits of determination lower than 5.0×10^{-8} $mol \cdot L^{-1}$. Furthermore, this method does not involve any complicated operation, and easily applied to real sample detection.

Acknowledgements

The authors herein thank the supports of the National Science Foundation for Preeminence Youth of China (NSFC-PY no. 20425517), the National Natural Science Foundation of China (NSFC no. 20275032), the Program for New Century Excellent Talents in University (NCET) and Chun Hui Program directed under the Ministry of Education of PRC, and the Municipal Science and Technology Committee of Chongqing.

References

[1] P.B. Miranda, Y.R. Shen, J. Phys. Chem. B 103 (1999) 3292～ 3307.
[2] A. Rao, A. Dhinojwala, Langmuir 19 (2003) 8813.
[3] M.A. Jones, P.W. Bohn, Anal. Chem. 72 (2000) 3776.
[4] K. Fujiwara, H. Watarai, Langmuir 19 (2003) 2658.
[5] J.-W. Benjamins, B. Jonsson, K. Thuresson, T. Nylander, Langmuir 18 (2002) 6437.
[6] J.S. Salafsky, K.B. Eisenthal, J. Phys. Chem. B 104 (2000) 7752.
[7] T. Uchida, A. Yamaguchi, T. Ina, N. Teramae, J. Phys. Chem. B 104 (2000) 12091.
[8] P.B. Miranda, Y.R. Shen, J. Phys. Chem. B 103 (1999) 3292.
[9] R.R. Naujok, H.J. Paul, R.N. Corn, J. Phys. Chem. 100 (1996) 10497.
[10] S.R. Green, T.J. Su, J.R. Lu, J. Penfold, J. Phys. Chem. B 104 (2000) 1507.
[11] L.A. Bottomley, Anal. Chem. 70 (1998) 425R.
[12] R.F. Pasternack, C. Bustamante, P.J. Collings, A. Giannetteo, E.J. Gibbs, J. Am. Chem. Soc. 115 (1993) 5393.
[13] R.F. Pasternack, P.J. Collings, Science 269 (1995) 935.
[14] C.Z. Huang, K.A. Li, S.Y. Tong, Anal. Chem. 6819 (1996) 2259.
[15] Q.F. Li, X.G. Chen, H.Y. Zhang, C.X. Xue, Y.Q. Fan, Z.D. Hu, Fresenius J. Anal. Chem. 368 (2000) 715.
[16] L.J. Dong, R.P. Jia, Q.F. Li, X.G. Chen, Z.D. Hu, Anal. Chim. Acta 459 (2002) 313.
[17] W. Lu, C.Z. Huang, Y.F. Li, Anal. Chim. Acta 475 (2003) 151.
[18] S.P. Liu, P. Feng, Microchim. Acta 140 (2002) 189.
[19] P. Feng, W.Q. Su, C.Z. Huang, Y.F. Li, Anal. Chem. 73 (2001) 4307.
[20] P. Feng, C.Z. Huang, Y.F. Li, Anal. Biochem. 308 (2002) 83.

[21] W. Lu, C.Z. Huang, Y.F. Li, Analyst 127 (2002) 1392.

[22] M.A.S. Vigeant, M. Wagner, L.K. Tamm, R.M. Ford, Langmuir 17 (2001) 2235.

[23] H. Watarai, F. Funaki, Langmuir 12 (1996) 6717.

[24] V. Thamlikitkul, S. Kobwanthanakun, S.J. Pruksachatvuthi, Int. Med. Res. 20 (1992) 20.

[25] B.D. Karlberg, Anal. Chim. Acta 83 (1976) 309.

[26] E. Verdon, P. Couedor, J. Chromatogr. B 705 (1998) 71.

[27] P.H. Chan, H.B. Liu, Y.W. Chen, K.-C. Chan, C.W. Tsang, Y.C.

[28] Leung, K.Y. Wong, J. Am. Chem. Soc. 126 (2004) 4074.

[29] B. Morelli, Talanta 47 (1994) 479.

[30] I. Benjamin, Chem. Rev. 96 (1996) 1449.

[31] P. Taboada, D. Attwood, J.M. Ruso, F. Samiento, V. Mosquera, Langmuir 15 (1999) 2022.

[32] X.Y. Zheng, Y. Peng, D.Q. Ren, et al., The National Pharmacopoeia of People's Republic of China-2000 Edition, vol. 2, Chemical Industry Press, Beijing, 2000, p. 353.

[33] M.X. Jiang, New Practical Pharmacology, Science Press, Beijing, 2000, p. 526.

[34] F.S. Ruan, S. Hou, L. Li, J. Med. Univ. 20 (1997) 60.

(Cheng Zhi Huang, Ping Feng, Yuan Fang Li, Ke Jun Tan, Hui Ying Wang,
published in *Analytica Chimica Acta*, 2005, 538, 337～343)

4.5 Pharmacokinetic Detection of Penicillin Excreted in Urine Using a Totally Internally Reflected Resonance Light Scattering Technique with Cetyltrimethylammonium Bromide

Abstract: A quantitative analysis method for penicillins including ampicillin (AmP), benzyl penicillin (BP), oxacillin (OA) and amoxycillin (AmO) is proposed that makes use of the totally internally reflected resonance light scattering (TIR-RLS) signal from the penicillin at the H_2O/CCl_4 interface in the presence of cetyltrimethylammonium bromide (CTMAB), and enables the pharmacokinetics of penicillin taken orally and excreted through urine to be monitored. Penicillin is coadsorbed with CTMAB at the H_2O/CCl_4 interface in neutral solution, resulting in the formation of ion associates that display greatly enhanced TIR-RLS signals (maximum at 368～372 nm). This enhanced TIR-RLS intensity was found to be proportional to the penicillin concentration over the range 0.2×10^{-6} to 2.2×10^{-6} mol·L^{-1}, with limits of determination (3σ) of 5.0×10^{-6} to 7.0×10^{-6} mol·L^{-1}. Pharmacokinetics studies performed using the present method show that the excretion of orally-taken ampicillin through urine has a half-time of 1.05 h and an excremental quantum over 8 h of 49.3%, respectively.

Keywords: Totally internally reflected resonance light scattering (TIR-RLS) • Penicillin • Cetyltrimethylammonium bromide

4.5.1 Introduction

Since the introduction of a resonance light scattering (RLS) technique by Pasternack et al[1, 2], where a common spectrofluorometer was used to measure light scattering signals, such techniques have generated great interest amongst researchers. One important application of this technique is to assay trace amounts of nucleic acids[3～6], proteins[7～9], metallic ions[10, 11] and drugs[12, 13], based on the enhanced RLS signals from molecular recognition or aggregation assemblies that form in supramolecular interactions. However, although they possess high sensitivity and simplicity, RLS methods suffer from drawbacks such as their low tolerance to interference from other components, and they are difficult to use if we wish to directly quantify trace amounts of analyte in complicated samples such as human urine. In this case, pretreatment techniques have been generally been used, such as 1000-fold dilution of the sample with water, use of standard addition methods, and prior separation [7～11].

It is well known that total internal reflection (TIR) of light occurs when a light beam encounters the interface between a medium with a higher refractive index (through which it has been moving) and a medium with a lower refractive index at an angle of incidence that is greater than the critical angle (θ_c). Although all of the visible light is reflected from the interface, electromagnetic energy is carried across the interface in the form of an evanescent wave, which decays exponentially with the depth from the interface, falling to undetectable levels within less than one wavelength[14], meaning that chemical species in the interfacial region could be highly and selectively excited, and so it is possible to construct a TIR analysis method that has high sensitivity and selectivity[15]. Although such total internal reflection (TIR) techniques are not novel, any method that may be used to detect the non-fluorescent signals arising from the interface is worthy of further investigation. We previously applied the RLS technique in order to measure the light scattered from the species present at a liquid/liquid interface, which in turn enabled us to study the molecular recognition and assembly processes that occurred at the interface[16], and we proved that this TIR-RLS coupled technique has better selectivity and sensitivity than aqueous phase RLS methods, since the liquid/liquid interface enriches analytes and separates coexisting substances from the aqueous or organic phases[6~18]. In order to further explore the enrichment and separation processes that occur at interfaces using RLS signal measurements, in this paper we propose a method for detecting an analyte in urine, using penicillin as the model analyte, noting that a typical clinical sample of human urine has a strong light scattering background.

Penicillins have found wide application as additives in food, feed and aquiculture, and in antibacterial medicines, and so it is very important to quantify the penicillin present in pharmaceutical preparations, biological samples, and food products. Various ways of determining penicillin have been reported, including microbiological [19], titrimetry [20], high performance liquid chromatography (HPLC) [21], fluorimetry [22] and spectrophotometry [23, 24]. These methods, however, lack specificity [19], sensitivity [20], and complicated pretreatments are generally necessary [21, 22]. Herein we propose a TIR-RLS method for determining penicillin that does not involve complicated pretreatments, based on measuring the enhanced TIR-RLS signal produced from the ion associate species at the H_2O/CCl_4 interface, which can be applied to monitor the penicillin excretion from urine. The principle of the method proposed here is based on the electrostatic interaction between the negatively-charged penicillin and cationic surfactant in weakly acidic aqueous medium. Ionic associates are the result of the electrostatic attractions between closelypacked monolayers at the liquid/liquid interface and the hydrocarbon chains of surfactant molecules oriented away from the aqueous phase[25, 26].

4.5.2 Experimental

4.5.2.1 Apparatus

We employed a Hitachi F-2500 spectrofluorometer (Tokyo, Japan) equipped with a 150-W Xe lamp to measure the TIR-RLS spectra and intensities; the sample compartment of the spectrofluorometer was modified as illustrated as our previous reports [16, 17]. In order to make the inside wall hydrophobic and afford a flat H_2O/CCl_4 interface, the bottom 1.0 cm of the inside of the optical quartz cell (the total depth of the cell is about 3.5 cm) was treated with 2% dichlorodimethylsilane in benzene.

4.5.2.2 Reagents

Penicillins used in this study include ampicillin (AmP), benzyl penicillin (BP), oxacillin (OA) and amoxycillin (AmO). 1.0×10^{-3} mol·L^{-1} stock solutions were prepared by dissolving the penicillin sodium salts (all are commercially available from Chongqing Institute ofPharmacology, China) in doubly-distilled water. 1.0×10^{-3} and 1.0×10^{-4} mol·L^{-1} working solutions were prepared by successive dilution with doubly-distilled water.

2.0×10^{-5} mol·L^{-1} cetyltrimethylammonium bromide (CTMAB) was prepared by dissolving its crystal product (Merck, Germany) in doubly-distilled water. 0.1 mol·L^{-1} KH_2PO_4–NaOH buffer solution (pH 6.6) was used to control the acidity of the aqueous system. All other reagents were of analytical-reagent grade and doubly-distilled water was used throughout.

4.5.2.3 Human urine samples

Human urine samples were collected from three healthy volunteers 0.5, 1.0, 1.5, 2.0, 3.0, 4.0, 5.0, 6.0, 7.0, 8.0, and 9.0 h after they each took a single 750-mg ampicillin capsule orally with a glass of drinking water. Then 0.10 mL of the urine sample was pipetted, and detections were performed according to standard procedures. If the penicillin concentration was too high, appropriate dilutions with doubly distilled water were made.

4.5.2.4 Standard procedure

1.0 mL tetrachloromethane and 0.10 mL of the working or sample solution of the penicillin to be determined were placed into an optical quartz cell, and then 0.50 mL CTMAB solution and 0.5 mL KH_2PO_4–NaOH buffer solution (pH 6.6) were added. The aqueous phase mixture was diluted to 2.0 mL with doubly-distilled water and mixed thoroughly. Then the mixture was allowed to stand for 15 min prior to TIR-RLS measurements. TIRRLS spectra were taken for this mixture and then compared to the spectra obtained for a blank mixture treated in the same way without individual penicillin.

The TIR-RLS spectra were obtained by simultaneously scanning the excitation and emission monochromators of the F-2500 spectrofluorometer from 220 to 700 nm with $\lambda_{ex}=\lambda_{em}$. The TIR-RLS intensities were measured at 370 nm with a slit width of 5.0 nm for both the excitation and the emission monochromators.

4.5.3 Results and discussion

4.5.3.1 Spectral characteristics and interaction

Curves 1 and 2 in Fig. 1 display the TIR-RLS features for BP and CTMAB, respectively. It is apparent that the TIR-RLS signals from BP and CTMAB at the H_2O/CCl_4 interface are very faint over the whole scanning region. However, greatly enhanced TIR-RLS signals could be observed, with the maximum signal observed at 368～372 nm for a trace amount of BP mixed with CTMAB.

Penicillin has an amphiphilic structure [27]. Since the pK_{a1} values of AmP, BP, OA, and AmO are 2.5, 2.8, and 2.4, respectively [28], these penicillins are negatively charged in aqueous medium at pH 6.6 since they are fully ionized. Therefore, they can form ionic associates with positively-charged surfactant through electrostatic attraction. The electrostatic interaction between the penicillin and CTMAB at the H_2O/CCl_4 interface reduces the net charge on both the penicillin and the CTMAB molecules, and thus encourages the movement of these penicillin-CTMAB ion associates in the aqueous phase towards the interface, where coadsorption occurs. This concentrates the levels of penicillin-CTMAB ion associates at the interface, resulting in greatly enhanced TIR-RLS signals from it, while other coexisting substances (including some commonly-used clinical drugs such as brucine, theobromine, niacin, and so on) that cannot form ion associates with CTMAB remain in the aqueous medium.

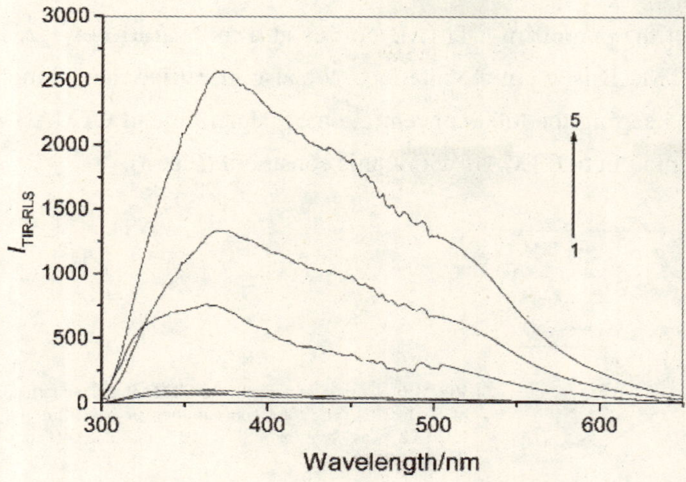

Fig. 1 TIR-RLS spectra for BP (curve 1), CTMAB (curve 2), BPCTMAB (curves 3–5) at the H_2O/CCl_4 interface. BP (curves 3 to 5, × 10^{-6} $mol \cdot L^{-1}$) 0.5, 1.0, 2.0; CTMAB 5.0 × 10^{-6} $mol \cdot L^{-1}$; pH 6.6

4.5.3.2 Effect of pH

Since the binding of penicillin to CTMAB depends upon the electrostatic attraction, factors that influence the charge density of the aqueous medium could also exert influence over this electrostatic binding. For amphiphilic molecules, pH is an important influence on the distribution of charge density over the molecular structure. We employed KH_2PO_4-NaOH buffer (pH 6.6) to control the pH of the aqueous medium. As shown in Fig. 2, the TIR-RLS intensity of penicillin-CTMAB varies greatly as the pH of the aqueous phase is varied. The TIR-RLS intensity of CTMAB remains constant with pH. The TIR-RLS intensities of BP-CTMAB, OACTMAB, AmP-CTMAB, and AmO-CTMAB all vary greatly with pH and reach their maximum values at pH values of 6.2～6.8, 6.4～6.8, 6.4～7.0, and 6.4～7.0, respectively. It is noticeable from Fig. 2 that the enhanced TIR-RLS signals of BP-CTMAB and OA-CTMAB are less than those of AmP-CTMAB and AmO-CTMAB above pH 7.2; this is probably due to the second proton becoming dissociated at around this pH for AmP and AmO (p K_{a2}-values are 7.2 for AmP and 7.4 for AmO) [28], whereas there is no dissociation of the second proton from BP and OA molecules at this pH.

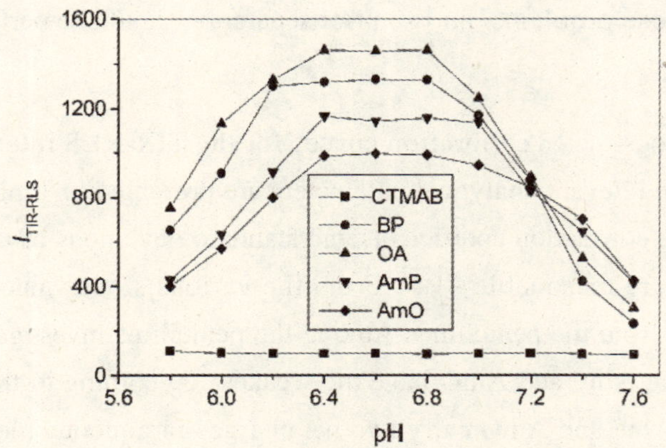

Fig. 2 The dependence of the TIR-RLS signal intensity on the pH value of the aqueous phase. Concentration: CTMAB 5.0 × 10^{-6} $mol \cdot L^{-1}$, Penicillin 1.0 × 10^{-6} $mol \cdot L^{-1}$. $\lambda_{ex}=\lambda_{em}$=370 nm

4.5.3.3 Molar ratio of penicillin-CTMAB at H_2O/CCl_4

It has shown that the CTMAB concentration influences the TIR-RLS intensity. When the concentration of penicillin was kept constant at 1.0 × 10^{-6} $mol \cdot L^{-1}$, the TIR-RLS intensity increased with the CTMAB concentration until turning points occurred on each of the penicillin-CTMAB curves at a molar ratio of 1:2, indicating that the binding ratio of penicillin to CTMAB is 1:2 at the interface. We also identified the 1:2 molar ratio of the penicillin-CTMAB ion associates by keeping the total concentration of penicillin and CTMAB as 3.0 × 10^{-6} mol·L^{-1},and varying the molar ratio of penicillin to CTMAB within this constraint (Fig. 3).

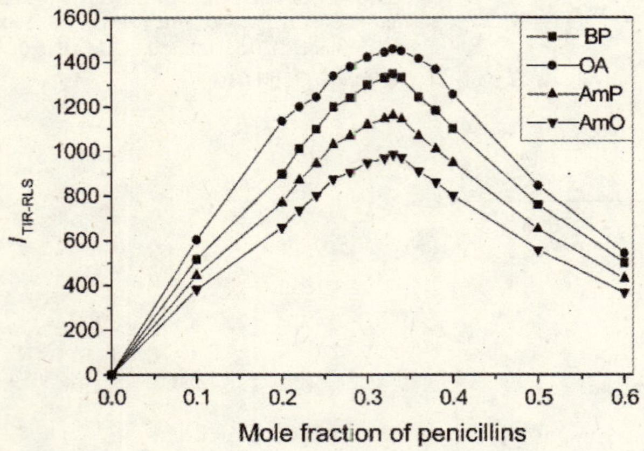

Fig. 3 Molar ratio of penicillin to CTMAB at the interface of H_2O/ CCl_4. The total concentration of penicillin and CTMAB was kept as 3.0 × 10^{-6} mol·L^{-1}. pH 6.6, $\lambda_{ex}=\lambda_{em}$=370 nm

4.5.3.4 Interferences from coexisting foreign substances

Influences of coexisting foreign substances on the determination of 1.0 × 10^{-6} mol·L^{-1} BP were investigated, and the results are listed in Table 1. Common metal ions such as NH_4^+, Ca(II), Mg(II), Cu(II), Fe(III), Se(IV), Zn(II), Pb(II), Al(III), and Cd(II) can be tolerated with concentrations of > 1.0 × 10^{-3} mol·L^{-1}. 1.0 × 10^{-3} mol·L^{-1} of many organic components, including glucose, lactose, sucrose, maltose, L-phenylalanine, L-glycine, L-tryptophane, L-histidine, glycine, and ascorbic acid, do not cause any interference. Drugs, including 5.0 × 10^{-5} mol·L^{-1} brucine, theobromine, niacin, D-pantothenic acid calcium, thiamine hydrochloride nicotinamide, pyridoxine hydrochloride, and quinine sulfate can also be tolerated. In addition, high concentrations of urea, up to 0.5 mol·L^{-1}, are also tolerable. Thus, this method provides good selectivity even with a background of metal ions and common organic components, and could be applied to the direct determination of trace amounts of penicillin in the complicated background described above. However, due to their similar interaction mechanisms, interference from penicillin metabolites may pose problems, and so prior separation should be performed.

4.5.3.5 Calibration curves

Following the general procedure, we then constructed calibration curves for the TIR-RLS intensity versus the individual penicillin concentration. All of the relevant analytical parameters are presented in Table 2. It is apparent that these regression results, including the correlation coefficients and standard deviations of the residuals, and the errors in the slopes and intercept values are reasonable[29, 30]. From the various slope values it was possible to compare the TIR-RLS signal intensities from the penicillins. Among the penicillins investigated, BP and OA have the strongest TIR-RLS responses, while AmP and AmO have the weakest. According to the molecular structures and the pKa values of the penicillin, AmP and AmO carry two net charges in aqueous medium at pH 6.6, while BP and OA carry only one net charge. Therefore, BP and OA are not as hydrophilic as AmP and AmO[31], which favors their movement toward the interface, resulting in stronger TIR-RLS signals. The limits of detection (3σ) are 4.87, 5.30, 5.84, and 7.07 × 10^{-8} mol·L^{-1} for BP, OA, AmP, and AmO, respectively.

4.5.3.6 Sample determination and pharmacokinetic study

Artificial samples containing various penicillins as well as metal ions, carbohydrates and organic compounds were determined, and the results are given in Table 3. It is apparent that the penicillins in the synthetic samples can be determined with recoveries of 96.7%~102.0% and RSD of 1.5%~3.3%. In order to check that this method can measure the penicillin content in a urine sample, a standard addition method was employed using AmP as a typical analyte and a series of standard AmP solutions were added into the urine taken from the volunteers 30 min before and after taking AmP capsules orally. Fig. 4 shows the results of this determination. It is apparent that the present method can detect the Amp contents in the urine sample, and the detected content of AmP found using the standard method (4.85×10^{-7} mol·L^{-1}) is almost identical to the value found using the present TIR-RLS method, which was 4.41×10^{-7} mol·L^{-1} ($n = 3$, RSD, 1.9%).

Following the general procedure, we performed pharmacokinetic studies using the present method to monitor the excretion of penicillin in urine, using AmP as a model analyte. None of the human urine samples underwent pretreatment. Data for the amount of AmP present at different times in the urine are shown in Table 4. These data were then used to calculate the pharmacokinetic parameters according to the following equation[32]:

$$\log\frac{\Delta X_u}{\Delta t} = -\frac{Kt_c}{2.303} + \log\frac{k_e k_a F X_0}{k_a - k}$$

where ΔX_u and tc are the amount of AmP in the urine and the time halfway through collecting the urine (the "midpoint time"), k is the excremental quantum (the percentage of the drug excreted through urine over a given time period). The plot of $\log(\Delta X_u/\Delta t)$ against tc gave a straight line of $\log(\Delta X_u/\Delta t) = 2.4539 \sim 0.2879$tc with a correlation coefficient (r) of -0.9983 (the standard deviation of the residual $(S_y/_x)_=$ 0.0342, slope error = 0.0050, intercept error = 0.0220 when the degrees of freedom n-2 = 7). Therefore, there is good correlation and linearity between $\log(\Delta X_u/\Delta t)$ and the midpoint time [29, 30]. Using the slope values, it was then possible to determine k. The curve conforms to the one compartment model of first-order elimination kinetics. The half time ($t_{1/2}$) of the penicillin (the time taken for the drug concentration in the body (generally in blood plasma) to drop from the

Table 1 Influences of various foreign substances

Foreign substance	Concentration tolerated ($\times 10^{-4}$ mol·L^{-1})	Foreign substance	Concentration tolerated ($\times 10^{-4}$ mol·L^{-1})	Foreign substance	Concentration tolerated ($\times 10^{-4}$ mol·L^{-1})
NH_4^+, Cl	440	Starch	60.1 mol·L^{-1}	Ascorbic acid	11.5
Mg^{2+}, NO_3^-	180	Sucrose	100	Quinine sulfate	0.6
Ca^{2+}, Cl	100	Maltose	101	Brucine	1.4
Al^{3+}, Cl	15.5	Lactose	201	Thiamine hydrochloride	0.8
Cu^{2+}, Cl	15.1	Glucose	102	Niacin	1.2
Zn^{2+}, Cl	38.0	L-lysine	21.4	D-pantothenic acid calcium	0.75
Se (IV)	25.7	L-phenylalanine	30.6	Nicotinamide	1.1
Fe^{3+}, Cl	18.5	L-glycine	18.1	Pyridoxine hydrochloride	1.4
Cd^{2+}, NO_3^-	11.2	L-tryptophane	24.1	Urea	5000
Pb^{2+}, NO_3^-	24.4	L-histidine	28.6		

pH 6.6, Concentration: BP 1.0×10^{-6} mol·L^{-1}, CTMAB 5.0×10^{-6} mol·L^{-1}, $\lambda_{ex}=\lambda_{em}$=370 nm

Table 2 Calibration curve linear regression equations, linear ranges and detection limits for the penicillins

Penicillin	Linear range ($\times10^{-6}$ mol·L^{-1})	Linear regression equation (c,$\times10^{-6}$ mol·L^{-1})	Correlation coefficient (r, n=9)	Standard deviation of residuals ($S_{I/c}$)	Errors of intercepts and slopes	Detection limit (3σ, 10^{-8} mol·L^{-1})
BP	0.15–2.2	Δ I=29.5+1216.8 c	0.9988	44.07	28.76; 22.39	4.87
OA	0.10–2.0	ΔI=47.6+1334.4 c	0.9966	83.42	48.81; 41.50	5.30
AmP	0.15–2.2	ΔI=35.7+1057.2 c	0.9968	62.60	35.67; 31.77	5.84
AmO	0.2–2.2	ΔI=42.9+911.2 c	0.9945	70.26	46.44; 36.10	7.07

pH 6.6, Concentration: *CTMAB* 5.0 × 10^{-6} mol·L^{-1}. $\lambda_{ex}=\lambda_{em}$=370 nm

Table 3 Results from the synthetic sample determinations

Penicillin in the sample ($\times10^{-6}$ mol·L^{-1})	Coexisting substances ($\times10^{-4}$ mol·L^{-1})	Found ($\times10^{-6}$ mol·L^{-1}, n=5)	Recovery (%)	RSD (%)
BP 1.5	$Mg(NO_3)_2$,10; $CuCl_2$,4; $ZnCl_2$,5; $Pb(NO_3)_2$,5; $CaCl_2$,10; $AlCl_3$,1; $FeCl_3$,4	1.45	96.7	3.3
OA 2.0	Nicotinamide, 0.2; Ascorbic acid, 2.0; Quinine sulfate, 0.1; Thiamine chloride, 0. 2	2.03	101.5	1.5
AmP 1.0	Starch, 25; Maltose, 25; Glucose, 25; L-phenylalanine, 10	1.02	102.0	2.0

*mg·L^{-1}. pH 6.6, Concentration: CTMAB 5.0 × 10^{-6} mol·L^{-1}. $\lambda_{ex}=\lambda_{em}$=370 nm

maximum concentration to half of the maximum concentration) and the excremental quantum over 8 h were obtained from k via the procedure described in[32]. The values of $t_{1/2}$ and the excremental quantum within 8 h were 1.05 h and 49.3%, respectively, which are in good agreement with that reported by other authors[33] (half time and excremental quantum within 8 h were 1 h and 50.6%, respectively). This result indicates that our TIR-RLS technique for determining penicillin in human urine sample is reliable, sensitive and practical.

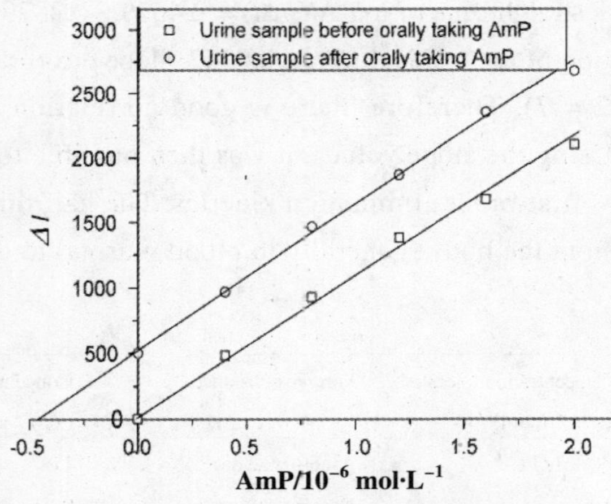

Fig. 4 AmP in urine sampled half an hour before and after taking AmP capsules orally, determined using the standard addition method. Linear regression equations are ΔI= 55.0 + 1038.4 c (n = 6, r=0.9978, SI/c=57.78, intercept error 41.86; slope error 34.53) and DI= 535.4 + 1103.1 c (n = 6, r= 0.9985, Sy/x = 49.94, intercept error 36.14; slope error, 29.85) for urine sampled half an hour before (open squares) and after (open diamonds) taking AmP capsules orally, respectively. An amount of 0.10 mL (diluted 100-fold) of the urine sample was applied for the detection. $\lambda_{ex}=\lambda_{em}$=370 nm. pH 6.6, Concentration: CTMAB 5.0×10^{-6} mol·L^{-1}

Table 4 Amount of AmP excreted via urine within 8 h

Urine collection time (hours after penicillin was ingested)	t_c(h)	Δt	ΔX_u (mg)	$\Delta X_u/\Delta t$	$\log(\Delta X_u/\Delta t)$
0.5	0.25	0.5	58.71	117.42	2.0697
1.0	0.75	0.5	89.90	179.80	2.2548
1.5	1.25	0.5	63.13	128.32	2.1013
2.0	1.75	0. 5	39.44	92.04	1.897
3.0	2.5	1.0	62.10	55.35	1.7931
4.0	3.5	1.0	25.73	28.21	1.4104
5.0	4.5	1.0	14.43	14.43	1.1593
6.0	5.5	1.0	7.23	7.57	0.8591
7.0	6.5	1.0	3.92	3.74	0.5929
8.0	7.5	1.0	1.99	1.99	0.2989

pH 6.6, Concentration: CTMAB 5.0×10^{-6} mol·L^{-1}. $\lambda_{ex}=\lambda_{em}$=370 nm . These data were all fitted except for the first point (0.25, 2.0697). Linear regression gave $\log(\Delta Xu/\Delta t)$=2.4539-0.2879t_c with r=-0.9983, Sy/x=0.0342, slope error=0.0050, and intercept error=0.0220, when the degrees of freedom n-2=7

4.5.4 Conclusions

The present assay of penicillin based on enhanced TIRRLS measurements at the liquid/liquid interface is reliable, practical and sensitive. Compared with other methods stated in the "Introduction", the present method does not involve any complicated procedures. In particular, the present method provides a direct way of determining trace amounts of penicillin when high levels of interfering compounds are present too, and it does not need any pretreatment procedure. The method is therefore useful for studying the pharmacokinetics of the excretion of penicillin via urine.

Acknowledgements

This work has been supported by the National Natural Science Foundation of China (NSFC, Nos. 20425517 and 20275032), the Program for New Century Excellent Talents in University (NCET) and Chun Hui Program (No. (2004) 7–24) directed under the Ministry of Education of PRC, and the Municipal Science and Technology Committee of Chongqing.

References

[1] Pasternack RF, Bustamante C, Collings PJ, Giannetteo A, Gibbs EJ (1993) J Am Chem Soc 115:5393
[2] Pasternack RF, Collings PJ (1995) Science 269:935
[3] Huang CZ, Li KA, Tong SY (1996) Anal Chem 68:2259
[4] Huang CZ, Li KA, Tong SY (1997) Anal Chem 69:514
[5] Liu Y, Ma CQ, Li KA, Xie FC, Tong SY (1999) Anal Biochem 268:187
[6] Li YF, Shu WQ, Feng P, Huang CZ (2001) Anal Sci 17:693
[7] Ma CQ, Li KA, Tong SY (1997) Bull Chem Soc Jpn 70:129
[8] Yao G, Li KA, Tong SY (1999) Anal Chim Acta 398:319
[9] Cao QE, Ding ZT, Fang RB, Zhao X(2001) Analyst 126:1444
[10] Liu SP, Liu Q, Liu ZF, Huang CZ (2000) Anal Chim Acta 407:255
[11] Liu SP, Liu ZF, Huang CZ (1998) Anal Sci 14:799
[12] Liu SP, Luo HQ, Li NB, Liu ZF, Zheng WX (2001) Anal Chem 73:3907
[13] Liu SP, Feng P(2002) Microchim Acta 140:189
[14] Vigeant MAS, Wagner M, Tamm LK, Ford R M(2001) Langmuir 17:2235
[15] Watarai H, Funaki F(1996) Langmuir 12:6717
[16] Feng P, Su WQ, Huang CZ, Li YF (2001) Anal Chem 73:4307
[17] Feng P, Huang CZ, Li YF (2002) Anal Biochem 308:83
[18] Lu W, Huang CZ, Li YF (2002) Analyst 127:1392
[19] Thamlikitkul V, Kobwanthanakun S, Pruksachatvuthi SJ (1992) Int Med Res 20:20
[20] Karlberg BD (1976) Anal Chim Acta 83:309
[21] Verdon E, Couedor PJ (1998) Chromatogr B 705:71
[22] Jusko WJ (1971) J Pharm Sci 60:728
[23] Morelli B(1994) Talanta 47:479
[24] Besada A, Tadros NB (1987) Mikrochim Acta 2:225
[25] Naujok RR, Hillary JP, Corn RM (1996) J Phys Chem 100:10497
[26] Messmer MC, Conboy JC, Richmond GL (1995) J Am Chem Soc 117:8039
[27] Taboada P, Attwood D, Ruso JM, Samiento F, Mosquera V (1999) Langmuir 15:2022
[28] Chen MZ (1992) National basic medicines. Peoples Sanitation Press, Beijing, China, p 2

[29] Huber W(2004) J Quality 726:9

[30] Ning YN (2004) Applications of chemometrics in analytical chemistry. Science Press, Beijing, China, p 34–38

[31] Jiang MX (2000) New practical pharmacology. Science Press, Beijing, China, p 526

[32] Wei S(1997) Biopharmacology and pharmacokinetics. Union press of Beijing Medical University and Xiehe Medical University, Beijing, China, p 60

[33] Liu CX (1980) Pharmacokinetics. Hunan Science and Technology Press, Changsha, China, p 178

(Cheng Zhi Huang ,Ping Feng, Yuan Fang Li, Ke Jun Tan,
published in *Analytical and Bioanalytical Chemistry*, 2005,382, 85～90)

4.6 A Wide Dynamic Range Detection of Biopolymer Medicines with Resonance Light Scattering and Absorption Ratiometry

Abstract: Using the interaction of heparin with Janus Green Blue (JGB) as an example, herein a dual-wavelength resonance lighting scattering (RLS) ratiometric method and an absorbance ratiometric one are developed to detect biopolymer medicines based on their bindings with organic dyes. In aqueous solution, heparin could interact with JGB, displaying significantly enhanced RLS signals in UV–vis region. By measuring the RLS intensity ratio (R_{ratio}) and absorbance ratio (A_{ratio}) at the wavelengths of 285 nm over that at 345 nm, respectively, heparin over a wide dynamic range of content could be detected. Typically, when JGB concentration is kept at 1.00×10^{-5} mol·L^{-1}, using R_{ratio} could detect heparin over a range of 0.30～2000 ng·mL^{-1} with a limit of determination of 30 pg·mL^{-1}, while using A_{ratio} could detect heparin over the range of 0.01～2000.0 ng·mL^{-1} with a limit of determination of 1 pg ml^{-1}. The wavelength-dependent RLS and absorption ratiometric methods were found to have much better flexibility for a series of common influences, such as pH, and dye concentration, than that of RLS method at a single wavelength. The interaction nature was investigated through size measurements and RLS imaging detections.

Keywords: Heparin; Janus Green Blue (JGB); Resonance light scattering (RLS) ratiometry; Absorbance ratiometry

Abbreviations: RLS, resonance lighting scattering; $R_{ratio,}$ RLS intensity ratio; $A_{ratio,}$ absorbance ration; JGB, Janus Green Blue; PCS, photon correlation spectroscopy

4.6.1 Introduction

Light scattering is a very common phenomenon and has been widely applied in size measurements and distributions of colloid and pharmaceutical particles[1,2]. Resonance light scattering technique is a creative application of light scattering signals measured by simultaneously scanning the excitation and emission monochromators of a common spectrofluorometer[3,4]. It has proved that RLS technique could be used for the assignments of bio-assemblies of drugs and biopolymers[3～6]. For analytical purpose, RLS technique has the advantages of simplicity and high sensitivity for detecting biomolecules[7～11], nanoparticles[12], and drugs[13]. It has reported that the scattered light emission of gold particles is 10^5-fold than the fluorescence emission of a fluorescein molecule[14], and could act as highly fluorescent analogs and tracer labels in clinical and biological applications[15,16]. Thus, the RLS technique has shown high promise in analytical and biochemical sciences. In practical operation, however, the maximum RLS intensities at a single characteristic wavelength are not reliable to describe the properties for RLS spectra for their fluctuating variations at the single wavelength [17]. To overcome shortcomings RLS method, herein we propose a RLS ratiometry measured using a common spectrofluorometer using the interaction between heparin and Janus Green Blue (JGB) as an example, and a comparison is made with the corresponding absorbance ratiometric method.

Ratiometric method could date from 1985 when Tsien and co-workers reported a ratio fluorescent indicator for selective calcium detection[17]. Ever since, wavelength-dependent ratiometric methods were reported in fluorescence domains as more effective analytical methods including fluorescence ratiometry and ratio imaging technique to analyze intracellular oxygen[18], pH[19], metal ions[20], aminophenol[21], DNA[22], and membrane potential[23–29] in living cells. These ratiometric methods have proved to hold the advantages over the conventional ones of single wavelength-intensity since they account for variations in experiments[30].

Heparin is a high negatively charged sugaramic polysaccharide belonging to amylose family. It has been widely applied to prevent thrombosis of the extracorporeal circuit and to mediate activation of the hemostatic system during surgery, acting as anticoagulant, atrology, anti-inflammation, anti-knub and virus demurrer [31]. Quantifying trace amount of heparin is very important, and it has been frequently carried out using spectrophotometric[32], chromatographic, electrophoretic[33,34], and ion-selective electrode methods[35]. Our RLS ratiometric method of heparin, proposed herein based on the enhanced RLS signals resulting from its interaction with JGB through static attraction in neutral aqueous medium, is sensitive and reproducible compared to the common RLS method based on the measurements of scattered light intensities at a single wavelength.

4.6.2 Experimental

4.6.2.1 Apparatus

The RLS spectra were obtained using a Hitachi F-2500 spectrofluorometer (Tokyo, Japan) by simultaneously scanning the excitation and emission monochromators without wavelength difference, while the absorption spectra were measured using a Hitachi 3010 spectrophotometer (Tokyo, Japan). A N5 PCS submicron particle size analyzer (Beckman Coulter, Miami, USA) was used to detect the size of micro-particles in solutions based on photon correlation spectroscopy (PCS). A home-developed laser-powered optical imaging system was used for imaging detection[36].

4.6.2.2 Reagents

10.0 $\mu g \cdot mL^{-1}$ heparin stock solution was prepared by dissolving its sodium salt (160 $IU \cdot mg^{-1}$, Shanghai Organic Reagent Company, China) in water, and its working solution was further diluted with water to 0.01, 0.1,1.0 $\mu g \cdot mL^{-1}$. 2.0×10^{-4} $mol \cdot L^{-1}$ stock solution of Janus Green Blue (JGB, Shanghai Chemical Regent Company, Shanghai, China) was prepared by dissolving its crystal in water. Britton Robinson buffer (BR, pH 7.96) was prepared and used to control the acidity. All of other reagents were of analytical-reagent grade and doubly distilled water was used throughout.

4.6.2.3 Procedures

0.10 mL heparin sodium stock solution was pipetted into a 10.0 mL flask, then 1.0 mL BR buffer (pH 7.96) and 0.5 mL of 1.0×10^{-5} $mol \cdot L^{-1}$ JGB were subsequently added. The mixture was then diluted to the mark and mixed thoroughly. Ten minutes later, the mixture was used for RLS, absorbance, size distribution or imaging detection.

Size distribution was measured at a 90.0% scattering angle in 20.0 °C ambient temperature by taking viscosity and refractive index values of 1.002 centipoises and 1.333, respectively. 400 μL of the mixture was transferred to quartz cell (5.0 mm × 2.0 mm × 43.0 mm) for imaging detection. A 488 nm light beam emitted from an argon ion laser was used as the light source in this imaging detection, and the output power used to excite the solution was calibrated and monitored in every measurement to ensure that the power supply was stable.

4.6.3 Results and discussion

4.6.3.1 Spectroscopic characteristics of the interaction between heparin and JGB

Fig. 1 shows the RLS spectra of the interaction of heparin with JGB in weak basic medium. It could be seen that the RLS signals of both JGB and heparin are very weak. There is a characteristic RLS peak at 275 nm for heparin, and a characteristic RLS peak at 325 nm accompanied by a shoulder RLS peak at 280 nm for JGB. The weak RLS signals of JGB, however, could be greatly enhanced by heparin, showing a characteristic peak at 314 nm with several shoulder peaks in the region of 350.0～600.0 nm, indicating that the interaction between JGB with heparin has occurred. In other words, the enhanced light scattering signals might be attributed to the formation of heparin-JGB complexes.

Fig. 2 shows the absorption features of the interaction. JGB had three molecular absorption bands characterized at 285, 393, and 595 nm, respectively. Significant hypochromicity could be observed after JGB interacts with heparin in the 285 and 595 nm regions, and hyperchromicity at 393 nm with two isosbestic points at 300 and 567 nm. A ratio spectrum of absorbance could then be available (shown in square scatters in Fig. 2) from the quotients of absorbance at each corresponding wavelength, $A_{JGB\text{-}Hep}/A_{JGB}$. It could be seen obviously different ratio values at 285, 345, and 618 nm in the range of 220.0～700.0 nm. Thus, we coulduse RLS intensity ratio function of I_{285}/I_{345} orI_{618}/I_{345} and absorbance ratio functions of A_{285}/A_{345} or A_{595}/A_{345} to investigate the RLS and the absorption features ofthe interaction between heparin and JGB. Considering that the light scattering signals are easily affected by the presence of other particle substances in UV region, we deliberately choose the ratio function of I_{285}/I_{345} and A_{285}/A_{345} to identify the advantages of the RLS ratiometry.

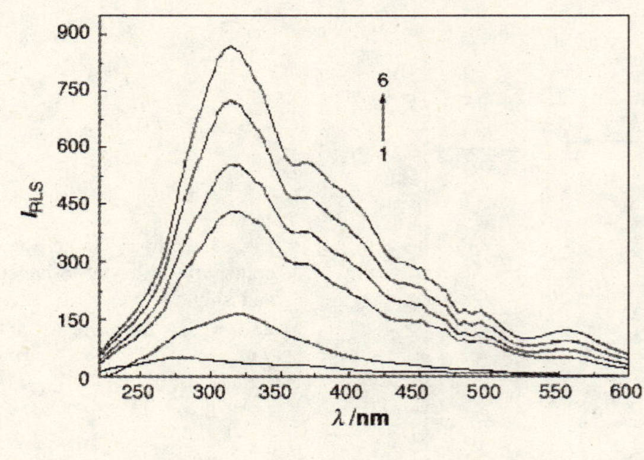

Fig. 1 RLS spectra ofthe interaction of JGB with heparin. Curves 1–6 represent 500, 0.0, 200, 400, 600, and 800 ng·mL^{-1} of heparin, respectively in the presence of 1.0 × 10^{-5} mol·L^{-1} JGB, except Curve 1 without any addition of JGB. pH 7.96.

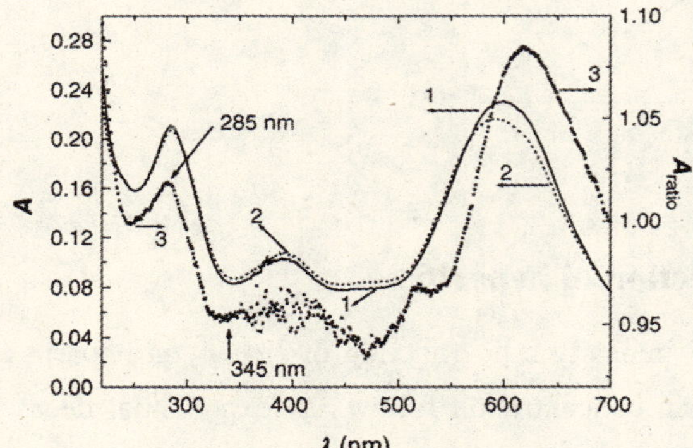

Fig. 2 The absorption spectrum of JGB (Curve 1) and its interaction with heparin (Curve 2) against buffer solution. The square scatters show the ratio spectra of absorbance at each corresponding wavelength. pH 7.96; c_{Hep}=1000 ng·mL^{-1}; c_{JGB} =1.0 × 10^{-5} mol·L^{-1}.

4.6.3.2 Flexibility of ratiometric method

Fig. 3 shows the dependence of RLS intensity ratio function of I_{285}/I_{345} and absorbance ratio functions of

A_{285}/A_{345} on pH-values of the medium. It could be seen that the ratio data show superior flexibility to pH variation compared to the enhanced RLS signals at a single wavelength. Over the wide pH ranges of 2.0～9.9 and 5.0～8.0, the ratios of I_{285}/I_{345} and A_{285}/A_{345} remain constant while the enhanced RLS intensities at a single wavelength remain constant only in the range of 7.0～9.9. On the other hand, the concentration of JGB has strong effects on the RLS ratio. Fig. 4 shows that the RLS intensities at 314 nm are constant when JGB varies over the range of 0.8～1.2×10^{-5} mol·L^{-1}, and the intensities then drop down out of this JGB concentration range. The absorbance ratios, however, get increased with increasing JGB concentration until 3.0×10^{-5} mol·L^{-1} in the aqueous medium, and then keep stable. It is obviously that the different dependence of RLS intensities and absorbance ratio on the JGB concentration could be applied for different purposes according to reality.

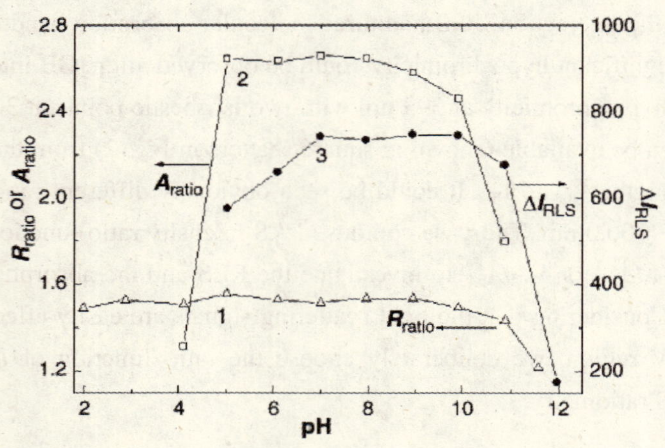

Fig. 3 The effect of pH on dual-wavelength RLS ratio (Curve 1, triangle), absorbance ratio (Curve 2, open square) and single wavelength RLS intensity (Curve 3, sold circle, λ = 314 nm). c_{Hep} = 500 ng·mL^{-1}, c_{JGB} =1.0 x 10^{-5} mol·L^{-1}.

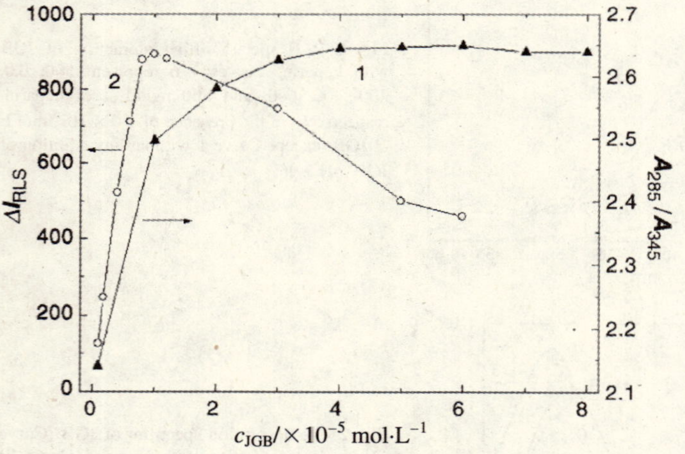

Fig. 4 Comparison of the effect of JGB concentration on absorbance ratio (Line 1) and single wavelength RLS intensity (Line 2, λ = 314 nm). c_{Hep} = 500 ng·mL^{-1}; pH 7.96.

4.6.3.3 Wide dynamic range detection of heparin

Fig. 5 shows the dependence of the RLS intensity ratio function of I_{285}/I_{345} on heparin concentration. The relationship between the RLS ratios and heparin concentration follows an exponential decay depending on the concentration of JGB. For 1.0×10^{-5} mol l^{-1} JGB, typically, the decay displays a dynamic range of 0.3 to 2000.0 ng·ml^{-1}. The inserted drawings show that the ratios are proportional to the logarithm of heparin content with good correlation coefficient. It could be seen from the figure that values of the $_{Ratio}$ tend to be larger with increasing JGB concentration.

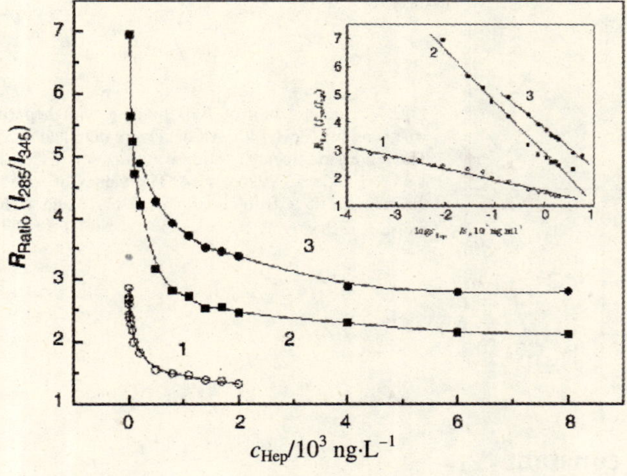

Fig. 5 RLS intensity ratio of I_{285}/I_{345} as a function of heparin concentration. pH 7.96. The inserted drawings show the relative RLS intensity ratio, I_{285}/I_{345}, as a function of the logarithm of heparin concentration of (10^3ng·mL^{-1}). Linear regression equations could be obtained at different JGB concentration: I_{285}/I_{345} =1.50~0.41 log c_{Hep} for 1.0 × 10^{-5} mol·L^{-1} JGB in the range of 0.3~2000 ng ml^{-1} heparin with the correlation coefficient *(r)* being -0.9866 (Curve 1), I_{285}/I_{345} =3.07~1.67 log c_{Hep} for 3.0 × 10^{-5} mol·L^{-1} JGB in the range of9.0~4000 ng·mL^{-1} with *r* = -0.9898 (Curve 2), andI_{285}/I_{345} = 3.81~1.46 log c_{Hep} for 4.0 × 10^{-5} mol·L^{-1} JGB in the range of 200.0~6000.0 ng·mL^{-1} with *r* = -0.9958 (Curve 3).

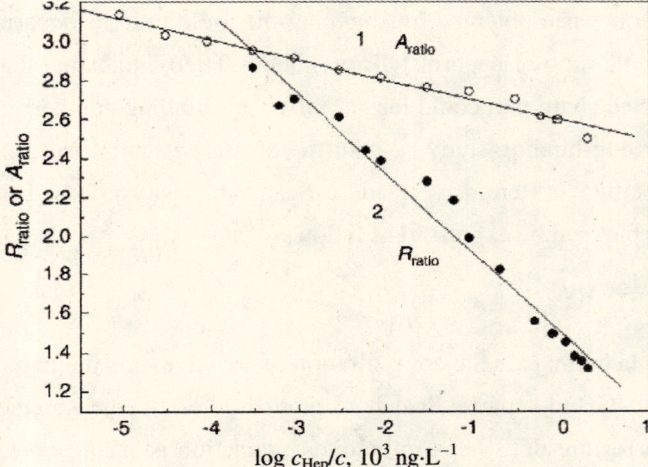

Fig. 6 Comparisons of the dependence of R_{ratio} and A_{ratio} on heparin concentration. c_{JGB} =1.0 × 10^{-5} mol·L^{-1}, pH 7.96. The values of A_{ratio} (Curves 1) and *I*ratio (Curves 2) were given as a function of the logarithm of heparin concentration (10^3 ng·mL^{-1}). Linear regression equations: Aratio=2.59–0.10 log*c* (*r* = -0.9875, Curves 1), I_{ratio} =1.50~0.41log *c*(*r* = -0.9866, Curves 2) in the range of 0.009~2000.0 and 0.3~2000.0 ng·mL^{-1}, respectively.

Compared to 5, Fig. 6 shows the relationships of A_{285}/A_{345} versus heparin concentration,, and an equation of *A*ratio = 2.59~0.10 log *c*(*r* = -0.9875) could be established over the heparin concentration range of 0.01~2000.0 ng ml^{-1}.

These two linear relationships provide the quantitative basis using both ratios of RLS and absorbance at 285 nm versus 345 nm. Compared with the RLS ratiometric method, the limit of determination of absorbance ratiometry was much lower (Table 1).

As to the RLS method at a single wavelength, the correlation was certified between the enhanced RLS in-ten-sity ($\triangle I_{RLS}$) and heparin concentration. At the maximum RLS wavelength 314 nm, $\triangle I_{RLS}$ has linear relationship with heparin content in the ranges of 100.0~1000.0 ng·mL^{-1}, 200.0~1000.0, 100.0~1000.0 ng·mL^{-1} when JGB concentrations were 1.0×10^{-5}, 3.0×10^{-5}, 4.0×10^{-5} mol·L^{-1}, respec-tively, and the corresponding detected limits were 8.87, 15.59, 22.13 ng·mL^{-1} in turn. It could be seen that above both ratiometric methods show superior analytical characteristics than RLS method at a single wavelength in terms of the dynamic range, and limits of determination.

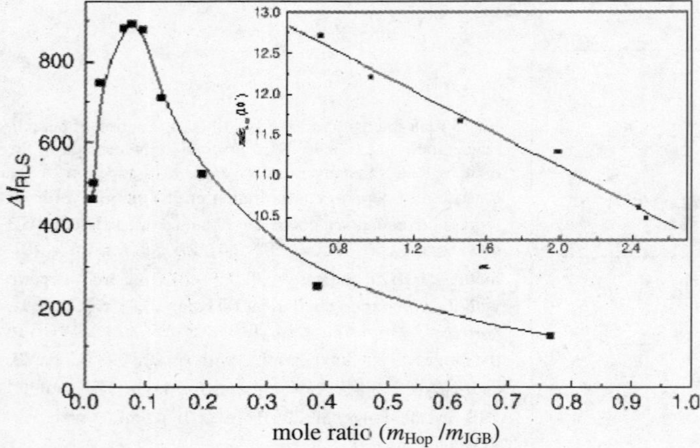

Fig. 7 Scatchard plot of JGB binding with heparin. c_{Hep} =1000 ng ml^{-1}. pH 7.96. All data were obtained at 314 nm. The regression linear equation was m/c_{JGB} =-1.15 × 10^5 m+ 1.34 × 10^6 (r =-0.9926, n= 6). The values of n and K for the reaction of JGB to heparin were 11.74 and 1.15 × 10^5 mol·L^{-1}, respectively.

4.6.3.4 Binding number and binding constant

Fig. 7 shows the binding number of JBG with heparin obtained by changing the mole ratio of heparin and JGB at 7.96. ΔI_{RLS} reaches a maximum when the mole ratio of heparin/JGB was about 0.076, indicating that one heparin could bind about 13 JGB molecules. Using Scatchard plot could further prove this binding number.

Scatchard plot has been widely employed for dug binding study [37], but the data are usually based on the measurements of absorbance or fluorescence intensity [37]. Herein we made a Scatchard analysis based on the measurement of RLS data. Generally, the Scatchard plot can be expressed as fellows [37]:

$$\frac{m}{c_f} = nK - mK$$

Where m is the mole ratio of the bound dye to heparin, c_f is the concentration of free dye; n is the maximum value of m, and K is the intrinsic binding constant of JGB to heparin. Scatchard plot based on the measurement of RLS data shows that the linear regression equation for this JGB-heparin binding interaction is $m/c_{JGB} = -1.15\times 10^5\, m + 1.34\times 10^6$ ($r = -0.9926$, n= 6). So we could deduce that the values of n and K for the interaction of JGB to heparin are 11.74 and 1.15×10^5 mol·L^{-1}, respectively. The n-value of 11.74 is close to the 13 obtained by the mole ratio variation method.

Table 1 Analytical parameters of RLS method at single wavelength, RLS and absorbance ratiometric methods

c_{JGB} (10^{-5} mol·L^{-1})	Method	Linear range (ng·mL^{-1})	Linear regression equations(c, ng·mL^{-1})	r	LOD (3σ, ng·L^{-1})
1.0	RLS*.	100.0～1000.0	ΔI =−2.87 + 0.88 c	0.9978	8.87
	R_{ratio}	0.3～2000.0	Iratio = 2.73−0.41 log c	−0.9866	0.03
	A_{ratio}	0.01～2000 0	Aratio = 2.59−0.10 log c	−0.9900	0.001
3.0	RLS	200.0～1000.0	ΔI =−41.62 + 0.48c	0.9988	15.59
	R_{ratio}	9.0～4000.0	Iratio = 8.43−1.83 log c	−0.9898	0.90
4.0	RLS	100.0～1000.0	ΔI =−22.97 + 0.38c	0.9981	22.13
	R_{ratio}	200.0～6000.0	Iratio = 8.18−1.46 log c	−0.9958	20.00

RLS method was made at 314 nm, and R_{ratio} and A_{ratio} were made at 285 nm and 345 nm, respectively. pH 7.96.

4.6.3.5 Nature of JGB and heparin interaction

The enhanced RLS signals of JGB induced by heparin are due to the large particles produced in the interaction[3～4]. These processes could be monitored by photo correlation spectroscopy (Fig. 8) and the RLS imaging detections (Fig. 9) to capture the size changes of micro-particles in the interacting system. These size distributions of micro particles in Fig. 8 were calculated using a Size Distribution Profile Deconvolution Algorithm. Fig. 8 shows that there are always two kinds of particles existed at any heparin concentration in the system we investigated. The upper and the lower part of Fig. 8 represent the changes of the small and the large particles, separately, with increasing heparin concentration.

With adding heparin into JGB solutions, interactions between JGB and heparin are developed through static attractions. The right and left of the diagonal columns in Fig. 8 present the sizes of certain sort of particles and their contributions to the total intensity of RLS, respectively. When JGB concentration was 1.0×10^{-5} mol·L^{-1}, and the heparin content was 100, 300, and 500 ng·mL^{-1}, respectively, the particles of small one decrease from 248.1 to 177.1 and 161.8 nm, while the particles of large one changes from 2913.4 to 1692.9, 1363.6 nm. From the Fig. 8, we could see that the small size particles in the presence of 1.0 μg·mL^{-1} heparin concentration made a contribution of 48% to the enhanced RLS signals.

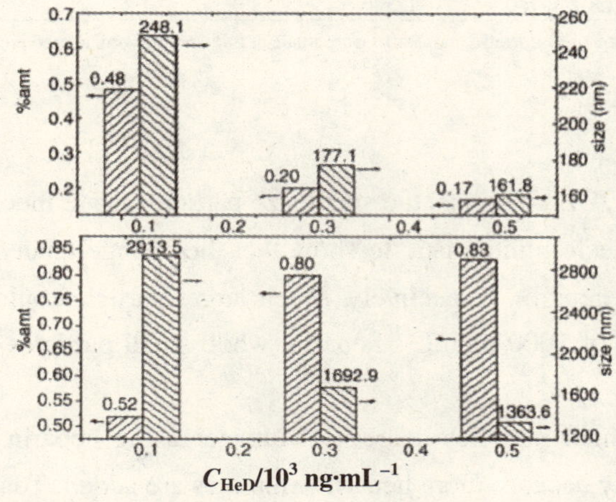

Fig. 8. Size distribution of JGB-heparin complex in the presence of different heparin concentration. There are always two kinds of particles exists at any heparin concentration, the upper part represents the small one and the lower part represents the larger one. The size distribution of micro particles is calculated by using a Size Distribution Profile Deconvolution Algorithm. %amt presents the attribution of particles with certain size to the total RLS intensity. JGB, 1.0×10^{-5} mol·L^{-1}, pH 7.96, temperature 20.0 °C, equilibration time, 5.0 min.

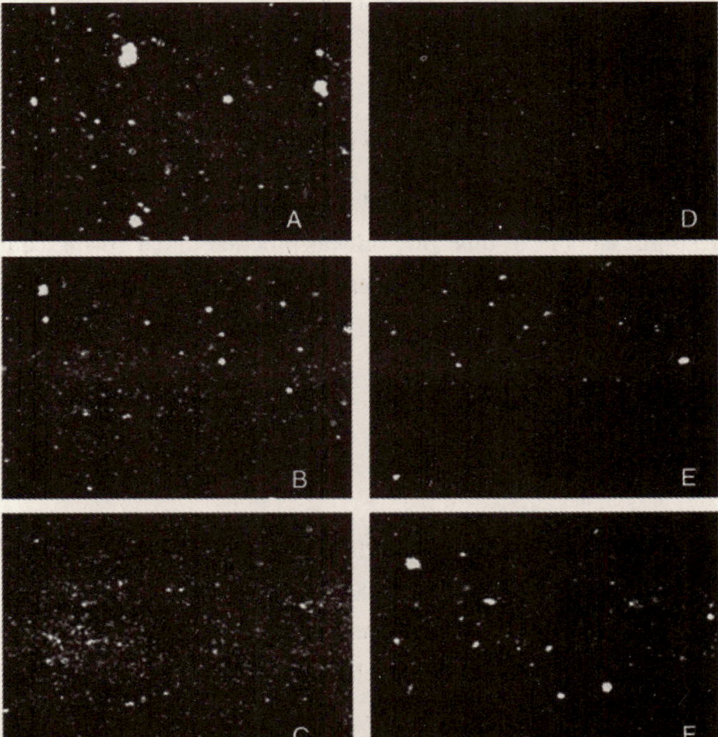

Fig. 9 Images of JGB-heparin micro particles formed at different heparin and JGB concentrations. Images of A, B, and C represent the images of micro particles at different heparin concentrations while JGB was kept as 1.0×10^{-5} mol·L^{-1}. The heparin concentrations were 100 ng·mL^{-1} (A), 300 ng·mL^{-1} (B), and 500 ng·mL^{-1} (C), respectively. Images of D, E, and F represent the images of micro particles at different JGB concentrations while heparin was kept as 50 ng·mL^{-1}. The JGB concentrations were 1.0×10^{-5} mol·L^{-1} (D), 3.0×10^{-5} mol·L^{-1} (E), 4.0×10^{-5} mol·L^{-1} (F), respectively. pH 7.96. The sub-frame area used for counts is 300 × 240 pixels (ca. 0.02 cm^2). Threshold, 30; rank filters, 3.

Table 2 Results for the determinations of heparin in heparin sodium injection

c_{JGB} (10^{-5} mol·L^{-1})	Method	Heparin found (IU 2mL^{-1})	Aver. (IU 2ml^{-1})	R.S.D. (%, n=4)
1.0	RLS[a]	12920 13100 12230 12490[b]	12685	3.1
		12990 12120 12580 12350[c]	12510	3.0
	R_{ratio}	12320 12650 12735 12890[b]	12648	1.9
		12490 12850 12960 12580[c]	12762	1.6
	A_{ratio}	12470 12660 12770 12530[b]	12608	1.1
		12410 12530 12860 12610[c]	12603	1.5
3.0	RLS	12150 12510 12740 12830[b]	12558	2.4
		12540 12730 12100 12840[c]	12553	2.6
	R_{ratio}	12690 12880 12470 12940[b]	12745	1.6
		12730 13010 12590 12610[c]	12735	1.5
4.0	RLS	12380 12880 12570 12940[b]	12693	2.1
		12150 12510 12740 12830[c]	12558	2.4
	R_{ratio}	12340 12690 12740 12630[b]	12600	1.4
		12440 12350 12810 12760[c]	12590	1.8

[a] Heparin specified (IU 2mL^{-1}), 12500. RLS method was made at 314 nm. *R*ratio and *A*ratio were made at 285 and 345 nm, respectively. pH 7.96.

[b] Xuzhou Wanbang Biochemical Pharmaceutical Factory, China.

[c] Tianjin Biochemical Pharmaceutical Co. Ltd., China.

Along with the increase of heparin content in JGB solutions, the small size particles made much smaller contribution to the enhanced RLS signals. Fig. 9 is much intuitionistic to show that the change tendency of particle size with the concentration variations of JGB and heparin, respectively. Much larger particle could be observed with increasing JGB concentration in the presence of 1000 ng·mL^{-1} heparin, while small particles get increased with increasing heparin content.

Although the sizes of both large and small particles decrease with increasing heparin concentration, the number of the bound particles increased rapidly because more heparin templates are added. That supplies the basis of the positive correlation between R_{ratio} values and the concentration of heparin. For this reason, quantitative detection method could be established.

4.6.3.6 Determination of heparin in heparin sodium injection samples

A 0.1 portion of heparin sodium injection was pipetted into a calibrated into a 1000 mL calibrated flask and was diluted to the mark with water. A 1.25 mL amount of this solution was pipetted into a 10-mL calibrated tube. The following procedure is the same as above. The results and recoveries were listed in Table 2. It could be seen that the RSD values of the ratiometric methods are lower than that of RLS methods at a single wavelength, thus the repeatability using ratiometric methods are got improved.

4.6.4 Conclusions

A dual wavelength ratiometric method herein is discussed and it provides a new generic approach, enlarging the applications of RLS and absorption methods. The analytical results of above data show that the advantages of the ratiometric methods seem obvious. At first, and the sensitivity and repeatability are much better than that of RLS method at a single wavelength. Secondly, not only does this dual-wavelength ratiometric method extend the linear relationship between the RLS and absorption ratios and the logarithm of heparin concentration but also it does not require imposing a strict control on the stability of the signals. Thirdly, the RLS ratiometric method allows the measurement of changes in the ratio of the RLS intensities at two wavelengths, and has become one answer to the problems posed by the former single-intensity measurement, and provided more precise measurement to normalize variation in path length, pH, dye concentration, etc. With some probes, larger extent quantitative detection is possible. These results indicate that the wavelengthdependent ratiometric method could be a new generic approach to enlarge the applications of RLS and absorption spectroscopy in biological, biomedical, environmental fields and would also be a useful way to deal with data so as to get more reliable information.

Due to the introduction of PCS measurements, certain correlations were found between the sizes of particles in solution and RLS ratiometric values. In general, existence of bigger particles could result in lager R_{ratio} values. For further research, we could take advantages of the potential simplicity of wavelength ratiometry to make a related device into reality by employing filters and fibers.

Acknowledgements

All authors herein are grateful to the supports from the National Natural Science Foundation of China (NSFC, No. 20425517, No. 20275032), the Program for New Century Excellent Talents in University (NCET-04-0852) and Chun Hui Program (No: [2004] 7-24) directed under the Ministry of Education of PRC, and the Municipal Science and Technology Committee of Chongqing.

Appendix A. Supplementary data

Supplementary data associated with this article can be found, in the online version, at doi:10.1016/j.aca.2005.07.062.

References

[1] M. Andersson, B. Wittgren, K.G. Wahlund, Anal. Chem. 73 (2001) 4852.
[2] A. Yethiraj, A. van Blaaderen, Nature 421 (2003) 513.
[3] R.F. Pasternack, C. Buatamante, P.J. Collings, A. Giannetto, E.J. Gibbs, J. Am. Chem. Soc. 115 (1993) 5393.
[4] R.F. Pasternack, P.J. Collings, Science 269 (1995) 935.
[5] R.F. Pasternack, J.I. Goldsimth, S. Szep, E.J. Gibbs, Biophys. J. 75 (1998) 1024.
[6] J.M. Ribo, J. Crusats, F. Sagues, J. Claret, R. Rubires, Science 292 (2001) 2063.
[7] C.Z. Huang, K.A. Li, S.Y. Tong, Anal. Chem. 68 (1996) 2259.
[8] C.Z. Huang, K.A. Li, S.Y. Tong, Anal. Chem. 69 (1997) 514.
[9] B.S. Liu, H.Y. Zhang, H.L. Zhang, Y. Zhao, Spectrosc. Spect. Anal. 23 (2002) 229.
[10] L.J. Dong, J. He, Q.F. Li, X.G. Chen, Z.D. Hu, Anal. Biochem. 315 (2003) 22.
[11] P. Feng, Y.F. Li, C.Z. Huang, Anal. Biochem. 308 (2002) 83.
[12] Z.L. Jiang, S.P. Liu, B.G. Zhao, S. Chen, J.A. Li, Spectrosc. Spect. Anal. 22 (2002) 615.
[13] P. Feng, W.Q. Shu, C.Z. Huang, Y.F. Li, Anal. Chem. 73 (2001) 4307.
[14] J. Yguerabide, E.E. Yguerabide, Anal Biochem. 262 (137) (1998) 157.
[15] P. Bao, A.G. Frutos, C. Greef, J. Lahiri, U. Muller, T.C. Peterson, L. Warden, X. Xie, Anal. Chem. 74 (2002) 1792.
[16] J. Yguerabide, E.E. Yguerabide, G. Bee, K. Yamout, L. Korb, J. Beck, T. Peterson, Nat. Genet. 23 (1999) 67.
[17] G. Crynkiewicz, M. Poenie, R. Tsien, Biol. Chem. 260 (1985) 3440.
[18] H. Xu, J.W. Aylott, R. Kopelman, T.J. Miller, M.A. Philbert, Anal. Chem. 73 (2001) 4124.
[19] T. Awaji, A. Hirasawa, H. Shirakawa, G. Tsujimoto, S. Miyazaki, Biochem. Biophys. Res. Commun. 289 (2001) 457.
[20] R.H. Yang, K.A. Li, K.M. Wang, F.L. Zhao, N. Li, F. Liu, Anal. Chem. 75 (2003) 612.
[21] X.D. Ge, L. Tolosa, G. Rao, Anal. Chem. 76 (2004) 1403.

[22] J. Ueberfeld, D.R. Walt, Reversible Anal. Chem. 76 (2004) 947.
[23] W. Tan, Z.Y. Shi, S. Smith, D. Birnbaum, R. Kopelman, Science 258 (1992) 778.
[24] H.A. Godwin, J.M. Berg, J. Am. Chem. Soc. 118 (1996) 6514.
[25] Z. Xu, A. Rollins, R. Alcaca, R.E. Marchant, J. Biomed. Mater. Res. 39 (1998) 9.
[26] A. Song, S. Parus, R. Kopelman, Anal. Chem. 69 (1997) 863–867.
[27] S. Deo, H.A. Godwin, J. Am. Chem. Soc. 122 (2000) 174.
[28] Y. Kawanishi, K. Kikuchi, H. Takakusa, S. Hizukami, Y. Urano, T.
[29] Higuchi, T. Nagano, Angew. Chem. Int. Ed. 39 (2000) 3438.
[30] G.J. Mohr, I. Klimant, U.K. Spichiger, O.S. Wolfbeis, Anal. Chem. 73 (2001) 1053.
[31] J.V. Mello, N.S. Finney, Angew. Chem. Int. Ed. 40 (2001) 1536.
[32] H.Q. Luo, S.P. Liu, Z.F. Liu, Q. Liu, N.B. Li, Anal. Chim. Acta 449 (2001) 261.
[33] I. Nemcova, P. Rychlovsky, M. Havelcova, M. Brabcova, Anal. Chim. Acta 401 (1999) 223.
[34] R. Malsch, J. Harenberg, C. Piazodo, G. Huhle, D.L. Heene, J. Chromatogr. B 685 (1996) 223.
[35] T. Hidenao, N. Tomoyo, H. Rerko, T. Toshihiko, I. Toshio, J. Chromatogr. B 704 (1997) 19.
[36] S.H. Ma, V.C. Yang, M.E. Meyerhoff, Anal. Chem. 64 (1992) 694.
[37] C.Z. Huang, Y. Liu, Y.H. Wang, H.P. Guo, Anal. Biochem. 321 (2003) 236.
[38] K.G. Strothkamp, R.E. Strothkamp, J. Chem. Educ. 71 (1994) 77.

(Yi Juan Long, Yuan Fang Li, Cheng Zhi Huang, published in *Analytica Chimica Acta*, 2005, 552, 175～181)

4.7 A resonance Light Scattering Ratiometry Applied for Binding Study of Organic Small Molecules with Biopolymer

Abstract: Resonance light scattering (RLS) technique is a creative application of light scattering signals detected by using a common spectrofluorometer, but it has drawbacks such as the fluctuation of signals caused by poorly quantified or variable factors. Herein we develop a RLS ratiometry to overcome the drawbacks of the technique and apply to measure the binding nature of organic small molecules (OSM) with biopolymer using the binding of cation porphyrins with heparin (HP) as an example. In near neutral solution, cationic porphyrins *meso*-tetrakis [(trimethylammoniumyl) phenyl] porphyrin (TAPP) and *meso*-tetra (4-methylpyridy) porphyrin (TMPyP-4) interact with heparin, resulting in hypochromatic effect, and enhanced RLS signals. Linear relationship could be established between the ratio of enhanced RLS signals at two wavelengths, where the maximum and minimum are available in the ratio curve of UV–vis spectrum of porphyrin to that of heparin –porphyrin complex, and the logarithm of heparin concentration, and thus a wide dynamic range detection method of biopolymers could be developed. In comparison with RLS method, this RLS ratiometric one is less affected by environmental conditions such as pH, ionic strength. The mechanism of these interactions was investigated based on the charge density distribution of the two porphyrin molecules and it could be concluded that the enhanced RLS intensity is proportionally promoted by the charge capacity of components in the complex. Additionally, the binding number and binding constant were measured scientifically by Scatchard plot.

Keywords: Resonance light scattering ratiometry; Organic small molecules (OSM); Biopolymers

4.7.1 Introduction

Binding study of organic small molecules (OSM) with biopolymers is very important in elucidating the nature of drugtargeted biomolecules [1,2]. In order to obtain the binding information in terms of kinetics and binding affinities, techniques such as X-ray diffraction, NMR spectroscopy, circular dichromism, ultraviolet–vis (UV–vis) molecular absorption and fluorescence spectroscopy have been traditionally available [3~5]. It has proved that Resonance Raman (RR) spectroscopy with ultraviolet excitation radiation is a valuable method [4,5], and its increased sensitivity is a good example to show that light scattering signals could have been applied sensitively to tissue studies [1], in vivo cancer diagnosis [2], immunocytology application [3], and DNA hybridization [4]. Similar to the enhanced RR spectroscopy, resonance light scattering (RLS) technique is a newly developed tool by using a common spectrofluorometer to detect enhanced light scattering signals in the assemblies of π-stacking molecules[5,6]. This technique has the advantages of simple operation and high sensitivity, showing high promise in studies ofbiochemistry [7~11], pharmacology [12], and molecular biology [4]. In practical application, however, the RLS signals suffer from fluctuation caused by many poorly quantified or variable factors in solution such as the incident light intensity, reagent concentration, and environmental conditions in the medium including pH, ionic strength, temperature, polarity [13]. Thus, it is necessary to improve the technique to compensate for these defaults.

Here we develop a RLS ratiometry considering that ratiometry is a good method to solve the problems posed by singlewavelength measurement because the ratiometry could provide precise data by taking the intensity ratio at two suitable wavelengths [14~17]. For example, fluorescent ratiometry has been commonly utilized in sensing physiological pH, oxygen and metal ion in cells [17~21]. We find that the RLS ratiometry could differentiate the binding difference of two cation porphyrins, *meso*-tetrakis [(trimethylammoniumyl) phenyl] porphyrin (TAPP) and *meso*-tetra (4-methylpyridy) porphyrin (TMPyP-4), with biopolymer, heparin (HP), a kind of sugaramic polysaccharide, which has widely applied to prevent thrombosis of extracorporeal circuit and to mediate activation of the hemostatic system during surgery [22,23]. Based on charge density distribution of the two porphyrin molecules, we try to discuss the binding dependence on molecular structure. Such knowledge then makes it possible to do systematic structural modifications of the drug molecule to optimize the binding interaction.

4.7.2 Experimental

4.7.2.1 Materials and apparatus

Heparin (HP) solution was prepared by dissolving heparin sodium (160 $IU \cdot mg^{-1}$, Shanghai Chemical Reagent Plant, Shanghai, China) in water. HP working solution is 10 $\mu g \cdot mL^{-1}$ (about 6.7×10^{-7} $mol \cdot L^{-1}$ with an average molecular weight of 15,000). Commercially available *meso*-tetrakis [(trimethylammoniumyl) phenyl] porphyrin (TAPP) and *meso*-tetra (4-methylpyridy) porphyrin (TMPyP-4) were purchased from Aldrich (St. Lewis, WO, USA), and their working solutions were 2.1×10^{-5} and 1.0×10^{-4} $mol \cdot L^{-1}$, respectively. Britton–Robinson buffer was used in this experiment to control pH value. All other reagents were of analytical-reagent grade without further purification or pretreatment. Millipore purified water was used throughout.

Absorption spectra were measured on a Techcomp 8500 UV–vis spectrophotometer (Hong Kong, China). RLS spectra were measured on a Hitachi F-2500 spectrofluorometer (Tokyo, Japan) by scanning simultaneously the excitation and emission monochromators of the spectrofluorometer from violet to visible region. Both the excitation and emission slits were set at 5.0 nm. An S-10A digital pH meter (Xiaoshan Scientific Instruments Company, Zhejiang, China) was used to measure the pH values. The charge distributions ofporphyrins are calculated using the Hyperchem Pro 7.0 (Hypercube, USA) software in AM1 mode.

4.7.2.2 General procedure

A 1.0 mL of porphyrin solution, 1.0 mL of Britton–Robinson buffer and a serial of heparin solution were added to a 10 mL volumetric flask successively. The mixture was diluted to 10.0 mL with water and shaken thoroughly. RLS spectra were then measured on the F-2500 spectrofluorometer by simultaneously scanning the excitation and emission monochromators with same starting wavelength and same scanning velocity. The RLS ratios were obtained by dividing the RLS intensity at 442 nm with 418 nm for HP/TAPP system and that at 448 nm with 418 nm for HP/TMPyP-4 system

4.7.3 Results and discussion

4.7.3.1 Wavelength for ratiometric measurement

Titrated with HP, the molecular absorptions of both TAPP and TMPyP-4 undergo hypochromism without significant shift of maximum wavelength, simultaneously resulting in enhanced RLS signals characterized at 437 and 452 nm maximum and at 412 and 416 nm minimum, respectively (Fig. 1). The enhanced RLS signals result from the aggregations in an absorption medium when the excitation wavelength is close to the absorption band,

and could be given as following equation [5,6]:

$$I(90)=\frac{16\pi^2 a^6 n_{\text{med}}^4 I_0}{r^2\lambda_0^4}\left|\frac{m^2-1}{m^2+2}\right| \qquad m=\frac{(n_{\text{real}}+in_{\text{im}})}{n_{\text{med}}} \quad (1)$$

Wherein $I(90)$ is the light scattering intensity detected at the right angle to the incident light beam, a is the size of the aggregation species, n_{med} is the refractive index of the medium, I_0 is the intensity of the incident light beam, r is the distance between the aggregation species and the detector, λ_0 is the wavelength of the incident light beam, and m is a complex index involving in the molecular absorption and the medium environments. There always is a wavelength (λ) which is close to λ_0 that makes the denominator m^2+2 in Eq. (1) equals zero, and leads up to strong enhanced values of $I\ (90)$.

It is well known that visible colors and absorption spectra of chromophores are the consequence of incident light through absorption and scattering [17], and enhanced RLS signals are strongly dependent on the absorption of aggregates [5,6]. Thus, it is necessary to simultaneously consider the molecular absorption and light scattering features in order to choose appropriate wavelengths for the light scattering ratiometric measurements. Our strategy is selecting the wavelengths at the peak and the valley of UV–vis spectral ratio curve, which couldbe obtainedby dividing UV–vis spectrum of the chromophoric component with that in the presence of the additives. Experiments showed that $\lambda_{\max}$ and $\lambda_{\min}$ in UV–vis ratio spectra are 418 and 442 nm for HP/TAPP system, and 418 and 448 nm for HP/TMPyP-4 system, respectively (Fig. 2). The wavelength of $\lambda_{\max}$ 418 nm in HP/TAPP system corresponds to the 412 nm minimum region of RLS spectrum, while that of $\lambda_{\min}$ 442 nm does to the 437 nm peak in RLS spectrum (Fig. 1). Similar phenomenon could be found for HP/TMPyP-4 system. From those features, it could confirm that the $\lambda_{\max}$ and $\lambda_{\min}$ in UV–vis ratio curve are of paramount importance related to RLS signals. Thus we choose the RLS ratio of $I(\lambda_{\min})/I\ (\lambda_{\max})$ for RLS ratiometric measurements.

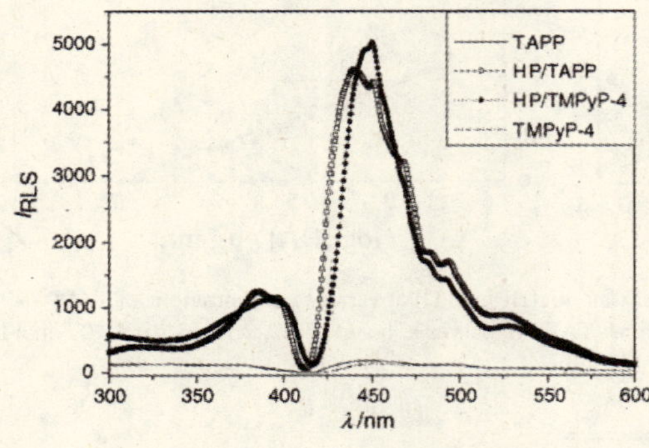

Fig. 1 Enhanced RLS signals of TAPP and TMPyP-4 by HP. c_{TAPP}, 4.2×10^{-6} mol·L^{-1}; $c_{\text{TMPyP-4}}$, 1.0×10^{-5} mol·L^{-1}; HP, 1.5 mg·mL^{-1}; pH, 7.2.

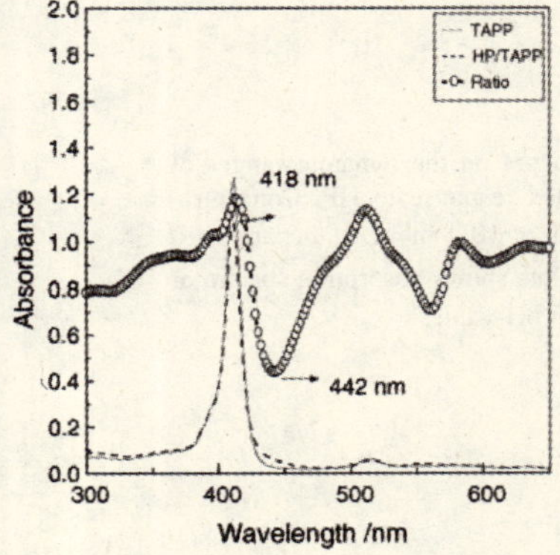

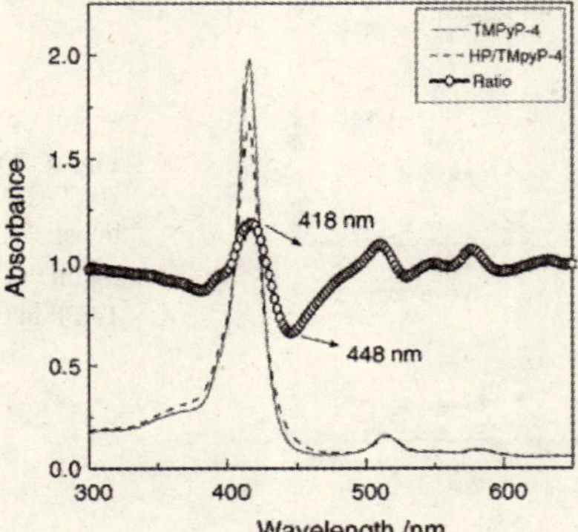

Fig. 2 Absorption spectra of TAPP, TMPyP-4 and their complexes with heparin. Dotted line with open circles represents the ratio of the absorption spectra of porphyrin to that of heparin–porphyrin complex. Concentrations: TAPP, 2.1×10^{-6} mol·L^{-1}; TMPyP-4, 1.0×10^{-5} mol·L^{-1}; Heparin, 0.2 μg·mL^{-1}; pH, 7.2.

4.7.3.2 Performance of heparin detection

It was found that RLS ratios decrease exponentially with HP concentration and have a perfect linear relationship with the logarithm of HP concentration in a wide range (Fig. 3). This constitutes the law to determine the binding extent between HP and porphyrins. By controlling the pH of the solution, different detection concentration ranges may be obtained (Fig. 4). At pH 1.8, the best detection range is from 0.01 to 3.2 μg·mL^{-1}. At pH 7.0 and 10.0, the detection range changes from 0.02 to 2.2 μg·mL^{-1}, respectively. In lower pH values, the higher acidic medium will lead to the protonation of nitrogen atom of TAPP molecule and TAPP form H_2TAPP^{2+} [7], which magnifies the binding capability of TAPP to HP. As shown in the inset plot of Fig. 4, the UV–vis spectrum of TAPP in pH 1.8 occurs to a red shift and hypochromism and has a shoulder in Soret band. This feature indicates that a change occurs in the form of TAPP, which is the reason why the detection range in pH 1.8 is magnified.

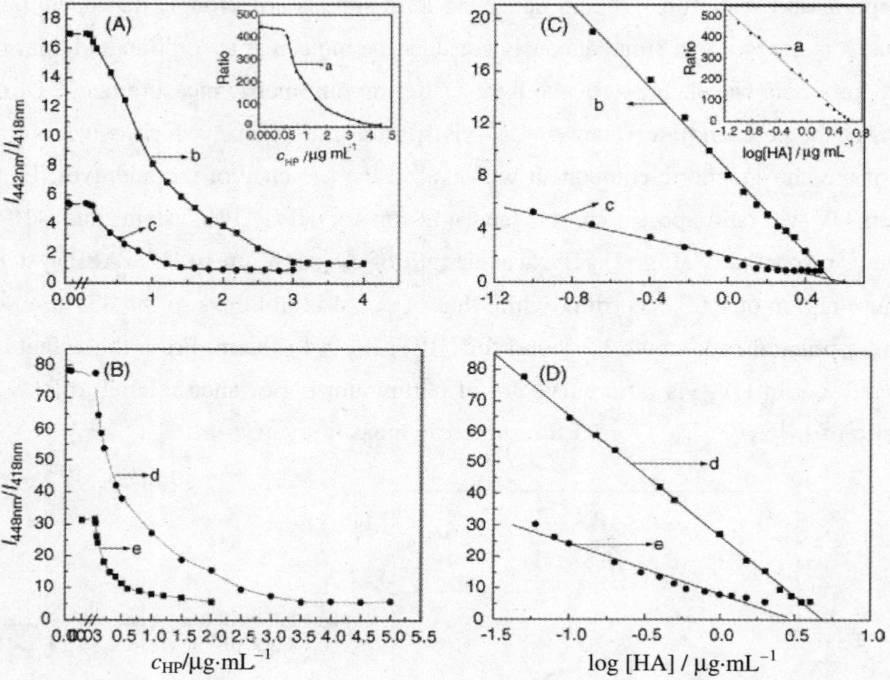

Fig. 3 Dependence of RLS ratios vs. HP concentration (A, B) and log[HP] (C, D) at various concentrations of TAPP (a, b and c in A and C) and TMPyP-4 (d and e in B and D). Concentrations: TAPP in curves a, b and c, 4.2, 2.1 and 1.0 × 10^{-6} mol·L^{-1}, respectively; TMPyP-4 in curves d and e, 1.0 and 0.8 × 10^{-5} mol·L^{-1}; pH, 7.2.

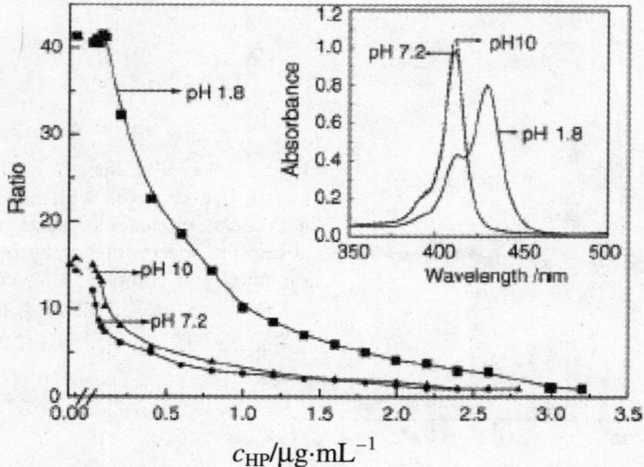

Fig. 4 Effects of pH on the dynamic ranges of HP/TAPP complex response to HP. Concentrations: TAPP, 2.1 × 10^{-6} mol·L^{-1}; heparin, 1.0 μg·mL^{-1}. Inset plots shows absorption spectra of TAPP in different pH-values.

Table 1 Results for the detection of heparin in the clinic injection solution by RLS ratiometric method

Sample number	Heparin specified (IU/2 mL)	Average (IU/2 mL) (n = 5)	R.S.D. (%) (n = 5)
011201[a]	12500	12712	1.73
010723[b]	12500	12657	1.45
020815[c]	12500	12469	1.54

Concentration: TAPP, 4.2×10^{-6} mol·L^{-1}; pH, 7.2.

[a] Xuzhou Wanbang Biochemical Pharmaceutical Factory of China.

[b] Changzhou Qianhong Biochemical Pharmaceutical Co. Ltd.

[c] Shanghai Biochemical Pharmaceutical Factory of China.

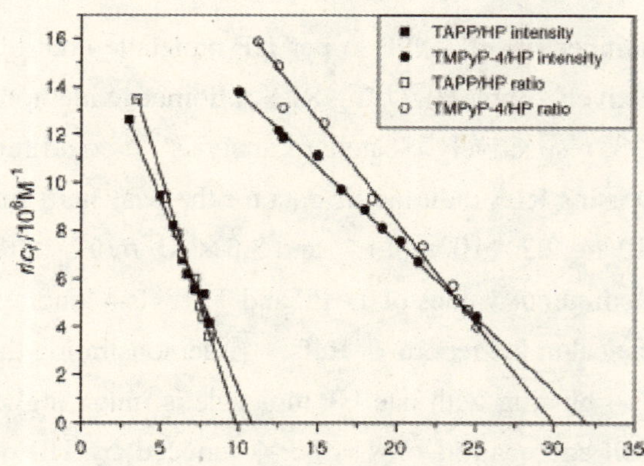

Fig. 5 Scatchard plots for the binding of TAPP and TMPyP-4 with heparin. Scatchard equations for HP/TAPP and HP/TMPyP-4 systems calculated by RLS intensity are $r/c_f = 1.6 \times 10^6$ (11.7 - r) (solid square) and $r/c_f = 6.2 \times 10^5$ (32.3 - r) (solid circle), while those calculated by RLS ratio are $r/c_f = 2.2 \times 10^6$ (9.7 - r) (open square) and $r/c_f = 8.5 \times 10^5$ (29.8 - r) (open circle). Titration of 2.67×10^{-7} mol·L^{-1} HP solutions was made with 0.20 ml aliquots of 5.0×10^{-6} mol·L^{-1} TAPP solution and aliquots of 1.0×10^{-4} mol·L^{-1} TMPyP-4 solution, respectively; pH, 7.2.

The effects of ionic strength on RLS ratio and RLS intensity were investigated in the range of 0.003～0.203 mol·L^{-1}. When the ionic strength gets increased from 0.003 to 0.113 mol·L^{-1}, the RLS ratios for HP/TAPP system remain consistent, and the ratios get increased beyond this range with increasing ionic strength. On the contrary, the RLS intensity of the system only remains constant when the ionic strength is lower than 0.053 mol·L^{-1}, and then decreases with increasing ionic strength. The same phenomenon was occurred in the HP/TMpyP-4 system. The constant and increasing RLS ratios with further ionic strength indicates that the ratiometric method has higher tolerance ability than RLS method has. On the other hand, the effect of ionic strength just on the complex means that the binding models of heparin and porphyrins are mainly ascribed to the electrostatic attraction since HP is highly negatively charged and the increasing Na^+ will compete with porphyrin to bind with HP [24,25].

To prove RLS ratiometric method feasible, clinic heparin sodium injections of three different trademarks were detected by the RLS ratiometric method. The clinic injections were just diluted without other pretreatments. The experimental results are listed in Table 1. The recoveries are in agreement with the results given by the manufactories at 95% confidence level. The RSD for the three samples (n = 5) is between 1.45% and 1.73%.

4.7.3.3 Mechanism of the interactions

Both TAPP and TMPyP-4 have the tendency to form stacking-type aggregation on biopolymer templates such as DNA [6,25]. Heparin is a highly negatively charged oligosaccharide with an average molecular weight of about 15,000 and an average charge of -70 [22]. The high negative charge of HP leads to strong repellence among the disaccharide units, and make it exist as a linear anionic polyelectrolyte [22]. In addition, one HP molecule contains 42 monosaccharide units and each tetrasaccharide unit has three O-sulfate groups, two N-sulfate groups, and two carboxyl groups [22], thus the total binding capacity per HP molecule is 73.5 in theory. Therefore, one HP molecule could theoretically bind with 18.4 porphyrin molecules in average through electrostatic attraction if taking the charges of one porphyrin molecule as +4.

Table 2 Average binding number of heparin with porphyrin calculated by RLS and RLS ratiometric method

Porphyrin	*c*porphyrin (10^{-6} mol·L^{-1})	RLS method		RLS ratiometric method	
		Linear range ($\times 10^{-7}$ mol·L^{-1})	*n*	Linear range ($\times 10^{-7}$ mol·L^{-1})	*n*
TAPP	4.2	0–3.33	14	0–4.0	10.5
	2.1	0–1.66	12.6	0–2.14	9.8
TMPyP-4	10	0–2.0	50	0–3.0	33.3
	8	0–2.1	48	0–2.42	33.1

n is the maximum binding number of heparin to porphyrin; pH, 7.2.

Using mole ratio variation method, the binding number *(n)* of TAPP to per HP molecule could be roughly calculated as 13 and that of TMPyP-4 to HP as 49, respectively (Table 2). Using RLS ratiometric method, however, the *n*-values of TAPP and TMPyP-4 to HP are 10 and 33, respectively. Scatchard analysis [26] could further prove the binding difference between HP and porphyrins. When using RLS radiometric data for the Scatchard analysis (Fig. 5), the binding constants of TAPP and TMPyP-4 with HP are 2.2×10^{6} mol·L^{-1} and 8.5×10^{5} mol·L^{-1}, respectively, with a binding affinity difference factor of 2.6, and the maximum *n*-values of TAPP and TMPyP-4 binding to per HP molecule are 10 and 30, respectively, which are much identical to the reports of Refs. [27], demonstrating that RLS ratiometry is much reliable. The *n*-value of 30 for TMPyP-4 binding with one HP molecule is much higher than the theoretical binding capacity of 18.4, indicating that self-aggregation of TMPyP-4 induced by HP occurs, and TMPyP-4 is highly stacked along the HP molecule. Thus, it is reasonable to deduce that hydrophobic interaction between TMPyP-4 molecules could exist in the presence of HP.

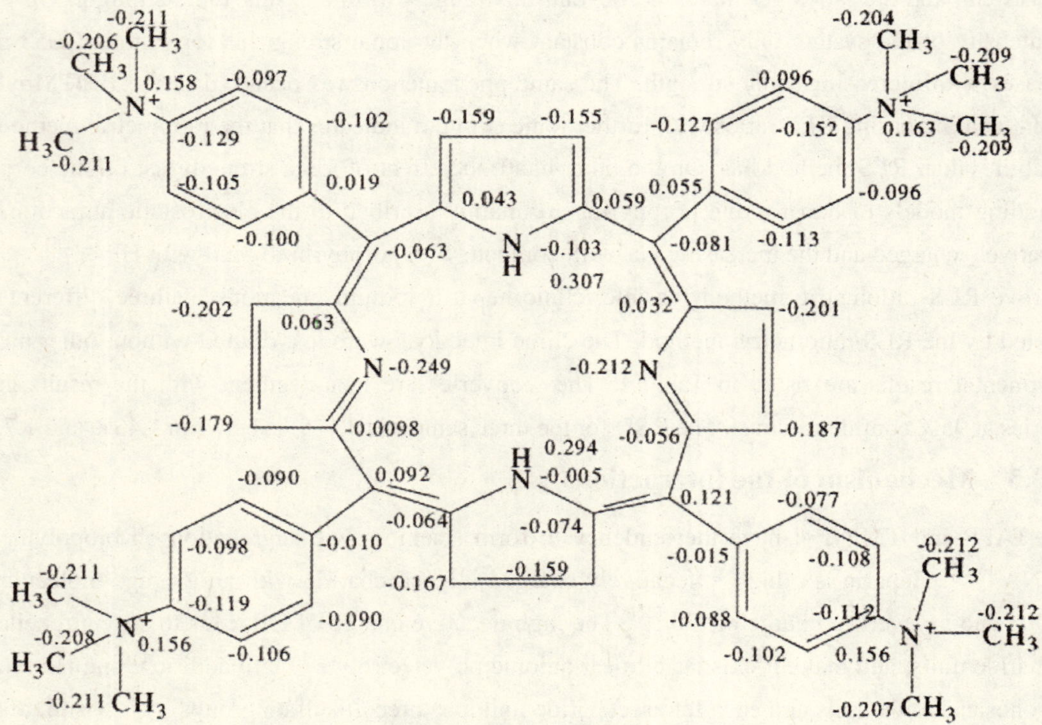

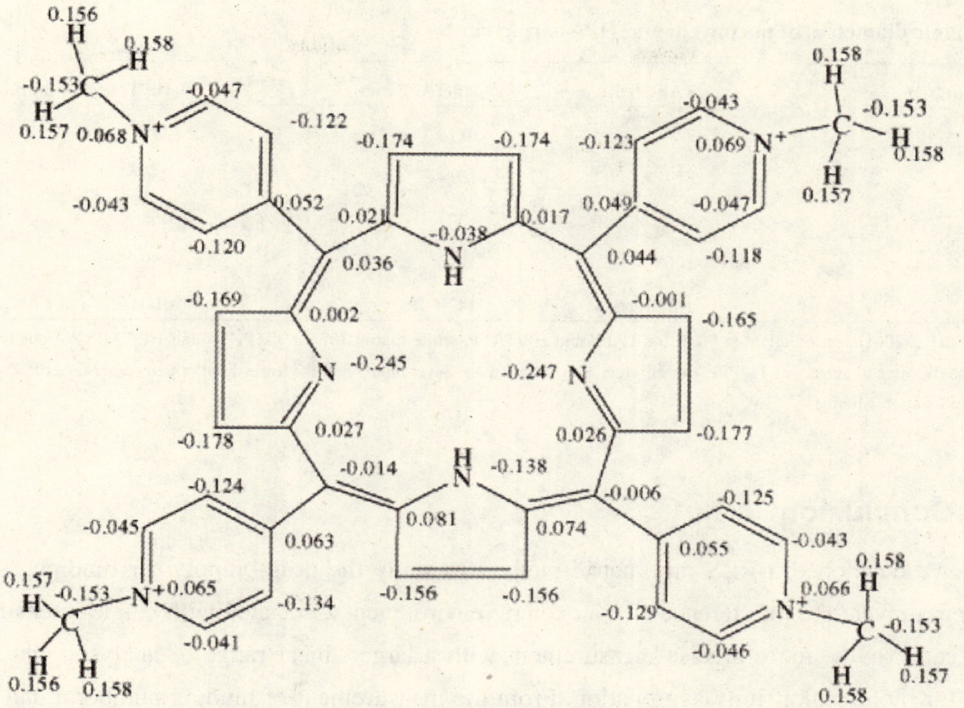

Fig. 6 Charge distribution of TAPP (top) and TMPyP-4 (bottom) calculated by the Hyperchem Pro 7.0 software in AM1 method.

As improved above, HP-porphyrin involves electrostatic attraction and hydrophobic affinity. When TAPP and TMPyP-4 of same concentration were mixed with heparin, the RLS intensity of HP/TAPP was much greater than that of HP/TMPyP-4. Therefore, TAPP has higher affinity than TMPyP-4 toward HP. This difference can be referred to the less net charge of TMPyP-4 than that of TAPP. Though two porphyrins have same cationic charge of four ammonium ions, the cationic charge of ammonium ions in TMpyP-4 is greatly lessened by the conjugative effect of pyridine. To enforce the conclusion, the charge distributions of TAPP and TMPyP-4 were calculated in AM1 mode using Hyperchem Pro 7.0 software (Fig. 6). The results show that the net charge of nitrogen atom in ammonium ions in TAPP molecule is +0.158 in average, while that in ammonium ions in TMPyP-4 molecule is +0.067 in average since the charge of ammonium ions in TMPyP-4 is greatly lessened by the conjugative effect of pyridine. The 2.4-fold net charge difference between the nitrogen atoms in ammonium ions of the two porphyrins is much close to the binding affinity difference factor of 2.6. Thus, it could deduce that the charge difference mainly decides the electrostatic attraction and hydrophobic affinity, which decides the size, shape of the HP –porphyrin complexes, and the HP –porphyrin complexes display enhanced RLS spectra.

Based on the measurements of photon correlation spectroscopy, the dynamic diameter of TAPP gets increased from 730 to 1075 nm in the range of $0.4\sim1.2\times10^{-5}$ mol·L^{-1}, and that of TMPyP-4 is smaller than 3 nm. Experiments have shown that TAPP is easier to induce a superhelical structure of DNA than TMPyP-4 does in aqueous medium due to its aggregation tendency [7], thus the values of TAPP diameters in Table 3 are perhaps referred to the molecular associates rather than single molecules, while the small diameters of TMPyP-4 samples and their weak scattering are the single-molecular signatures. Therefore, their bindings with HP then result in larger dynamic diameter, for example, with an increasing factor of 1.3 for TAPP (Table 3). The dynamic diameters get increased with porphyrin concentrations, indicating that aggregation ofporphyrin induced by HP really occurs. These data prove that the enhanced light scattering signals, which greatly dependent on the size and numbers of aggregate particles in medium [5,6], could differentiate the binding difference of porphyrins with biopolymers.

Table 3 Dynamic diameters of porphyrin and HP –porphyrin

$c_{porphyrin}$ (10^{-5} mol·L^{-1})	TAPP (nm)	HP/TAPP (nm)	HP/TMPyP-4 (nm)
0.4	729	917	298
0.6	829	1034	356
0.8	968	1324	468
1.0	1068	1416	580
1.2	1075	1420	1003

HP, 1.0 μg·mL^{-1}; pH, 7.20. Detection angle is 90.0° for TAPP and HP/TAPP, while that is 30° for TMPyP-4 and HP/TMPyP-4 due to their weak scattering signals at 90.0° The dynamic diameters of TMPyP-4 in different concentration are lower than 3 nm, the lower limit of detection range of N5 Submicon particle size analyzer (Beckman Coulter, Miami).

4.7.4 Conclusion

Herein, we developed a RLS ratiometric method to study the drug-biopolymer binding. The newly assay method can circumvent the interferences from exoteric environment associated with single-intensity measurement. The method can provide more precise measurement with a larger linear range of analysis, which is a good dynamic range for biological affinity aggregation. From the measurement of binding number n and investigation of reaction mechanism, it can conclude that the RLS ratiometric method is a new tool of dynamics to measure the extent of association reactions. The mechanism of the interacting system, heparin and porphyrins, demonstrated that the electrostatic attraction and hydrophobic affinity plays a dominant role in HP–porphyrin interaction and the enhancement of RLS intensity is proportionally promoted by the charge capacity of components in complex.

Acknowledgements

All authors herein are grateful to the supports from the National Natural Science Foundation of China (NSFC, no: 20425517), and the Municipal Science and Technology Committee of Chongqing.

References

[1] R.S. Gurjar, V. Backman, L.T. Perelman, I. Georgakoudi, K. Badizade-gan, I. Itzkan, R.R. Dasari, M.S. Feld, Nature 7(2001) 1245.

[2] V. Backman, R.S. Gurjar, K. Badizadegan, I. Itzkan, R.R. Dasari, L.T. Perelman, M.S. Feld, IEEE J. 5(1999) 1019.

[3] S. Schultz, D.R. Smith, J.J. Mock, D.A. Schultz, PNAS 97 (2000) 996.

[4] P. Bao, A.G. Frutos, C. Graat, J. Lahiri, U. Muller, T.C. Peterson, L. Warden, X. Xie, Anal. Chem. 74 (2002) 1792.

[5] R.F. Pasternack, P.J. Collings, Science 269 (1995) 935.

[6] R.F. Pasternack, C. Bustamante, P.J. Collings, A. Giannetto, E.J. Gibbs, J. Am. Chem. Soc. 115 (1993) 5393.

[7] C.Z. Huang, K.A. Li, S.Y. Tong, Anal. Chem. 68 (1996) 2259.

[8] H. Zhong, J.J. Xu, H.Y. Chen, Talanta 67 (2005) 749.

[9] R.P. Jia, H.L. Zhai, Y. Shen, X.G. Chen, Z.D. Hu, Talanta 64 (2004) 355.

[10] H. Zhong, N. Li, F.L. Zhao, K.A. Li, Talanta 62 (2004) 37.

[11] C.Z. Huang, K.A. Li, S.Y. Tong, Anal. Chem. 69 (1997) 514.

[12] P. Feng, W.Q. Shu, C.Z. Huang, Y.F. Li, Anal. Chem. 73 (2001) 4307.

[13] C.Z. Huang, Y.F. Li, Anal. Chim. Acta 500 (2003) 105.

[14] W. Tan, Z.Y. Shi, S. Smith, D. Birnbaum, R. Kopelman, Science 258 (1992) 778.

[15] S. Maruyama, K. Kikuchi, T. Hirano, Y. Urano, T. Nagano, J. Am. Chem. Soc. 124 (2002) 10650.

[16] D. Roll, J. Malicka, I. Gryczynski, Z. Gryczynski, J.R. Lakowicz, Anal. Chem. 75 (2003) 3108.

[17] J.R. Lakowicz, in: J.R. Lakowicz (Ed.), Topic in Fluorescence Spectroscopy, vol. IV, Plenum Press, New York, 1994, p. 3.

[18] S. Deo, H.A. Godwin, J. Am. Chem. Soc. 122 (2000) 174.

[19] R. Yang, K. Li, K. Wang, F. Zhao, N. Li, F. Liu, Anal. Chem. 75 (2003) 612.

[20] H. Xu, J.W. Aylott, R. Kopelman, T.J. Miller, M.A. Philbert, Anal. Chem. 73 (2001) 4124.

[21] E.J. Park, M. Brasuel, C. Behrend, M.A. Philbert, R. Kopelmon, Anal. Chem. 75 (2003) 3784.

[22] T. Katayama, E.I. Takai, R. Kariyama, Y. Kanemasa, Anal. Biochem. 88 (1978) 382.

[23] S. Mathison, E. Bakker, Anal. Chem. 71 (1999) 4614.

[24] S.C. Liu, F.Y. Zhou, M. Hook, D.D. Carson, PNAS 94 (1997) 1739.

[25] Q.C. Jiao, Q. Liu, C. Sun, H. He, Talanta 48 (1999) 1095.

[26] K.G. Strothkamp, R.E. Strothkamp, J. Chem. Educ. 71 (1994) 77.

[27] Y.J. Wei, A Ph.D. Dissertation of Peking University, Beijing, 1997.

(Cheng Zhi Huang, Xiao Bing Pang, Yuan Fang Li, Yi Juan Long, published in *Talanta*, 2006, 69, 180～186)

4.8 A Light Scattering and Fluorescence Emission Coupled Ratiometry Using the Interaction of Functional CdS Quantum Dots with Aminoglycoside Antibiotics as a Model System

Abstract: Any signals, if their intensities have simple functional relationship with analyte concentration, can be applied to analytical purposes. Rayleigh light scattering signals and fluorescence signals are twins in flurospectroscopy, so the light scattering signals are the major interference when the Stokes shift is small. Herein, we propose a light scattering and fluorescence emission (LS–FL) coupled ratiometry using CdS quantum dots (QDs) as a fluorescence probe to detect aminoglycoside antibiotics (AGs). As model analytes, AGs, when attached to the surface of CdS-QDs *via*electrostatic interaction in aqueous medium, result in strong enhanced light scattering (LS) emission characterized at 376 nm and fluorescence quenching of CdS-QDs at 500 nm. Thus, a ratiometry using the coexistent light scattering and fluorescent emission signals has been proposed. Based on the linear relationship between logarithm of light scattering and fluorescence emission ratio (R) and logarithm of AGs concentration, a novel assay of AGs is established with the limits of detection (3σ) being $58 \sim 190$ nmol·L^{-1}, and applied successfully to detect AGs injection and serum samples.

Keywords: Light scattering and fluorescence emission coupled ratiometry; CdS quantum dots (CdS-QDs); Aminoglycoside antibiotics

4.8.1 Introduction

Spectrofluorometry has shown a high promise in modern detection science. However, light scattering signals often coexist with fluorescence and act as interference roles, reducing the determination sensitivity in spectrofluorometry [1]. Efforts have been made to reduce the interference effects of light scattering emission such as low-temperature frozen and magnetic field-resolved techniques [2]. On the other hand, among the different ways of signal transduction for analytical applications, fluorescence signaling and light scattering signaling are of particular interest because they could offer the advantage of high sensitivity over the other employed signaling mechanisms [3~5]. However, those measurements employing fluorescence or light scattering signals are generally restricted in single-wavelength responses, which suffer from poorly quantified or variable factors such as the apparatus response, probes concentration, and environment around the probes (pH, polarity, temperature, and so forth) [1]. Dual-wavelength fluorescent ratiometry and dual-wavelength light scattering ratiometry, which allows the measurement of changes in the ratio of the fluorescence and lightscattering intensities at two wavelengths, respectively, have been one answer to the problems posed by the single-wavelength measurements [5~13]. These occur to us to make simultaneously use of fluorescence and light scattering emission signals in the hope of constructing a method holding the advantages of both fluorescence and light scattering techniques, for we believe it is a challenge area how to make simultaneously use of the fluorescence signaling and light scattering signaling for analytical purpose.

Considering that a obtained three-dimensional(3D) emission spectrum using a common spectrofluorometer could display the details of fluorescence and light scattering emissions simultaneously, herein, we measure the nature of the coexistence of fluorescence and light scattering emissions based on the interaction of quantum dots (QDs) with organic small molecules (OSMs), and then propose a light scattering–fluorescence emission (LS–FL) ratiometry, which allows measuring the ratio of enhanced scattering intensity at the excitation wavelength and fluorescence quenching at the emission wavelength.

Quantum dots (QDs) have attracted great interests because of quantum confinement and surface properties, the size-tuned absorption and emission spectra and achievable large Stokes shifts [14,15]. As fluorescence probes, QDs have been applied to the detection of biomacromolecules [16~18], metal ions [19], pharmaceuticals [20,21], and so on. Besides, as nanoparticles, QDs have unique light scattering signals, and they are likely to be used as effective light scattering emission probes just like golden nanoparticles, which could be used in microarrays RLS technique to detect DNA hybridization and proteins [22,23].

Aminoglycoside antibiotics (AGs), such as tobramycin (TOB), kanamycin (KANA), and gentamicin (GEN) are widely used in human and veterinary medicine against both Gram-positive and Gram-negative bacterial infections [24]. However, it is well known that they cause damage to the kidneys and cranial nerves [25]. Methods have been developed including microbiological assay [26], high performance liquid chromatography (HPLC) [27,28], immunoassay [29,30], resonance Rayleigh scattering (RRS) assay [31], and so forth. These methods, however, are limited due to the bad reproducibility, time-consuming, or the purity of the enzyme. Thus, in this work, we choose AGs as model analytes by making use of their interactions with our home prepared water soluble CdS-QDs capped with thio-glycolic acid. In the Britton-Robinson (BR) buffer at pH 5.02, AGs are adsorbed on the surface of CdS-QDs *via* electrostatic interaction to form much larger aggregation species, leading to strong enhanced light scattering signals and fluorescence quenching of CdS-QDs. Based on these properties, derivative equation for light scattering and fluorescence emission ratio has theoretically been drawn and actually identified for AGs detection.

4.8.2 Experimental

4.8.2.1 Apparatus

The fluorescence spectra and RLS spectra were obtained using a Hitachi F-4500 fluorescence spectrophotometer (Tokyo, Japan), while a N5PCS submicron particles size analyzer (Beckman coulter, Miami, USA) was used to detect the size of micro-particles in solution based on photo correlation spectroscopy (PCS). A pHS-3D digital pH meter (Leici, Shanghai, China) was used to adjust the pH values of the solutions, and an MVS-1 vortex mixer (Beide Scientific Instrumental Ltd., Beijing, China) was used to blend the solutions.

4.8.2.2 Materials

Typical aminoglycoside antibiotics (AGs) used in this study were purchased from Chongqing Institute of Pharmacology (Chongqing, China) including tobramycin (TOB), gentamicin (GEN) and kanamycin (KANA). Stock solutions of these AGs and $Cd(NO_3)_2$ (Tingxin Chemical Reagents Co., Shanghai), Na_2S (Shanghai Chemical Reagents Co., Shanghai), thioglycolic acid (TGA, Chengdu Kelong Chemical Reagents Co., Chengdu) were prepared by dissolving these commercial products into doubly distilled water. Working solutions of TOB,GEN and KANA were 42.9, 41.9 and 41.3 $\mu mol \cdot L^{-1}$, respectively, while that of $Cd(NO_3)_2$ and Na_2S were 0.1 $mol \cdot L^{-1}$. Britton-Robinson buffer solution (0.04 $mol \cdot L^{-1}$, pH 5.02) was used to control the acidity of the aqueous medium. All reagents used are of analytical grade without further purification. Water used throughout was doubly distilled.

Aqueous colloids of CdS solution were prepared according to previously published methods [32] using TGA as the stabilizing agent, and the preparation was starting with appropriate TGA to titrate a 2.0×10^{-4} mol·L^{-1} $Cd(NO_3)_2$ solution until 1:1 molar ratio of TGA:Cd^{2+}. After thoroughly mixing, the pH value of the mixture was adjusted about 6 by using 0.2 mol·L^{-1} NaOH solution, and then an appropriate volume of 0.1 mol·L^{-1} Na_2S was added with agitation until the S^{2-}/Cd^{2+} molar ratio of 0.7:1 in a final volume of 500ml. After thoroughly mixing, the mixture was incubated for 12 h at 0℃. The CdS-QDs made according to this procedure is about 4 nm [33], and has the fluorescence at 500 nm when excited at 376 nm.

4.8.2.3 Methods

In a dry 10-ml volumetric flask were added 0.10 ml of standard AGs or sample solution and 1.00 ml of above prepared CdS solution with different affluxes along the wall of the volumetric flask. The mixture was vortexed, and 1.0 ml of Britton-Robinson buffer solution was added. After diluted to 10-mL with water and mixed thoroughly, the mixture was transferred for light emission measurements. Three-dimensional (3D) spectra were made from 200 to 700 nm using the 3D function of the spectrofluorometer. The emission spectra were scanned over the range of 350～700 nm with the excitation wavelength at 376 nm, so that both the LS and FL signals could be simultaneously obtained in one scanning. RLS spectrum was obtained by simultaneously scanning the excitation and emission monochromators of the spectrofluorometer from 225 to 450 nm.

4.8.2.4 Pretreatment of samples

All the sulfate injections of TOB, GEN and KANA (commercially purchased from Southwest Pharmaceutical Industrial Ltd., Chongqing) were measured without special treatment except dilution with doubly distilled water.

Three human serums were sampled from the Hospital of Southwest University (Chongqing, China). A 2.0 mol·L^{-1} trichoroacetic acid solution was added to human serums to remove the proteins through high-speed centrifugation. The supernatant solution mixed with appropriate amount of AGs solution. The mixture was adjusted to weak acid medium with 0.2 mol·L^{-1} NaOH solution, and then diluted to 100-fold with doubly distilled water before being transferred for detection.

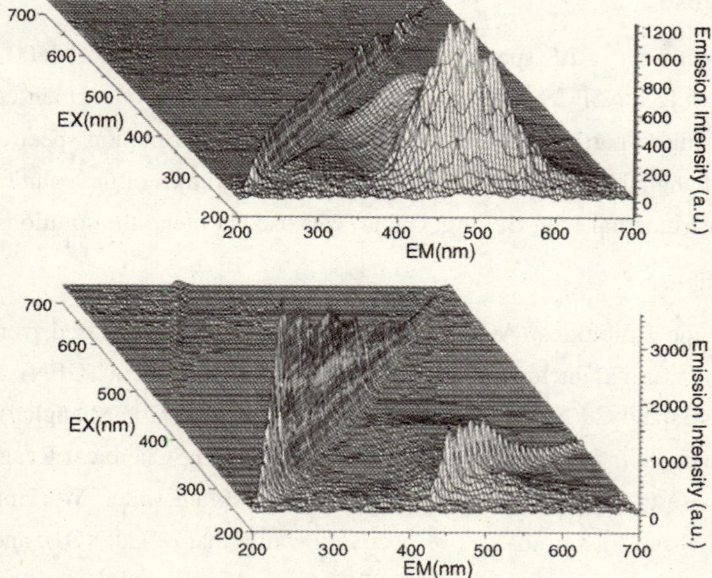

Fig.1 Three-dimensional emission spectra of CdS-QDs in the absence (up) and presence (down) of TOB. pH 5.02; concentration: CdS-QDs, 4.0×10^{-5} mol·L^{-1}; TOB, 0.64 μmol·L^{-1}

4.8.3 Results and discussion

4.8.3.1 Emission features of the interaction between CdS-QDs and AGs

As Fig. 1 shows, CdS-QDs could emit characteristic fluorescence of 500 nm excited at 376 nm, in the form of "mountain peak". At the same time, Rayleigh scattering signals are always existent, displaying a form of "extending mountainous band" with the $\lambda_{ex} = \lambda_{em}$ [1]. By carefully observation, another two weak "extending mountainous bands" could be found at $2\lambda_{ex} = \lambda_{em}$, and $\lambda_{ex} = 2\lambda_{em}$, which are possibly ascribed to the second-order light scattering and anti-second-order light scattering signals, respectively [34]. It should be noted that the band of $2\lambda_{ex} = \lambda_{em}$ gets immerged into the "major mountain" characterized at 500 nm fluorescence emission when excited at 250 nm, where the fluorescence emission is much stronger than the second-order light scattering.

The presence of TOB, however, greatly changes the emission features of CdS-QDs. The fluorescence quenching of CdS-QDs makes the two fluorescence mountainous peaks disappear, while the enhanced light scattering signals could be observed including the strong light scattering band of $\lambda_{ex} = \lambda_{em}$ characterized at 376 nm and the two light scattering bands of $2\lambda_{ex} = \lambda_{em}$ and $\lambda_{ex} = 2\lambda_{em}$.

Fig.2 shows excitation and emission spectra of CdS-QDs and those of its interaction with TOB. Both TOB and CdS-QDs have weak LS signals characterized at 376 nm. However, the mixture of TOB with CdS-QDs has very strong LS signals characterized at 376 nm, and the fluorescence of CdS-QDs characterized at 500 nm is quenched without special changes in the spectra shape. Similar phenomena could be found in GEN and KANA when they interact with CdS-QDs. All of these strong enhanced LS and fluorescence quenching percentage were found to increase with increasing AGs.

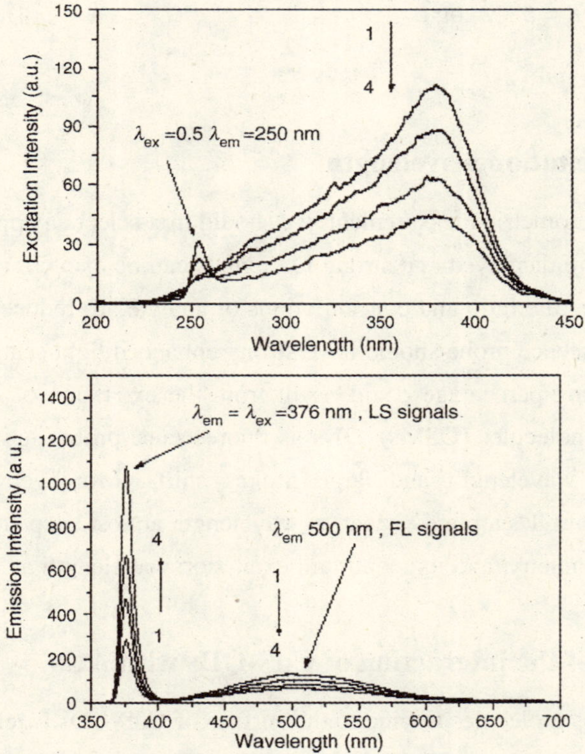

Fig. 2 Fluorescence excitation and anti-second-order light scattering (up) and fluorescence emission and Rayleigh light scattering (down) spectra of CdS-QDs in the absence and presence of different concentrations of TOB. pH 5.02; λem, 500nm(up); λex, 376 nm (down). Concentration: CdS-QDs, 4.0×10^{-5} mol·L^{-1}; TOB: 1, 0; 2, 0.21 μmol·L^{-1}; 3, 0.43 μmol·L^{-1}; 4, 0.64 μmol·L^{-1}.

4.8.3.2 Theory

If fluorescence quenching of probes can match the Stern-Volmer equation, either dynamic or the static mechanism, following equation could be drawn:

$$\frac{F_0}{F} - 1 = K_{sv}c \quad (1)$$

where F_0 and $F$are the fluorescence intensities at λ_{em} when excited at λ_{ex} in the absence and presence of analyte, respectively, $c$theconcentrationofanalyte,and K_{sv} is the Stern-Volmer quenching constant. The enhanced light scattering intensities (I) measured at the wavelength of λ_{ex} with the concentration of analyte obeys the following equation [3,4]:

$$\Delta I = I - I_0 = kc \quad (2)$$

where I_0 and I are the light scattering intensities in the absence and presence of analyte at λ_{ex}, respectively, c the concentration of analyte, and k is expressed as the slope.
Defineratio $R=[(F_0-F)\times I]/F$, then R could be expressed as $R=kK_{sv}c^2$, thus we can draw following equation:

$$\log R = \log(kK_{sv}) + 2\log c \quad (3)$$

Therefore, a linear relationship could be expected between log R and log c with the value of slope as 2. The intercept in Eq. (3) indicates that the proposed LS–FL ratiometry should have the properties of both the fluorescence and light scattering emissions. However, a deviation resulted from Eqs. (1) and (2) leads to the slope of Eq. (3) not being always the coefficient "2":

$$\log R = b + a\log c \quad (4)$$

where a and b are coefficients.

4.8.3.3 Choice of excitation wavelength

To carry out the LS–FL ratiometric measurement, we should first select an appropriate excitation wavelength (λ_{ex}) where strong LS signals are displayed and strong FL signals can be excited, and then create an equation exhibiting the relationship between the ratio and concentrations of analyte. To reduce the interferes of the noise and spectra overlay, an ideal fluorescence probe should have strong enhanced light scattering emission at λ_{ex} and large Stokes shift, and large quenching percentage could result from the excitation of λ_{ex} when reacted with analyte. Compared with organic small molecules (OSMs), QDs as fluorescence probes have strong light scattering emission at maximum excitation wavelength and large Stokes shifts. Moreover, light scattering signals and fluorescence excitation signals of QDs around excitation wavelength almost keep constant (Figs. 2 and 3). So QDs are ideal probes for LS–FL ratiometry, and its maximum excitation wavelength at 376 nm is chosen as excitation wavelength.

4.8.3.4 Mechanism of the interaction of CdS-QDs with AGs

It is therefore easy for AGs molecules to bind to the surface of CdS-QDs *via*electrostatic interaction for AGs contain positive charge while the surface of TGA-capped CdS-QDs contain negative charge at the pH 5.02. With the AGs bounded on the surface of CdS-QDs increasing,

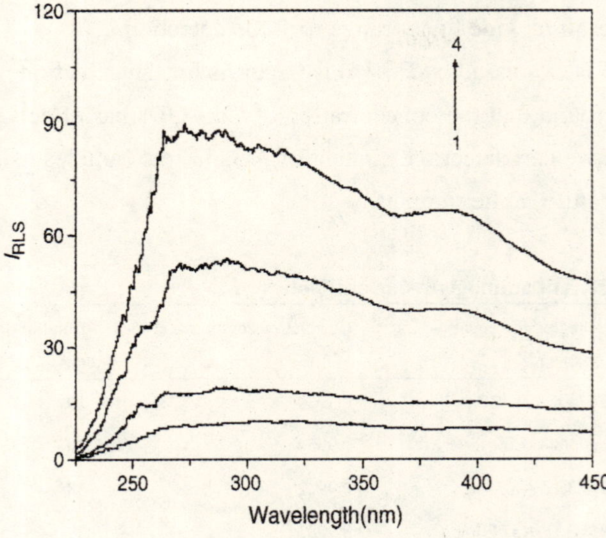

Fig. 3 Light scattering (LS) spectra of the system following $\lambda ex = \lambda em$ in the absence and presence of different concentration of TOB. pH 5.02; concentration: CdS-QDs, 4.0×10^{-5} mol·L^{-1}; TOB: 1, 0; 2, 0.21 μmol·L^{-1}; 3, 0.43 μmol·L^{-1}; 4, 0.64 μmol·L^{-1}.

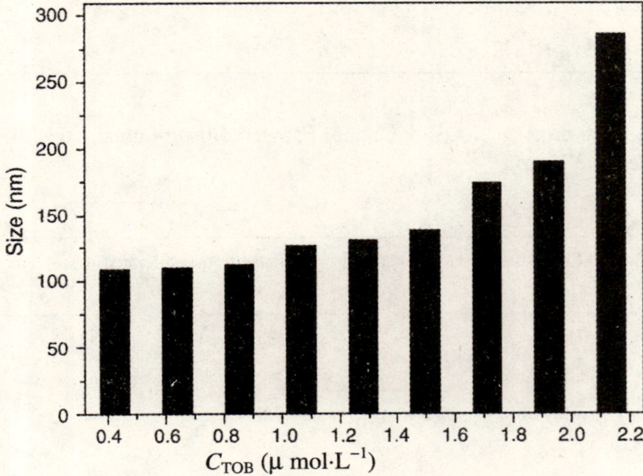

Fig. 4 Dependence of CdS-TOB size on the different concentration of TOB at a90° scattering angle in the ambient temperature of 20 °C. pH 5.02. Concentrations: CdS-QDs, 8.0 × 10^{-5} mol·L^{-1}. Owing to the weak light scattering (LS) signals and small size of CdS-QDs and TOB alone, it is difficult to accurately measure their size and data do not display.

the surface of CdS-QDs would gradually show positive charge property and be prone to bind to another negatively charged CdS-QDs, which would finally cause the aggregation and quench fluorescence of CdS-QDs [35]. Dynamic light scattering (DLS) measurements show that the interaction between CdS-QDs and AGs result in large particles, and the particle size gets increased with increasing AGs concentrations for a given amount of CdS-QDs. According to Mie and Rayleigh scattering theory, enhanced LS signals should be ascribed to the formation of large particles and their number (Fig. 4) [36]. These processes could be monitored through the DLS measurements, and it was found that the size got greatly increased only after the concentration of TOB was higher than 1.07 μmol·L^{-1}, with the apparent molar ratio of 1:80 (TOB/Cd). That is to say, the assembly between CdS-QDs and TOB could mainly result in large size particles.

4.8.3.5 Calibration curves and sample determinations

It could be found that the overall quenching percentage(Fo/F) as a function of AGs concentration matches the Stern-Volmer equation, whereas the enhanced scattering intensity(I) had linear relationship with AGs concentration (Table 1), thus Eqs. (1) and(2) could be obeyed.Therefore, log R as a function of log c of AGs concentration could match Eq. (4) in the complete concentration range, and experimental data are more reproducible and reliable. As Table 1 shows, the fluorescence quenching method has higher sensitivity than light scattering method in this assay, but the use of the LS–FL ratio, R, could result in wide linear range for AGs detection.

The relationship between log R and log c of AGs as expressed by Eq. (4) is the basis for the detection of AGs in aqueous solution using the LS–FL ratiometry. It is found that the concentration of CdS-QDs has effects on the linear range and sensitivity of determination, and thus we can detect the content of AGs in real samples using appropriate concentration of CdS-QDs according to the nature of the samples.

Table 1 Analytical parameters for the determination of different aminoglycoside antibiotics

Methods	Analytes	Linear range ($\mu mol \cdot L^{-1}$)	Linear regression equation (c, $\mu mol \cdot L^{-1}$)	Correlation coefficient (r)	Limit of detection (3σ, $nmol \cdot L^{-1}$)
LS method	TOB[a]	0.43~2.14	$I = -2674.8 + 5522.3c$	0.9939	19
FL method	TOB[a]	0.17~1.50	$F_0/F = 0.90 + 0.76c$	0.9954	163
LS–FL ratiometry	TOB[a]	0.09~2.14	log R = 3.13 + 3.31 log c	0.9922	68
LS–FL ratiometry	TOB[b]	0.09~1.07	log R = 3.78 + 3.77 log c	0.9981	58
LS–FL ratiometry	KANA[b]	0.21~2.06	log R = 2.62 + 5.32 log c	0.9913	190
LS–FL ratiometry	GEN[b]	0.21~2.09	log R = 2.54 + 5.16 log c	0.9956	84

[a] Concentration of CdS-QDs was 8.0×10^{-5} $mol \cdot L^{-1}$.

[b] Concentration of CdS-QDs was 4.0×10^{-5} $mol \cdot L^{-1}$. pH 5.02, λ_{ex}, 376 nm; λ_{em}, 500 nm. Data of FL method were obtained at 500 nm when excited at 376 nm, and that of LS method were obtained at 376 nm.

Table 2 Tolerance levels of coexisting foreign substances

Coexisting foreign substance	Concentration tolerated (10^{-6} $mol \cdot L^{-1}$)	Change in R (%)	Coexisting foreign substance	Concentration tolerated (10^{-6} $mol \cdot L^{-1}$)	Change in R (%)
K(I), Cl^-	1000	+2.0	Urea	500	+5.7
Na(I), Cl^-	1000	+3.9	Glucose	100	+6.1
NH_4(I), Cl^-	200	+5.1	Amylum	100a	−3.0
Mg(II), F^-	111	+5.9	Lactose	150	+3.9
Ca(II), Cl^-	50	+2.3	Sucrose	200	−4.5
Al(III), Cl^-	60	+9.2	Maltose	100	−2.0
Co(II), Cl^-	3	−1.4	l-Lys	50	−3.1
Zn(II), SO_4^{2-}	8	−3.2	l-Arg	20	+3.9
Cu(II), Cl^-	0.2	+5.6	l-Gys	20	−3.0
Fe(III), SO_4^{2-}	0.5	+4.7	l-Ascorbic acid	20	−7.3
Mn(II), SO_4^{2-}	60	+6.8	HAS	0.4[a]	−4.8
Thiourea	50	+5.4	Creatinine	100	+7.4

Concentrations: CdS-QDs, 4.0×10^{-5} $mol \cdot L^{-1}$; TOB 0.43 $\mu mol \cdot L^{-1}$. pH 5.02, λ_{ex}, 376nm; λ_{em}, 500 nm.
[a] Represented by $\mu g \cdot mL^{-1}$.

Table 3 Determination results of aminoglycoside antibiotics sulfate injection and serum samples

Sample	Added ($ng \cdot mL^{-1}$)	Average founded ($ng \cdot mL^{-1}$)	Recovery (%) (n= 5)	RSD (%) (n=5)
TOB injection	400[a]	403	98.8–102.2	1.5
GEN injection	400[a]	397	97.5–101.2	1.6
KANA injection	500[a]	516	99.6–106.0	2.5
Serum 1	200[b]	203	95.5–104.5	3.0
Serum 2	300[b]	303	97.3–104.7	3.1
Serum 3	400[b]	399	96.3–102.8	2.9

Concentrations: CdS-QDs, 4.0×10^{-5} $mol \cdot L^{-1}$. pH 5.02; λ_{ex}, 376 nm; λ_{em}, 500 nm.

[a] Declared values of TOB, GEN and KANA injection were 40, 40, and 250 mg·mL^{-1}, respectively, andtheyweredilutedo 10000-, 10000- and 50000-fold, respectively.
[b] Concentration of added TOB in the serum samples after diluted 100-fold.

With a tolerance level of ±10%, the influences of coexisting foreign substances have been tested (Table 2). Except heavy metal ions such as Cu (II), Fe (III) and proteins, other metal ions and some organic small molecules could not interfere the detection. Copper ions and iron ions could quench fluorescence of CdS-QDs, and their interference could be eliminated using thiourea and fluoride ions, respectively. So this method may be applied to the direct determination of AGs injection and human serum samples by removing proteins and certain dilution.

In order to test the LS–FL ratiometry, real samples are detected, including the content of AGs in clinic injection and serum samples. Table 3 shows that the quantification results of clinic injections are in good agreement with the declared values, and the recoveries of 95.5～104.7% and RSD of 2.9～3.1% for serum samples indicate that the LS–FL ratiometry is reproducible and reliable.

4.8.4 Conclusions

In this contribution, a LS–FL ratiometry is discussed and the new generic approach can enlarge the applications of light scattering and fluorescence techniques. The analytical results show that it has obvious advantages. Firstly, this ratiometriy extends the linear relationship between log $R$and log c of analytes and it does not require imposing a strict control on the stability of the signals. Due to the use of dual-wavelength data, R-values are more reproducible and reliable. Secondly, since both the light scattering and fluorescence signals could be simultaneously obtained in one scanning, this ratiometriy has become one answer to the problems posed by the former single-intensity measurement. With some probes, quantitative detection is probable at an appropriate excitation wavelength. Since the concurrence of enhanced light scattering and fluorescence quenching is a common phenomenon, the LS–FL ratiometriy could be extensively applied in the biological, biomedical, and environmental fields.

Acknowledgement

All authors herein are grateful to the supports from the National Natural Science Foundation of China (NSFC, Nos.: 20425517; 30570465).

References

[1] J.R. Lakowicz, in: J.R. Lakowicz (Ed.), Topics in Fluorescence Spectroscopy, vol. IV, Plenum Press, New York, 1994, p. 3.
[2] L.J. Yu, Y.Q. Li, W. Sui, Spectrosc. Spect. Anal. 22 (2002) 819.
[3] C.Z. Huang, K.A. Li, S.Y. Tong, Anal. Chem. 68 (1996) 2259.
[4] C.Z. Huang, K.A. Li, S.Y. Tong, Anal. Chem. 69 (1997) 514.
[5] R.H. Yang, K.A. Li, K.M. Wang, F.L. Zhao, N. Li, F. Liu, Anal. Chem. 75 (2003) 612.
[6] G. Crynkiewicz, M. Poenie, R.Y.Tsien, J. Biol. Chem. 260 (1985) 3440.
[7] Y.J. Long, Y.F. Li, C.Z. Huang, Anal. Chim. Acta 552 (2005) 175.
[8] J. Ueberfeld, D.R. Walt, Anal. Chem. 76 (2004) 947.
[9] K. Aslan, P. Holley, L. Davies, J.R. Lakowicz, D. Geddes, J. Am. Chem. Soc. 127 (2005) 12115.
[10] Ajayaghosh, P. Carol, S. Sreejith, J. Am. Chem. Soc. 127 (2005) 14962.
[11] H. Hochreiner,I. Sanchez-Barragan, J.M. Costa-Fernandez, A. Sanz-Medel, Talanta 66 (2005) 611.
[12] R. Badugu, J.R. Lakowicz, C.D. Geddes, Talanta 66 (2005) 569.

[13] C.Z. Huang, X.B. Pang, Y.F. Li, Y.J. Long, Talanta 69 (2006) 180.

[14] L. Spanhel, M. Haase, A. Henglein, J. Am. Chem. Soc. 109 (1987) 5649.

[15] M.A. Hines, P. Guyot-Sionnest, J. Phys. Chem. 100 (1996) 468.

[16] C.M. Strohsuhl, H. Du, B.L. Miller, T.D. Krauss, Talanta 67 (2005) 479.

[17] Q. Ma, X.G. Su, X.Y. Wang, Y. Wan, C.L. Wang, B. Yang, Q.H. Jin, Talanta 67 (2005) 1029.

[18] M. Shingyoji, D. Gerion, D. Pinkel, J.W. Gray, F. Chen, Talanta 67 (2005)

[19] Y. Chen, Z. Rosenzweig, Anal. Chem. 74 (2002) 5132.

[20] Y. Ma, C. Yang, N. Li, X.R. Yang, Talanta 67 (2005) 979.

[21] J.G. Liang, S. Huang, D.Y. Zeng, Z.K. He, X.H. Ji, H.X. Yang, Talanta 69 (2006) 126.

[22] P. Bao, A.G. Frutos, C. Creef, J. Lahiri, U. Muller, T.C. Peterson, L. Warden, X. Xie, Anal. Chem. 74 (2002) 1792.

[23] Z. Wang, J. Lee, A.R. Cossins, M. Brust, Anal. Chem. 77 (2005) 5770.

[24] R.M. Shawar, D.L. MacLeod, R.L. Garber, J.L. Burns, J.R. Stapp, C.R. Clausen, S.K. Tanaka, Antimicrob. Agents Chemother. 43 (1999) 2877.

[25] C.A. Hammett-Stabler, T. Johns, Clin. Chem. 44 (1998) 1129.

[26] Omri, C. Beaulac, M. Bouhajib, M. Montplaisir,M. Sharkawi, J.

[27] LAGsc´e, Antimicrob. Agents Chemother. 38 (1994) 1090.

[28] M. Yang, S.A. Tomellini, J. Chromatogr. A 939 (2001) 59.

[29] D.A. Stead, R.M.E. Richards, J. Chromatogr. B 693 (1997) 415.

[30] W. Haasnoot, G. Cazemier, M. Koets, A.V. Amerongen, Anal. Chim. Acta 488 (2003) 53.

[31] H.H. Yang, Q.Z. Zhu, H.Y. Qu, X.L. Chen, M.T. Ding, J.G. Xu, Anal. Biochem. 308 (2002) 71.

[32] X.L. Hu, S.P. Liu, H.Q. Luo, Acta. Chim. Sin. 61 (2003) 1287.

[33] L. Jiang, X. Chen, W.S. Yang, J. Jin, B.Q. Yang, L. Xu, T.J. Li, Chem. J. Chinese Univ. 22 (2001) 1397.

[34] L.E. Brus, J. Phys. Chem. 90 (1986) 2555.

[35] G.Z. Chen, X.Z. Huang, Z.Z. Zheng, J.G. Xue, Z.B. Wang, Spectrofluorometry, 118, Science Press, Beijing, 1990, p. 153.

[36] Z.P. Wang, J. Li, J.Q. Hu, X. Yao, J.H. Li, J. Phys. Chem. B 109 (2005) 23304.

[37] R.F. Pasternack, C. Buatamante, P.J. Collings, A. Giannetto, E.J. Gibbs, J. Am. Chem. Soc. 115 (1993) 5393.

(Qie Gen Liao, Yuan Fang Li, Cheng Zhi Huang, published in *Talanta*, 71-2007, 567～572)

4.9 Resonance Light Scattering Imaging Determination of Heparin

Abstract: A laser-induced resonance light scattering (RLS) imaging method to determine heparin is described based on the high light scattering emission power of the aggregation species of heparin with α, β, γ, δ-tetra (4-trimethylaminoniumphenyl) prophyrin (TAPP) in solution. By imaging the light scattering signals of the aggregation species, we proposed the method to determine the heparin with a detection range of 0.02～0.6 μg·mL^{-1} and the detection limit (3σ) of 1.3 ng·mL^{-1}.

Keywords: Heparin, α, β, γ, δ-tetra(4-trimethylaminonium phenyl)prophyrin (TAPP), resonance light scattering (RLS) imaging.

Light scattering submicroscopic particles such as metallic particles and particles of other composition have high-producing power and can be used as fluorescent analogs and tracers labels in clinical and biological applications[1～3]. Their light scattering signals are not prone to quenching and photobleaching. So the use of light scattering particles in DNA microarray hybridization[4] and protein assay[5] has yielded the significant increase in sensitivity over fluorescent labels. In this work, we display our studies to determine the heparin with high sensitivity by light scattering imaging method.

4.9.1 Experimental

RLS images were obtained with an Olympus IX70 inverted microscope (Olympus, Tokyo, Japan). The 441.6 nm laser line from a He-Cd laser source (Shanghai Laser Technology Institute, China) was used for excitation. The schematic of the experimental setup for RLS imaging is similar to the earlier report[5]. The right-angled RLS signals of the aggregations were collected through a microscope objective (4×, NA = 0.10, Olympus), and RLS images were captured by a Cohu 4910 series cooled CCD camera (Cohu, CA). Scion image software (Scion Image, Scion Corp) was used to count the number of aggregations species. Mean particle size and size distribution were measured at room temperature by a N5 Submicro Particle Size Analyzer (Bechman Coulter, Inc, Miami, USA).

4.9.2 Results and Discussion

Under the experimental conditions, heparin exists in a big polyvalent anionic state with its anionic groups –O–SO_3^-, –$NHSO_3^-$, and –COO^-. The cationic prophyrin, TAPP, hence, can assemble on the heparin template by electrostatic attractions and the hydrophobic interactions. The interaction of TAPP with heparin can generate the small aggregation species and the greatly enhanced scattering light can be observed by guiding the 441.6 nm laser line to excite the scatterers of TAPP-heparin complex. Fig. 1 displays the RLS images of TAPP-heparin complex particles captured by CCD camera. The 3-D image (Fig. 1B) demonstrated the intensities of the particles on Fig. 1A.

The digital analysis for these RLS images showed that the imaged aggregation species were related to the concentrations of heparin. Fig. 2 shows the relationship of the RLS images of aggregation species in solution expressed by bright squares labeled with the serial numbers of particle counts with the different concentrations of heparin. The counts of bright squares in these images are related to the setup of threshold value. In this experiment, the threshold value was setup to be 30 according to a value of three times the standard deviation above the average of photoelectron counts for 8～10 images of reagent blank solution[8]. It is demonstrated that there are too much bright squares could be counted possibly originated from background or the other aggregation species out of the focus plane when smaller threshold values are setup. It can be seen from Fig. 2 that only a few bright squares were displayed in the images of TAPP and heparin solution alone, while many bright squares can be observed when TAPP coexisted with traces of heparin under the same experimental conditions, and the counts of particles increased with increasing heparin concentration (Fig. 2C, 2D). Considering that more than 99.7% of the pixels have lower intensity counts than the threshold value if there are no aggregation species in the solution[8], we concluded that these bright squares in the images indeed corresponded to the light scattering signals from the aggregation of TAPP on heparin in solution.

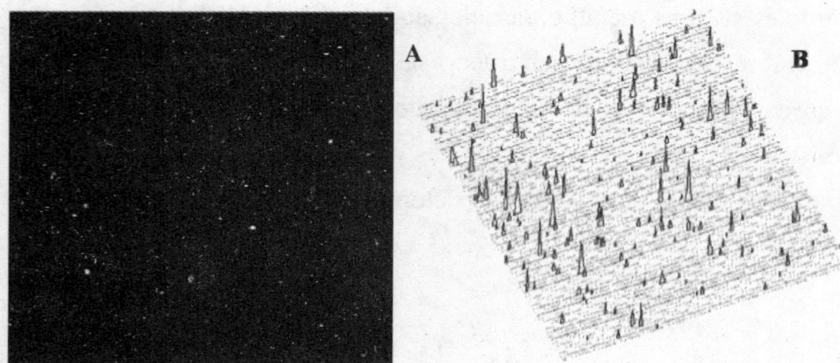

Fig. 1 RLS images of TAPP-heparin complex particles captured by CCD camera (A) and the 3-D image (B) demonstrating the intensities of the particles on image A.

The subframe area is 300 × 300 pixels. TAPP, 1.0×10^{-6} mol·L^{-1}, heparin, 0.3 μg·L^{-1}, pH 6.80, ionic strength, 0.012 mol·L^{-1}.

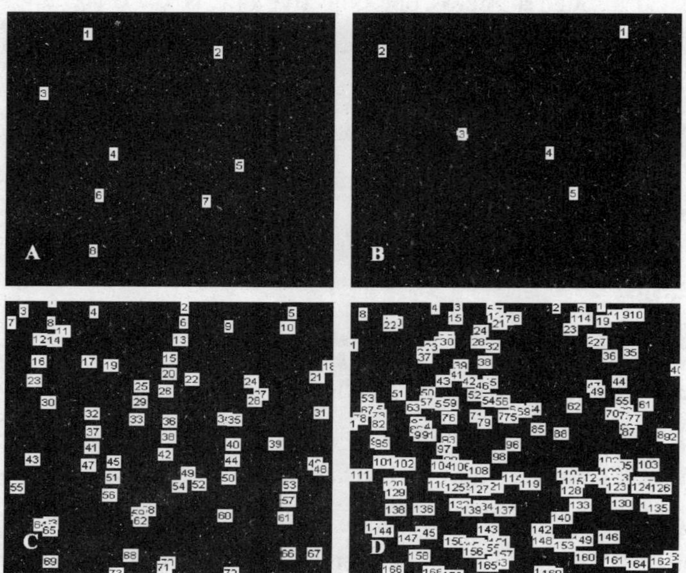

Fig. 2 Counts of TAPP-heparin aggregation species in different heparin concentrations.

The subframe area is 300 × 300 pixels, threshold = 30. TAPP, 1.0 × 10^{-6} mol·L^{-1} except that B is no TAPP added, heparin (μg·mL^{-1}), A, 0, B, 0.3, C, 0.15, D, 0.225. pH 6.80, ionic strength, 0.012 mol·L^{-1}. The bright squares labeled with serial number display the counts of the particles.

Table 1 Change of the sizes of aggregation species with heparin concentrations

Added heparin (μg·mL^{-1})	0	0.1	0.2	0.3	0.4	0.5	0.6	0.7
Mean particle sizes (nm)	1062	1753	1994	2172	2070	2038	1827	756

The results were obtained by unimodal analysis at 25°C. TAPP, 1.0 × 10^{-6} mol·L^{-1}, pH 6.80, ionic strength, 0.012 mol·L^{-1}.

At room temperature, we studied the relationship of the sizes of light scattering aggregation species in solution with the concentration of heparin. As Table 1 shown, the mean sizes of aggregation species become larger when trace amount of heparin was added. With increasing the heparin concentrations the mean sizes of particles reached to maximal and no longer varied, which is possibly related to the saturation of the assembly of TAPP on heparin. However, at further grown of heparin concentration the particles became smaller due to the porphyrin deaggregation. It demonstrated that the adding of heparin could influence the number and size of aggregation species responsible for the scattering light emitting. Thus, RLS imaging can be used to investigate the interaction of heparin with TAPP.

The effects of pH, ionic strength and the concentrations of TAPP on imaging have also been investigated. The results showed that RLS imaging method could be greatly influenced by these conditions, which can influence the interaction of heparin with TAPP and the scattering features of the scatterers in solution. As the common RLS method, however, the present method also has the disadvantage of bad selectivity. Under the optimum conditions, the influences of coexisting foreign substances were investigated.

Common metal ions, sugars, surfactants can be allowed with high concentrations, except to proteins the tolerance was lower. So the method can be applied to direct determination of heparin samples which do not contain proteins such as heparin sodium injection samples.

According to the general procedure, a linear relationship between the counts of aggregation species and heparin concentrations was constructed. The counts *(N)* of bright squares in 300 × 300 pixels area were proportional to the heparin concentrations in the ranges of 0.02 - 0.6 μg·mL^{-1}, and the linear regression equation was N = -59.52 + 756.4 c (μg·mL^{-1}, r = 0.9963, n = 7) with the limit of determination (3σ) of 1.3 ng·mL^{-1}. The determination results for three heparin sodium injection samples with the proposed method were examined by t statistical test and the acceptable data were displayed in Table 2. It can be seen that the results found by the present method are identical to the reference values, indicating that the present method is reliable.

Table 2 Results for the determination of heparin in heparin sodium injection solutions

Sample	Heparin specified (IU/2 mL)	Heparin found (IU/2 mL)	Average (IU/2 mL)	RSD (%)
1[a]	12500	12833,12265, 12750, 12208, 12327	12477	2.34
2[b]	12500	12388, 12750, 12327, 12633, 12572	12534	1.40
3[c]	12500	12449, 12265, 12695, 12388, 12750	12509	1.65

Heparin sodium injection solutions were purchased respectively from [a] Jiangsu Wanbang Biochemical Pharmaceutical Co. Ltd of China, [b] Nanjing Xinbai Pharmaceutical Co. Ltd of Chian and [c] Shanghai Biochemical Pharmaceutical Factory of China. The subframe area is 300 × 300 pixels, threshold = 30. TAPP, 1.0 × 10^{-6} mol·L^{-1}, pH 6.80, ionic strength, 0.012 mol·L^{-1}.

Acknowledgments

Herein we are grateful to the supports from the National Natural Science Foundation of China (No. 20425517, No. 20275032), the Program for New Century Excellent Talents in University (NCET-04-0852) and Chun Hui Program (No: [2004] 7-24) directed under the Ministry of Education of PRC, and the Municipal Science and Technology Committee of Chongqing.

References

[1] S. Schultz, D. R. Smith, J. J. Mock, et al., Proc. Natl. Acad. Sci. U.S.A., 2000, 97(3), 996.

[2] T. A. Taton, C. A. Mirkin, R. L. Lesinger, Science, 2000, 289, 1757.

[3] T. A. Taton, G. Lu, C. A. Mirkin, J. Am. Chem. Soc., 2001, 123(21), 5164.

[4] P. Bao, A. G. Frutos, C. Greef, et al., Anal. Chem., 2002, 74(8), 1792.

[5] C. Z. Huang, Y. Liu, Y. H. Wang, et al., Anal. Biochem., 2003, 321, 236.

[6] J. Yguerabide, E. E. Yguerabide, Anal. Biochem., 1998, 262, 137.

[7] J. Yguerabide, E. E. Yguerabide, Anal. Biochem., 1998, 262, 157.

[8] X. H. Fang, W. H. Tan, Anal. Chem., 1999, 71(15), 3101.

(Hong Ping GUO, Cheng Zhi HUANG, Jian LING, published in *Chinese Chemical Letters*, 2006,17, 53～56)

4.10 Visual Detection of Sudan Dyes Based on the Plasmon Resonance Light Scattering Signals of Silver Nanoparticles

Abstract: A visual light scattering detection method of Sudan dyes is reported in food products based on the formation of silver nanoparticles (NPs) in this contribution. Sudan dyes including I, II, III and IV have reducibility due to the nitrogen-nitrogen double bond and phenol group in their molecular structure, and redox reaction could occur with $AgNO_3$. Owing to the formation of silver NPs as a result of the redox reaction, color changes could be observed by net eyes from the red of Sudan to the brown of silver NPs during the redox reactions, resulting in strong plasmon resonance light scattering (PRLS) signals characterized at 452 nm, which could be measured using a common spectrofluorometer. It was found that the PRLS intensities were proportional to the dye concentrations over the range of 0.2～2.4 μmol·L^{-1} Sudan I, 0.1～2.4 μmol·L^{-1} Sudan II, 0.1～2.4 μmol·L^{-1} Sudan III and 0.2～3.0 μmol·L^{-1} Sudan IV, with the corresponding limits of determination (3σ) of 3.2 nmol·L^{-1}, 3.0 nmol·L^{-1}, 3.2 nmol·L^{-1} and 2.9 nmol·L^{-1}, respectively. Using hot chili as a model sample, detections could be made with the recovery of 90.8%～103.3% and RSD of 4.0%～4.9%, and the results are identical with that of liquid chromatographic method proclaimed by European Commission. In order to make such PRLS method much more practical, we could visually detect the quantity of Sudan dyes based on the PRLS signals using simple devices such as a portable laser pointer (653 nm) and a light emitting diode (LED, 458 nm). Mechanism investigations show that the functional group of Sudan oxidized by $AgNO_3$ is the phenol group, not the nitrogen-nitrogen double bond.

Key Words: Sudan Dyes, Plasmon Resonance Light Scattering, Silver Naroparticles

Metal nanoparticles (NPs) have been of interest for centuries, and they have been paid much attention in recent years due to their special optical and electronic properties, which are not present in the bulk metal.[1] One important optical phenomenon is that the particle suspensions display brilliant colors giving rise to plasmon absorption and scattering.[2, 3] It is for these particular features that metal NPs have wide and potential applications in many aspects involving in the developments of optical sensors, [4～8] the detections of DNA hybridization,[9, 10] the studies of protein folding,[11] aptamer-protein complexes.[12]

In principle, the plasmon absorption and scattering properties are due to electron oscillations in the metallic particles. The irradiation of light to a small metallic NP would lead to coherent oscillation of the conduction electrons, which is called plasmon resonance of particles.[13] Subsequently, the oscillating electrons radiate electromagnetic wave with the same frequency as that of the incident light beam, and thus the small metallic NPs are often referred to as plasmon scatterer. [13] The oscillation frequency is determined by the factors of the density of electrons, the effective electron mass, the shape and size of the charge distribution.[14, 15] In general, dipole plasmon resonance occurs for small particles less than the incident wavelength, whereas a quadrupole mode or higher order multipole resonance would be observed as the particle size increases.[16] As an example of metallic particles, silver NPs exhibit characteristic optical properties in the visible range due to the plasmon resonance. In fact, single silver NPs could interact with photon more efficiently than any other particle of the same dimension. Such high efficiency together with the optical properties makes silver NPs very attractive for a lot of optical applications.[17] We expect that the light scattering signals resulting from the plasmon scatterer could be detected using a common spectrofluorometer, and we herein propose a visual light scattering detection method of Sudan dyes in food products based on the measured plasmon resonance light scattering (PRLS) signals.

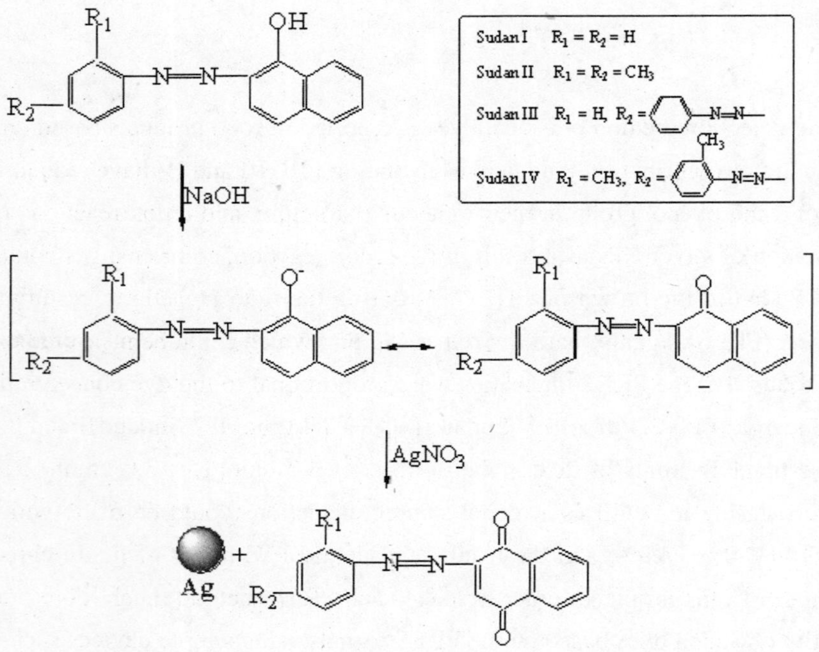

Sudan I $R_1 = R_2 = H$

Sudan II $R_1 = R_2 = CH_3$

Sudan III $R_1 = H$, $R_2 =$ C_6H_5–N=N–

Sudan IV $R_1 = CH_3$, $R_2 =$ $CH_3C_6H_4$–N=N–

Fig. 1 The molecular structures of Sudan and the chart of their reactions with $AgNO_3$.

Sudan I, II, III and IV (Figure 1 shows the molecular structure) are a series of artificial 'azo' dyes usually used in oil paint, printing, waxes, plastics and dyeing[18, 19] since their bright and vivid colors could improve the luster of commercial products. Sudan is not permitted to use in food productions for being classified as a category carcinogen by the International Agency for Research on Cancer (IARC). [20] There is evidence that Sudan I is potentially carcinogenic in rodents and cause damage to genetic material since it can react with given sequence of DNA *in vitro*. The major DNA adduct formed in this reaction has been characterized and identified as the 8-(phenylazo) guanine adduct. [21] In addition to microsomal enzymes, Sudan I and its C-hydroxylated metabolites are also oxidized by peroxidases, as a consequence, DNA, RNA, and protein adducts are formed. [22, 23]

However, the family of Sudan dyes, especially Sudan I, has been found in food products containing hot chili in some parts of areas around the world, which is a crucial risk to human health. In May 2003, the French Food Authority (AFFSA) discovered that a number of products containing chilli powder imported from India contained Sudan I. [24] In China, Sudan was also found in batches of roast chicken wings and chicken burgers on sale, and in some commercial products like piccalilli and chili sauce.

To date, the standard used to detect the Sudan family is based on liquid chromatographic method proclaimed by European Commission, [25] and other approaches like HPLC-UV, [26] HPLC/APCI-MS [27] and HPLC-DAD detections[28] have also been made. Whichever method is used, separation with HPLC is needed first, which is time-consuming and brings about inconvenience to analysis in real time. Thus, the safety quality control of Sudan dyes in food products is very crucial and developing simple detection method is urgent. Herein, we propose a new simple method to detect Sudan directly based on the formation of silver NPs.

4.10.1 Experimental Section

4.10.1.1 Apparatus

The plasmon resonance light scattering (PRLS) spectrum and intensity were measured with a F-4500 fluorescence spectrophotometer (Hitachi, Tokyo, Japan). The plasmon absorption was measured with a U-3010 spectrophotometer (Hitachi, Tokyo, Japan). A TecNai-10 electron microscope (FEA, America) was used to measure the TEM images of silver NPs. A vortex mixer QL-901 (Haimen, China) was used to blend the solution. Besides, a LC system (Hitachi, Tokyo, Japan) with diode array detector L-2450, column oven L-2300 and pump L-2130 was applied for sample detection for comparison. A low speed of 800-Model Centrifuge (Shanghai Operational Instrumental Limit, Shanghai, PRC) was used for the real sample pretreatment. The IR spectrums were obtained with a SPECTRUMGX spectrophotometer (Perkin Elmer, USA). In order to construct a simple and practical procedure, a laser pointer (653 nm, 2.0 mW) and a LED (458 nm, 0.5 mW), whose output power has been calibrated with a WL-4 Power Meter (Laser Institute of Physics, Southwest University, Chongqing, PRC), were used for visual light scattering detection. For safety consideration, special attention should be paid for the safe use of laser pointer, which is harmful to eyes.

4.10.1.2 Reagents

Sudan I and II were commercially purchased from Chemical Reagent Company (Shanghai, China), while Sudan III and IV from Kasei Kogyo Co. LTD (Tokyo, Japan). 1.0×10^{-3} mol·L^{-1} stock solutions of Sudan I to IV were prepared respectively by directly dissolving their commercial products in DMF. The working solution was obtained by diluting the stock solution with DMF to 1.0×10^{-5} mol·L^{-1}.

0.1 mol·L^{-1} stock solution of $AgNO_3$ was prepared by dissolving solid $AgNO_3$ in doubly distilled water and the working solution was obtained by diluting the stock solution to 1.0×10^{-3} mol·L^{-1} with water. 0.1 mol·L^{-1} NaOH, 0.4% $NH_3 \cdot H_2O$, and 0.2% TritonX-100 working solutions were used. All the reagents were of analytical grade without further purification. Water used throughout was doubly distilled.

4.10.1.3 General Procedure

2.25 mL of 1.0×10^{-3} mol·L^{-1} $AgNO_3$, 0.4 mL of 0.1 M NaOH and 0.25 mL of 0.4% $NH_3 \cdot H_2O$ working solution were added in a 10-mL test tube. The mixture was vortexed thoroughly, and then an appropriate volume of the Sudan solution and 0.3 mL of TritonX-100 were added. At last, the mixture was diluted to 5 mL with doubly distilled water and mixed thoroughly again. 20 minutes later, the PRLS spectra and the intensities were measured against the reagent blank solution treated in the same way without Sudan.

The PRLS spectrum was obtained by scanning simultaneously the excitation and emission monochromators of the F-4500 spectrofluorometer from 320 to 700 nm (namely, $\Delta\lambda$=0 nm), and all PRLS measurements were made with 10.0 nm slit-width of the excitation and the emission of the spectrofluorometer. The PRLS intensity was measured at the maximum PRLS peak.

4.10.1.4 Preparation of Quinone Products

In order to understand the reaction mechanism, the products of the redox reaction were separated and characterized by using following procedures. 10.0 mL of 0.1 mol·L^{-1} $AgNO_3$, 10.0 mL of 1.0 mol·L^{-1} NaOH and 1.8 mL of 28% ammonia were at first placed into a 200-mL conical flask. After the mixture was vortexed thoroughly, 100 mL of 1.0×10^{-3} mol·L^{-1} Sudan I solution was added dropwise. The reaction mixture was then stirred for 30 min at room temperature, filtered and extracted with $CHCl_3$ (30 mL × 3). The combined organic phase was dried by anhydrous sodium sulfate and evaporated under reduced pressure to give an oily residue. The residue was purified at last by silica gel column using acetic ether/petroleum ether (distillate of 60°C~90°C) (1: 50 (v/v)), evaporated, and dried in vacuum, giving a yellow product.

4.10.1.5 Pretreatment of Samples

Real samples including cayenne oil, chili sauce and redeye were commercially purchased from supermarket (Beibei Chongbai, Chongqing, PRC). 1.0 g of the real samples were placed respectively into a 10-mL volumetric flask, and then dissolved into 10 mL with DMF. The mixture was vortexed thoroughly, and centrifugal sedimentation was carried out for 2 min at the speed of 3600 rpm. 10 min later the top pellucid liquid was transferred for detection according to the general procedure. For comparison, standard liquid chromatographic detection for Sudan proposed by European Commission was made. [25] The real samples for liquid chromatographic detections were prepared by dissolving 20 g of cayenne oil or chili sauce in 100 mL acetonitrile. The mixture was vortexed thoroughly, and filtrated 1 h later, and the filtrate was used directly for sample injection.

4.10.2 Results And Discussion

4.10.2.1 Spectral Features of the Redox Reactions of Sudan with $AgNO_3$

Sudan I, II, III or IV alone in the alkaline condition has different color and absorption spectra (shown in Fig. 1S in Supporting Information). The characteristic absorptions are located at 376 nm and 486 nm for Sudan I, 396 nm and 502 nm for Sudan II, 344 nm and 524 nm for Sudan III, and 374 nm and 518 nm for Sudan IV, respectively. The absorption features, however, only characterized at 398.0 nm, are greatly changed after reacting with $AgNO_3$ (shown in Fig. 2). The insert picture in Fig. 2 shows the colorimetric response of the sensing detection of Sudan I. The color change reactions of Sudan II, III or IV with $AgNO_3$ are the same as Sudan I.

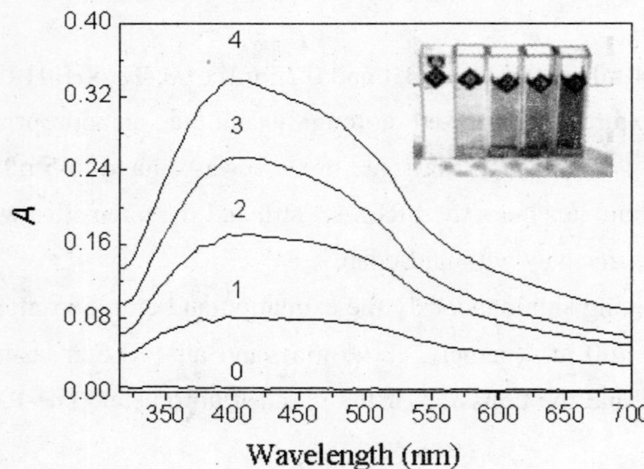

Fig. 2 The plasmon absorption of silver NPs resulting from the reaction of $AgNO_3$ and Sudan I (The insert picture shows the color change for the visible sensing detection in response to different quantity of Sudan I). Concentrations: $AgNO_3$, 4.5 × 10^{-4} mol·L^{-1}; NaOH, 8.0 × 10^{-3} mol·L^{-1}; $NH_3{\cdot}H_2O$, 0.02%; Sudan I (Curves 0 to 4, μmol·L^{-1}), 0, 1.0, 2.0, 3.0, 4.0; TritonX-100, 0.012%.

The four Sudan dyes possess two reducible groups, which are a nitrogen-nitrogen double bond and a phenol group. More precisely, the latter turns into a phenate ion at a high enough pH and becomes reducible (Fig. 1), and thus could be oxidized by $AgNO_3$. As a result, $AgNO_3$ is deoxidized and present as brown silver NPs.[29, 30] Fig. 3

shows the TEM images of silver NPs formed in the presence of 0.4 $\mu mol \cdot L^{-1}$ (A), 1.2 $\mu mol \cdot L^{-1}$ (B), and 2.0 $\mu mol \cdot L^{-1}$ Sudan I (C), respectively. These silver NPs are nearly of the same size. The average dimensions are about 17.9 ± 2.0 nm (A), 17.2 ± 2.0 nm (B) and 17.5 ± 1.5 nm (C), which are calculated by averaging all the observed particles of the picture in Fig. 3 (3 for A, 16 for B, and 22 for C). However, the number of the silver NPs generated at a high concentration of Sudan I is more than that at a low concentration. Namely, the concentration of silver NPs is increased with increasing Sudan. Thus, the absorption band of the formed silver NPs over the range of 350～525 nm (Fig. 2), characterized at 398 nm, should be ascribed to the plasmon absorption of silver NPs according to references.[30–32] Since the size of the formed silver NPs is much less than the wavelength, this plasmon absorption should be mainly ascribed to the dipole plasmon resonance.[16]

The light scattering signals of Sudan or $AgNO_3$ alone detected using a common spectrofluorometer are very weak. When silver NPs are formed from the mixture of Sudan and $AgNO_3$, the light scattering signals get enhanced, and increase with increasing Sudan concentration (shown in Fig. 4). The light scattering signals with the characteristic peak being in the region of absorption band should be ascribed to the "resonance light scattering".[33～34] It is no doubt that the characteristic light scattering signals displayed at 452 nm (Fig. 4), over the 350～525 nm plasmon absorption range of silver NPs (Fig. 2), should be ascribed to RLS ones.[17] Thus, the light scattering signals measured using the common spectrofluorometer should indeed be ascribed to the plasmon resonance light scattering (PRLS).[13] In general, the intensity of light scattering depends on the volume and number of the species, the wavelength of incident light, and the real and imaginary parts of the scatterer's polarizability.[33～35] In this experiment, the more Sudan was added, the more silver NPs were formed, whereas, the size or the volume stayed nearly the same when the concentration of Sudan I is relatively low (Fig. 3, A, B and C). So, the enhanced PRLS signals could be mainly due to the increasing number of silver NPs, whereas, the silver NPs begin to aggregate if the concentration of Sudan I becomes higher (Fig. 3, D and E).

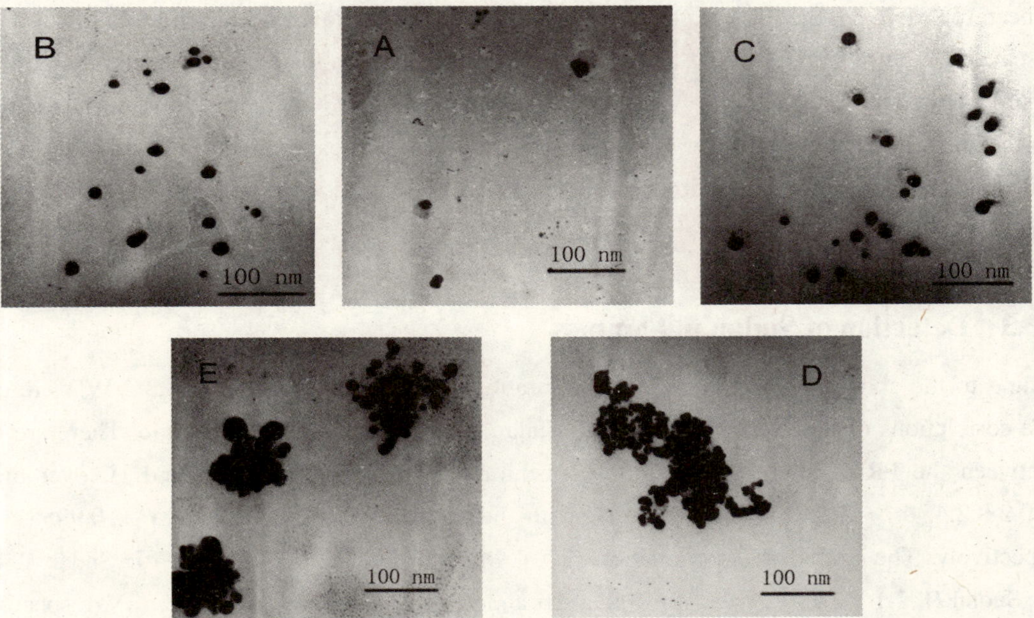

Fig. 3 TEM images of silver NPs resulting from the reaction of $AgNO_3$ and Sudan I. The average dimensions are about 17.9 ± 2.0 nm (A), 17.2 ± 2.0 nm (B) and 17.5 ± 1.5 nm (C), which are calculated by averaging all the observed particles of the picture in Fig 3 (3 for A, 16 for B, and 22 for C). Concentrations: $AgNO_3$, $4.5 \times 10^{-4} mol \cdot L^{-1}$; NaOH, $8.0 \times 10^{-3} mol \cdot L^{-1}$; $NH_3 \cdot H_2O$, 0.02%; Sudan I, 0.4 $\mu mol \cdot L^{-1}$ (A), 1.2 $\mu mol \cdot L^{-1}$ (B), 2.0 $\mu mol \cdot L^{-1}$ (C), 5.0 $\mu mol \cdot L^{-1}$ (D), 8.0 $\mu mol \cdot L^{-1}$ (E); TritonX-100, 0.012%.

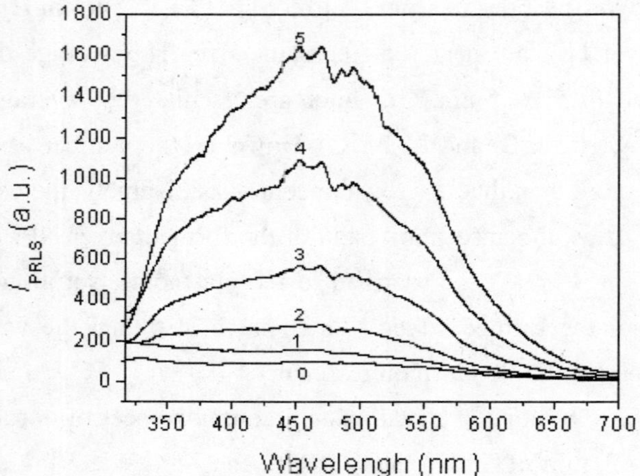

Fig. 4 The PRLS spectra of silver NPs resulting from the reaction of $AgNO_3$ and Sudan I. Concentrations: $AgNO_3$, 4.5×10^{-4} mol·L^{-1}; NaOH, 8.0×10^{-3} mol·L^{-1} except Curve 0; $NH_3 \cdot H_2O$, 0.02%; Sudan I (from Curves 0 to 5, μmol·L^{-1}), 0, 1.0 (without $AgNO_3$), 0.2, 0.5, 1.0, 1.5; TritonX-100, 0.012%.

4.10.2.2 Optimal Conditions for the Redox Reactions

We carried out the reaction in the alkaline condition since it was observed that silver NPs could not be formed under neutral or acidic pH conditions. Inspired by Tollens' reagent, we employed silver ammonia ion as an oxidant. It is pity that no silver NPs were formed and no color changes were observed. Considering that the formation of silver NPs is dependent on the ionization of the phenol group at a high pH,[30] we added NaOH solution in order to provide high enough alkalinity. [36, 37] The addition of NaOH, although provide high alkalinity for the ionization of the phenol group, makes silver cation deposit and greatly weaken the oxidation capacity of $AgNO_3$. Therefore, the synergistic effect of ammonia and NaOH should be detected. Fig.s 5a and 5b show the dependence of the PRLS intensity on the concentrations of NaOH and ammonia. As NaOH and ammonia increase until 8.0×10^{-3} mol·L^{-1} and 0.02%, respectively, the PRLS intensity gets increased correspondingly.

It has been reported that the dispersions of NPs could be much improved by the addition of surfactants, [38, 39] and the presence of a physically adsorbed layer of nonionic surfactant on the surface of colloidal gold could prevent irreversible aggregation of gold NPs. [40] In order to make the silver NPs more stable, surfactants, especially nonionic surfactants are used as stabilizer in aqueous medium. [41] Our experiments showed that the addition of TritonX-100 could indeed improve the stability of formed silver NPs, and would not influence the PRLS intensity of the system.

4.10.2.3 Detection of Sudan in Samples

According to the above general procedures, calibration curves of Sudan I, II, III and IV were constructed (Fig. 6). The correlations of PRLS intensity with all Sudan dyes were obtained at 452 nm. There are linear relationships between the PRLS intensities and the concentrations of Sudan I, II, III, and IV over the range of (μmol·L^{-1}) 0.2～2.4, 0.1～2.4, 0.1～2.4, 0.2～3.0 with the correlation coefficient, 0.9973, 0.9958, 0.9969 and 0.9990, respectively. The limits of determination (3σ, LOD) are 7.9×10^{-4} μg·mL^{-1} for Sudan I, 8.3×10^{-4} μg·mL^{-1} for Sudan II, 1.1×10^{-3} μg·mL^{-1} for Sudan III and 1.1×10^{-3} μg·mL^{-1} for Sudan IV, respectively. Compared to the LOD of Sudan I of the standard liquid chromatographic method (1.3×10^{-2} μg·mL^{-1}) proclaimed by European Commission, [25] the present method is much more sensitive.

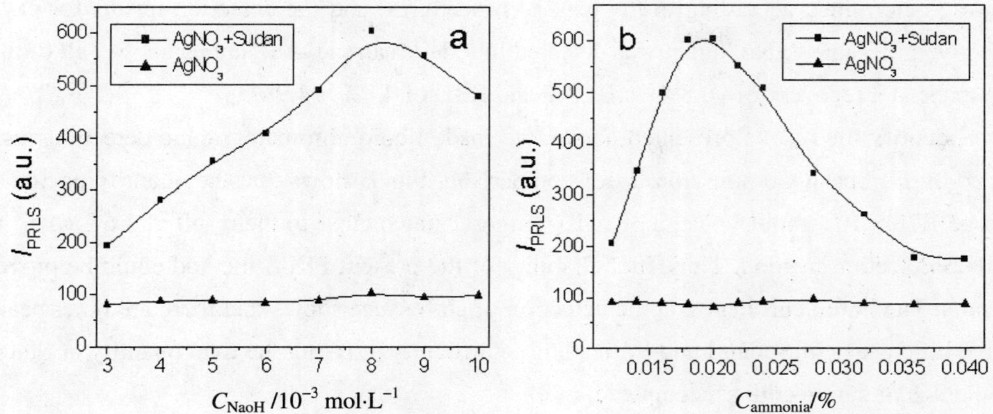

Fig. 5 Dependence of the PRLS intensity on the concentrations of NaOH (a) and ammonia (b). λ, 452 nm. Concentrations: (a), $AgNO_3$, 4.5×10^{-4} mol·L^{-1}; $NH_3 \cdot H_2O$, 0.02%; Sudan I, 0.6 μmol·L^{-1}; TritonX-100, 0.012%; (b), $AgNO_3$, 4.5×10^{-4} mol·L^{-1}; NaOH, 8.0×10^{-3} mol·L^{-1}; Sudan I, 0.6 μmol·L^{-1}; TritonX-100, 0.012%.

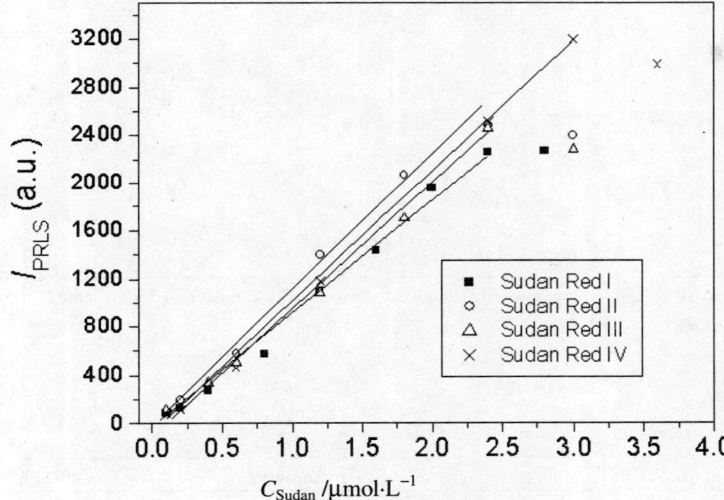

Fig. 6 Calibration curves for Sudan dyes. Linear regression equation (c, μmol·L^{-1}), ΔI = -130.4 + 1005.5 c, ΔI = 1.74 + 1082.6 c, ΔI = −67.9 + 1016.7 c, and ΔI = −108.9 + 1092.9 c for Sudan I, II, III and IV over the corresponding range of 0.2～2.4, 0.1～2.4, 0.1～2.4, 0.2～3.0 μmol·L^{-1} with the correlation coefficient of 0.9973, 0.9958, 0.9969 and 0.9990, respectively. Limits of determination (3σ) are 3.2, 3.0, 3.2 and 2.9 nmol·L^{-1}, respectively (corresponding to 7.9×10^{-4}, 8.3×10^{-4}, 1.1×10^{-3} and 1.1×10^{-3} mg·mL^{-1}, respectively). Concentrations: $AgNO_3$, 4.5×10^{-4} mol·L^{-1}; NaOH, 8.0×10^{-3} mol·L^{-1}; $NH_3 \cdot H_2O$, 0.02%; TritonX-100, 0.012%. λ, 452 nm.

The influences of foreign coexisting substances such as proteins, glucide, amino acid, surfactant and metal ions were tested (Data were shown in Table 1S in Supporting Information). Of these tested substances, Al^{3+}, Ca^{2+}, Cu^{2+}, Ba^{2+}, Mg^{2+}, Ni^{2+}, K^+, glucide, SDBS, amylose and formaldehyde, could be allowed to be higher than 1.0×10^{-5} mol·L^{-1} given the tolerance level of 10%. Amino acids but lysine could be allowed to be higher than 1.0×10^{-3} mol·L^{-1}. The tolerances of ethanol, acetone, BSA and HSA are relatively high. On the contrary, heavy metal ions including Pb^{2+}, Cr^{3+}, Fe^{3+}, surfactants including CTMAB, Tween-80, and Vitamin C could be allowed lower. For a real sample, however, it showed that the interferences created by the latter were not significant.

As the four Sudan dyes have the same redox reactions with $AgNO_3$, thus it is difficult to separately detect one of them in a mixture. However, it is possible to detect the total quantity of Sudan in a real sample for the four calibration curves in Fig. 6 have the similar slopes. The problem is that errors will take place resulting from their own slight different responses whichever one is chosen as the standard. Table 1 lists the detection error of Sudan IV with increasing Sudan I. It can be seen that all the detection errors are less than ±10%, namely, it is feasible that the approximate calculation of total quantity of Sudan using one of them as the standard.

To test the present method, three real samples including cayenne oil, chili sauce and redeye sampling from supermarket were determined according to the general procedures, and the detection results for cayenne oil and chili sauce are given in Table 2. No Sudan was detected in redeye sample. As Table 2 shows, all of the determinations could be made at a recovery of 90.8%～103.3% and RSD of 4.0%～4.9%.

To further identify the results presented above, we made liquid chromatographic detections using the standard proclaimed by European Commission[18] for comparison. Fig 7 shows that the quantity of Sudan IV in cayenne oil could be 1.78×10^{-5} mol·L^{-1}, i.e. 3.38×10^{-2} mg·g^{-1}, much close to the result of 1.64×10^{-2} mg·g^{-1} using the present PRLS detection method. Thus, the reliability of the present PRLS method could be proved further by the similar results. The liquid chromatographic detection of chili sauce shows that there are other peaks coexisting with the relative little peaks of Sudan I and IV, leading to difficulty in fixing the total quantity of Sudan. However, it proves that there is Sudan in chili sauce indeed.

Table 1 Detection error of Sudan IV with increasing Sudan I.

	Added (μmol·L^{-1})	Found (μmol·L^{-1})	
No.	Sudan I	Sudan I +Sudan IV	DR (%)
1	0.2	1.22	1.7
2	0.4	1.35	-3.6
3	0.6	1.55	-3.1
4	0.8	1.63	-9.4
5	1.0	1.91	-4.5
6	1.2	2.11	-4.1
7	1.4	2.27	-5.4
8	1.6	2.41	-7.3
9	1.8	2.61	-6.8
10	2.0	2.89	-3.7

Data were obtained by using Sudan IV as the standard. Quantity of Sudan IV in sample is 1.0 μmol·L^{-1}. Concentrations: $AgNO_3$, 4.5×10^{-4} mol·L^{-1}; NaOH, 8.0×10^{-3} mol·L^{-1}; $NH_3 \cdot H_2O$, 0.02%; TritonX-100, 0.012%. λ, 452 nm.

Table 2 Total quantity of Sudan in real samples (*n*=5)

Sample	Found (μmol·L^{-1})	Added (μmol·L^{-1})	Total Found (μmol·L^{-1})	Recovery (%)	RSD (%)
Cayenne oil	0.43	0.80	1.16	90.8～102.5	4.0
Chili sauce	0.20	0.30	0.49	93.3～103.3	4.9

All the values were the average of five measurements obtained using Sudan IV as standard. Each sample was prepared by dissolving 1.0g to 10 mL with DMF, and then diluted 10-fold to detect. Concentrations: $AgNO_3$, 4.5×10^{-4} mol·L^{-1}; NaOH, 8.0×10^{-3} mol·L^{-1}; $NH_3 \cdot H_2O$, 0.02%; TritonX-100, 0.012%. λ, 452 nm.

To make detections much easier, we could directly detect the quantity of Sudan *via* observing intuitively the phenomenon of scattered light. Using a laser pointer [*Caution! Laser is harmful to people's eyes. It should be handled with extreme care.*] and a light emitting diode (LED) to irradiate solutions respectively (Figure 8), we could obviously see that scattered light signals are enhanced gradually as the concentration of Sudan IV increases, and thus roughly detection could be made using such simple devices, which could be much more practicable. Although the wavelength of the laser pointer (653 nm) is located at the right edge of the PRLS spectra (Fig 4), it could be used for this PRLS signals based visual detention since its output power (2.0 mW) is much higher than that of LED (0.5 mW). The two devices thus could complement each other in terms of the wavelength and the output power. In addition, the visible light scattering detection using the laser pointer could determine much lower quantity of Sudan, although the color change of solutions with relatively high concentrations could be directly observed. Namely, the sensitivity is improved further for the light scattering sensing detection. The concentration of a cayenne oil sample, the one in the last cell in Fig. 8, could be easily detected to be close to 0.4 μmol·L^{-1}, which is consistent with the result in Table 2.

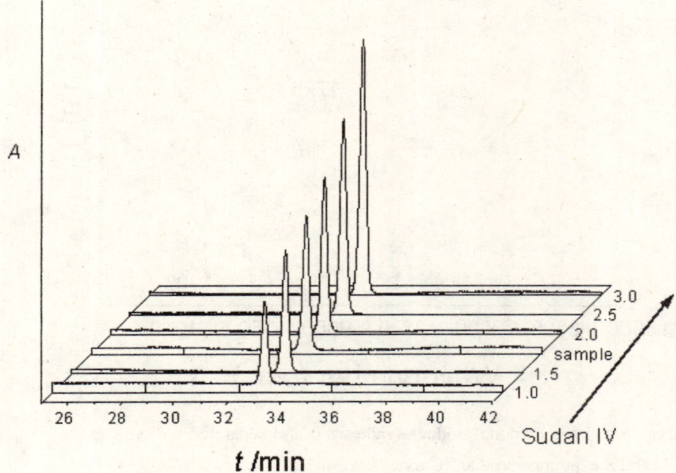

Fig. 7 Liquid chromatographic detection of Sudan in cayenne oil sample. Liquid chromatographic conditions: mobile phases, Reagent A, acidic solution (165 mL acetic acid dissolved in 1000 mL water); Reagent B, acetonitrile; Gradient program, 0~20 min (eluent B composition, 70%~95%), 20~30 min (B, 95%~100%), 30~42 min (B, 95%~100%); flow rate, 0.7 mL/min; the wavelength of detection, 520 nm; Column temperature, 25 °C. Concentration of standard, Sudan IV (from front to back, × 10^{-5} mol·L^{-1}): 1.0, 1.5, 2.0, 2.5 and 3.0. Linear regression, $A = 3.46 \times 10^4 + 4.06 \times 10^5 c$ (where A is the peak area, c is the concentration of Sudan IV). The correlation coefficient is 0.9992. From the standard curve and linear regression, the quantity of Sudan IV in cayenne oil is 1.78×10^{-5} mol·L^{-1} (i.e. 3.38×10^{-2} mg/g). RSD is 3.6%.

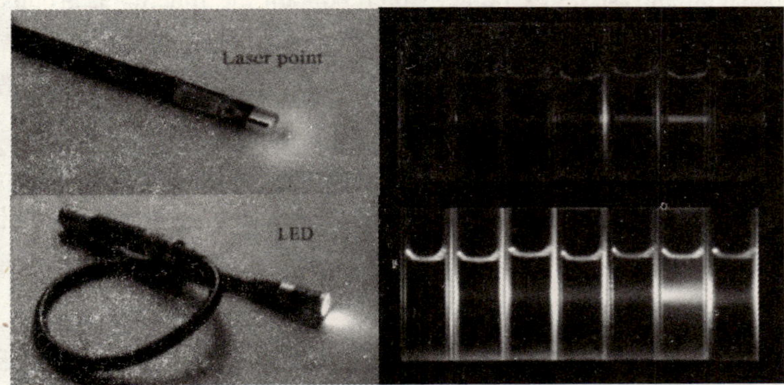

Fig. 8 PRLS signals based visual detection of Sudan IV using a portable laser pointer (653 nm, 2.0 mW, up) and a light emitting diode (LED, 458 nm, 0.5 mW, down) as irradiated light sources. Concentrations: $AgNO_3$, 4.5×10^{-4} mol·L^{-1}; NaOH, 8.0×10^{-3} mol·L^{-1}; $NH_3{\cdot}H_2O$, 0.02%; Sudan IV (from left to right, μmol·L^{-1}), 0, 0.1, 0.2, 0.4, 0.6, 1.2, and a real sample of cayenne oil consistent with the one in Table 2. Triton X-100, 0.012%.

4.10.2.4 Mechanism Investigations

The principle of the present method is to detect the PRLS signals of silver NPs resulted from redox reaction. Sudan I, II, III and IV have reducibility for the functional groups of nitrogen-nitrogen double bond and the phenol group, thus $AgNO_3$ can be reduced to silver NPs, resulting in the color change of the mixture to brown and displaying strong PRLS signals. From Fig. 6, we can see that the slopes of four calibration curves are quite close to each other, indicating that these reactions concerning Sudan I, II, III, and IV could produce similar response. In other words, the reaction mechanism is the same. As Fig. 1 shows, there is only one phenol group in each molecule of Sudan, whereas the number of nitrogen-nitrogen double bond in Sudan III and IV is twice as many as in Sudan I and II. Thus, it is deduced that the functional group oxidized by $AgNO_3$ is the phenol, instead of the nitrogen-nitrogen double bond. Suppose that the functional group was the nitrogen-nitrogen double bond, then the number of silver NPs produced by Sudan III and VI would be much more than that by Sudan I and II for a given Sudan concentration, resulting in different PRLS response and inconsistent slope. However, the similar slope values indicate no such dependence. Thus, we could deduce that the functional group oxidized by $AgNO_3$ is the phenol group, not the nitrogen-nitrogen double bond.

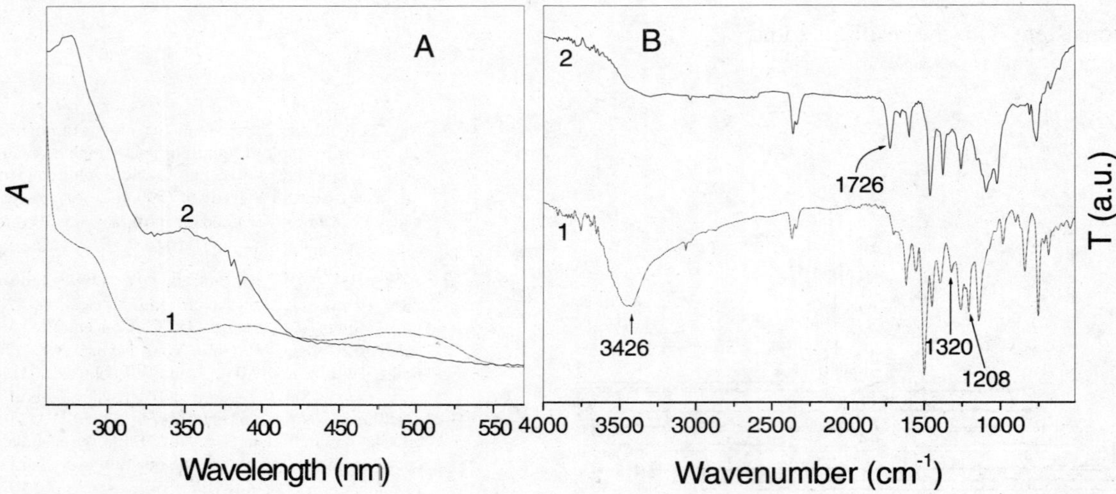

Fig. 9 (A) UV-vis absorption spectra of Sudan I (Curve 1) and the quinone product synthesized and separated *via* organic approach (Curve 2). (B) IR spectra of Sudan I (Curve 1) and the quinone product (Curve 2).

To validate the deduced mechanism, we measured the reaction between $AgNO_3$ with other azo-dyes including 4-[(5-chloro-2-pyridyl)azo]-1,3-diaminobenzene and Methyl Orange, which contain the functional groups of nitrogen-nitrogen double bond without phenol group. The results showed that the two dyes do not react with $AgNO_3$ under above NaOH and ammonia controlled experimental conditions. More exactly, the functional group of Sudan is not the nitrogen-nitrogen double bond indeed.

In order to confirm the reaction mechanism, the products of the redox reaction were separated and characterized (shown in Fig. 9). Sudan I has the maximum absorptions at 376 nm and 486 nm, which are changed after reacting with $AgNO_3$. The maximum absorptions of the product, obtained *via* organic synthesis and separation, locate at 276 nm and 348 nm (Figure 9A), which are in great part due to the produced quinone structure.[42, 43] By comparing the IR features of pure Sudan I (Fig. 9B, curve 1) and the separated product (Fig. 9B, curve 2), we could find that the phenolic stretching vibration (ν_{OH}) at 3426 cm^{-1}, the phenolic bending vibration (δ_{OH}) at 1320 cm^{-1} and the C-O stretching vibration ($\nu_{C\text{-}O}$) at 1208 cm^{-1} in Sudan I disappear and the carbonyl stretching vibration ($\nu_{C=O}$) at 1726 cm^{-1} come into being in the synthetic product, validating the formation of quinone (Fig. 1). Whereas, Ar-H stretching and bending vibration, the benzene ring stretching vibration and N=N and Ar-N stretching vibration still exist (shown in Fig. 9) in the synthetic product (For further details of IR features, please see supporting information). Thus, we could draw the reaction principle shown in Fig. 1. The phenol group, at the high pH, first changes into a phenate group, and then is oxidized into a quinonic structure.

4.10.3 Conclusion

In this contribution, we propose a PRLS signals based sensing detection of Sudan dyes, avoiding the pretreatments of separation. The determination for real samples of cayenne oil and chili sauce shows that our method is sensitive, effective, simple, reliable and potential to be put into practice. The detection for solid samples including sausages and cayenne powder is ongoing, and we hope to extend farther applicable fields. We are trying our best to seek much simpler and easier devices such as test paper slip to detect one of them in real samples. Besides, this reaction may supply a new idea to synthesize stable silver NPs, when the appropriate condition is under control. This method may also be a valuable approach for the developments of detection of other food pigments.

Acknowledgements

All authors herein are grateful to the supports from the National Natural Science Foundation of China (NSFC, No: 20425517, 30570465), and Dr Xuebin Ma of the Organic Synthesis Laboratory, College of Chemistry and Chemical Engineering, Southwest University,

Reference

[1] Yu, Y. Y.; Chang, S. S.; Lee, C. L.; Wang, C. R. C. J. Phys.Chem. B 1997, 101, 1588～1593.

[2] Roll, D.; Malicka, J.; Gryczynski, I.; Gryczynski, Z.; Lakowicz, J. R. Anal. Chem. 2003, 75, 3440～3445.

[3] Link, S.; El-Sayed, M. A. Int. Rev. Phys. Chem. 2000, 19, 409～453.

[4] Mayes, A. G.; Blyth, J.; Millington, R. B.; Lowe, C. R. Anal. Chem. 2002, 74, 3649～3657.

[5] Kim, Y.; Johnson, R. C.; Hupp, J. T. Nano Lett. 2001, 1, 165～167.

[6] Storhoff, J. J.; Elghanian, R.; Mucic, R. C.; Mirkin, C. A.; Letsinger, R. L. J. Am. Chem. Soc. 1998, 120, 1959～1964.

[7] Elghanian, R.; Storhoff, J. J.; Mucic, R. C.; Letsinger, R. L.; Mirkin, C. A. Science 1997, 277, 1078～1081.

[8] Aslan, K.; Lakowicz, J. R.; Geddes, C. D. Anal. Chem. 2005, 77, 2007～2014.

[9] Storhoff, J. J.; Elghanian, R.; Mucic, R. C.; Mirkin, C. A.; Letsinger, R. L. J. Am. Chem. Soc. 1998, 120, 1959～1964.

[10] Storhoff, J. J.; Elghanian, R.; Mucic, R. C.; Mirkin, C. A.; Letsinger, R. L. J. Am. Chem. Soc. 1998, 120, 1959～1964.

[11] Aili, D.; Enander, K.; Rydberg, J.; Lundstrom, I.; Baltzer, L.; Liedberg, B. J. Am. Chem. Soc. 2006, 128, 2194～2195.

[12] Pavlov, V.; Xiao, Y.; Shlyahovsky, B.; Willner, I. J. Am. Chem. Soc. 2004, 126, 11768～11769.

[13] Aslan, K.; Holley, P.; Davies, L.; Lakowicz, J. R.; Geddes, C. D. J. Am. Chem. Soc. 2005, 127, 12115～12121.

[14] Kelly, K. L.; Coronado, E.; Zhao, L. L.; Schatz, G.C. J. Phys. Chem. B 2003, 107, 668～677.

[15] Zhao, L. L.; Kelly, K. L.; Schatz, G. C. J. Phys. Chem. B 2003, 107, 7343～7350.

[16] Kumbhar, A. S.; Kinnan, M. K.; Chumanov, G. J. Am. Chem. Soc. 2005, 127, 12444～12445.

[17] Malynych, S.; Chumanov, G. J. Am. Chem. Soc. 2003, 125, 2896～2898.

[18] Westmoreland, C.; Gatehouse, D. G. Carcinogenesis (Lond.) 1991, 12, 1403～1407.

[19] Moller, P.; Wallin, H. Mutat. Res. 2000, 462, 13～30.

[20] Stiborová, M.; Martínek, V.; Rydlova, H.; Hodek, P.; Frei, E. Cancer Res. 2002, 62, 5678～5684.

[21] Stiborová, M.; Asfaw, B.; Frei, E.; Schmeiser, H. H.; Wiessler, M. Chem. Res. Toxico.l 1995, 8, 489～498.

[22] Stiborova, M.; Frei, E.; Schmeiser, H. H.; Wiessler, M.; Hradec, J. Carcinogenesis (Lond.) 1990, 11, 1843～1848.

[23] Stiborová, M.; Schmeiser, H. H.; Frei, E. Cancer Lett. 1999, 142, 53～60.

[24] Donna, L. D.; Maiuolo, L.; Mazzotti, F.; Luca, D. D.; Sindona, G. Anal. Chem. 2004, 76, 5104～5108.

[25] European Commission, Health and Consumer Protection Directorate-General, Committee IV-Food Safety in Production and Currency, Part III—Physical and Chemical Harmful Substances Surveillance, New Method Declaration: 03/99

[26] Capitàn, F.; Capitan-Vallvey, L. F.; Fernàdez, M. D.; Orbe, I.; Avidad, R. Anal. Chim. Acta. 1996, 331, 141～148.

[27] Tateo, F.; Bononi, M. J. Agric. Food Chem. 2004, 52, 655～658.

[28] Yu, L. H.; Mu, D. H.; Li, G. X.; Yan, S. P. Chin. J. Spec. Lab. 2004, 21, 1131～1133.

[29] Sarkar, A.; Kapoor, S.; Mukherjee, T. J. Phys. Chem. B 2005, 109, 7698～7704.

[30] Selvakannan, P. R.; Swami, A.; Srisathiyanarayanan, D.; Shirude, P. S.; Pasricha, R.; Mandale, A. B.; Sastry, M. Langmuir 2004, 20, 7825～7836.

[31] Tokareva, I.; Hutter, E. J. Am. Chem. Soc. 2004, 126, 15784～15789.

[32] Liu, S. H.; Zhang, Z. H.; Han, M.Y. Anal. Chem. 2005, 77, 2595～2600.

[33] Pasternack, R. F.; Bustamante, C.; Collings, P. J.; Giannetteo, A.; Gibbs, E. J. J. Am. Chem. Soc. 1993, 115, 5393～5399.

[34] Pasternack, R. F.; Collings, P. J. Science 1995, 269, 935～939.

[35] Huang, C. Z.; Li, K. A.; Tong, S. Y. Anal. Chem. 1997, 69, 514～520.

[36] Saito, Y.; Wang, J. J.; Batchelder, D. N.; Smith , D. A. Langmuir 2003, 19, 6857～6861.

[37] Saito, Y.; Wang, J. J.; Smith , D. A.; Batchelder, D. N. Langmuir 2002, 18, 2959～2961.

[38] Ten Cate, M. G. J.; Crego-Calama, M.; Reinhoudt, D. N. J. Am. Chem. Soc. 2004, 126, 10840～10841.

[39] Pashley, R. M. J. Phys. Chem. B 2003, 107, 1714～1720.

[40] Aslan, K.; Pérez-Luna, V. H. Langmuir 2002, 18, 6059～6065.

[41] Nakano, M.; Nakatani, Y.; Sugita, A.; Kamo, T.; Natori, T.; Handa, T. Langmuir 2003, 19, 4604～4608.

[42] Tsuda, A.; Fukumoto, C.; Oshima, T. J. Am. Chem. Soc. 2003, 125, 5811～5822.

[43] Balakrishnan, G.; Mohandas, P.; Umapathy, S. J. Phys. Chem. 1996, 100, 16472～16478.

(Li Ping Wu, Yuan Fang Li, Cheng Zhi Huang, Qin Zhang,
published in *Analytical Chemistry*, 2006,78,5570～5577)